Communicable Disease Epidemiology and Control

A Global Perspective

This book is dedicated to Michael Colbourne (1919–1993), malariologist, teacher and previously Dean at the Universities of Hong Kong and Singapore, who while at the London School of Hygiene and Tropical Medicine gave me considerable help in its preparation.

Communicable Disease Epidemiology and Control

A Global Perspective

2nd Edition

ROGER WEBBER

Formerly of
London School of Hygiene and Tropical Medicine, UK

CABI Publishing

CABI Publishing is a division of CAB International

CABI Publishing
CAB International
Wallingford
Oxfordshire OX10 8DE
UK
Tel: +44 (0)1491 832111
Fax: +44 (0)1491 833508
E-mail: cabi@cabi.org
Website: www.cabi-publishing.org

CABI Publishing
875 Massachusetts Avenue
7th Floor
Cambridge, MA 02139
USA
Tel: +1 617 395 4056
Fax: +1 617 354 6875
E-mail: cabi-nao@cabi.org

A catalogue record for this book is available from the British Library, London, UK.

Library of Congress Cataloging-in-Publication Data

Webber, Roger.
  Communicable disease epidemiology and control: a global perspective /Roger Webber. - -2nd ed.
    p. cm.
  Includes index.
  ISBN 0-85199-902-6 (alk. paper)
  1. Communicable diseases- -Epidemiology. 2. Communicable diseases- -Prevention. I. Title.
RA643.W37 2005
614.5- -dc22

2004006925

ISBN 0 85199 902 6

Typeset by Kolam Information Services Pvt. Ltd, Pondicherry, India
Printed and bound in the UK by Biddles Ltd, King's Lynn

Contents

Introduction

Since the first edition of this book, communicable diseases have caught the attention of the world with the appearance of the severe acute respiratory syndrome (SARS), bovine spongiform encephalopathy (BSE or mad cow disease) and new variant Creutzfeld–Jakob disease (CJD), as well as the relentless increase in HIV infection. The vulnerability of the human population to these new diseases and the difficulty that the medical services have had in controlling them has revealed the seriousness of communicable diseases. Also, the use of anthrax as a weapon and the potential use of other microorganisms in this way has generated the fear and dread that developed when the great plagues forged their relentless passage across the world. But communicable diseases have always been with us – not a serious problem in developed countries, but the main cause of death and infirmity in the developing world. Lower respiratory infections are still the major cause of death, and malaria, despite all the efforts of control, causes considerable mortality every year.

The news is not all bad though. Since the first edition was published, poliomyelitis has been eradicated from Europe, the Americas and the Western Pacific, and continued good progress is being made in the rest of the world. Guinea worm has been cleared from most of the endemic area by simple improvements in water supply, a tribute to rudimentary health measures. Leprosy, the disease of antiquity, due to an active search and find programme has decreased to such a degree that it is no longer a health problem in many countries. Chagas' disease, the awful debilitating condition that has troubled South and Central America for such a long time, has been declared eradicated from Uruguay, Chile and Brazil, with Venezuela and Argentina soon to follow. This has been by simple control of the vector and improvement in standards of housing, attention to detail rather than some new invention.

The appearance of new diseases and the persistence of infections that have always been with us mean that a knowledge of communicable diseases is still necessary. Many developed countries felt that communicable diseases were no longer a health problem, but they are as important as they have ever been. This is no more so than in the developing world where the burden of communicable diseases has always been a major concern.

While individuals fall sick and require the expertise of the medical profession, it is the overall assessment of the cause of diseases and how to control them that will most rapidly solve the problem in the community. Indeed, communicable diseases are community problems and need to be looked at in this way. Epidemiology is the science of communities, looking at many individuals to try and discover common features in them. From this analysis, the cause and characteristics of a disease can be worked out. The emphasis in this book is, therefore, epidemiological.

Learning about these diseases one by one is a long and complicated process that the doctor needs to undertake in order to understand how to treat the individual. However, it is the method of transmission that is the key to control and several diseases often share the same method of transmission. This allows diseases to be grouped together so that knowing the characteristics of one means that any of the diseases in the group can probably be controlled in a similar way. While there are always exceptions, grouping them should make it easier to learn about all the many diseases that afflict us, and this is one of the intentions of this book. This seems to have been borne out, as the first edition has been used as a course book for several teaching programmes and it is hoped that changes made in this second edition will make it even more suitable.

Communicable diseases tend to behave in a similar pattern. Such generalizations determine the first chapters, which look at communicable disease theory, formulating common principles in both epidemiology and control. Classifying communicable disease can be by organism, clinical presentation or system of the body attacked, but the epidemiologist is interested in causation, which is the approach taken here.

Trying to find similarities can often be useful, well shown by grouping respiratory diseases into acute respiratory infections (ARI), which has produced an important advancement in the control of this familiar problem. Every effort has, therefore, been made to find common themes to make the understanding and learning of communicable diseases easier and as a consequence their management. Also, entomology and parasitology are often taught as separate disciplines, but since they form such an integral part of many communicable diseases, the essentials have been included.

The range of communicable diseases occurring throughout the world is considerable. A comprehensive list is given in Chapter 19, but only those of importance are covered in detail in the main part of the book. Emphasis is placed on the developing countries, as this is where most communicable diseases are found. It is hoped this selection of diseases provides a more representative perspective of the world situation (Table 1.1).

Whilst communicable diseases mainly affect the developing world, new and emergent diseases, such as new variant CJD and SARS have re-awakened the developed countries to the importance of these infections. This has now become a major issue, so a new chapter has been added to this second edition. Also, although most diseases arise within the same country, there is an international importance as more people travel to different countries and exotic diseases are imported. Concern has been raised that climate change due to global warming could provide conditions for diseases to increase their range and affect countries where they have not normally been a problem, so a new section has been added to this edition.

While the emphasis of this book is on diseases found in tropical and developing countries, it does seem to have found a useful place in the teaching programmes of developed countries and, therefore, a few more diseases, more common in developed countries, have been added. A balance has to be achieved though between attempting to cover everything superficially or concentrating on certain diseases in more depth, and within the constraints of trying to keep this book to a manageable size, it is hoped the right balance has been achieved.

Many of the examples are taken from my personal experience of working in the Solomon Islands and Tanzania, with shorter periods in South America and various Asian countries. Much of what I have learnt has come from the large number of people who have helped and worked with me in these countries. I owe them a considerable debt for their wisdom and assistance, help that I hope I pass on in the following pages.

Experience is invaluable, but organizing one's thoughts and developing a critical judgement comes from working in an academic environment and many people in the London School of Hygiene and Tropical Medicine (LSHTM) have helped me in the various drafts of this manuscript. I wish to particularly thank John Ackers, David Bradley, Sandy Cairncross, Michael Colbourne (who sadly died before the first edition was published), Janette Costello, Felicity Cutts, Paul Fine and Peter Smith. Andrew Tomkins of the Institute of Child Health and William Cutting of the University of Edinburgh, kindly read through sections on the childhood infections. Maurice King gave me considerable help in the layout of the book and encouragement to persevere with it. Sameen Sidiqi from the Pakistan Institute of Medical Sciences reviewed the text for use in Asia and wrote the section on rheumatic fever. Dr Julie Cliff, who has spent most of her working life in Africa and teaches at the University of Maputo, Mozambique, gave me much valuable advice as the manuscript was getting ready for publication. But, one person to whom I owe special thanks is Brian Southgate, who has been my mentor and friend for many years. He introduced me to many original concepts and has been a kindly guide to being more scientific.

In this edition, I particularly wish to thank Chris Curtis, Peter Godfrey-Faussett, Richard Hayes and David Warhurst from LSHTM for helping me update on material I could not find on the helpful websites of the World Health Organization (WHO) and by the publishers, CAB International, who have been my main source. The Internet has changed the whole way of researching for a book and I am most grateful to the many unknown writers who have contributed to the various sites I have used. But, the old-fashioned way of using books is still necessary and I wish to acknowledge the use of the library in LSHTM and, in particular, Brian Furner and John Eyers for all their assistance.

Many organizations assisted me and I am especially grateful to WHO for supplying print quality copies of their many figures. The Department for International Development (DFID) has been my employer in the Solomon Islands, Tanzania, and as a member of the Tropical Diseases Control Programme at LSHTM. They have given me considerable assistance in this entire endeavour and I would particularly like to thank the Health and Population Division Low Cost Book Programme for a generous grant towards publishing costs of the first edition.

In these days of rising prices and commercial competition, it is becoming increasingly difficult to produce books that are affordable in developing countries. Every effort has been made to produce this volume as cheaply as possible, without sacrificing quality, but even so the copy price is higher than I wished it to be. This is mainly to allow production at a lower cost for developing countries, so every copy bought is helping more copies to be made available where they are most needed.

Roger Webber

1

Elements of Communicable Diseases

1.1 What are Communicable Diseases?

A communicable disease is an illness that is transmitted from a person, animal or inanimate source to another person either directly, with the assistance of a vector or by other means. Communicable diseases cover a wider range than the person-to-person transmission of infectious diseases; they include the parasitic diseases in which a vector is used, the zoonoses and all the transmissible diseases. It is this element of transmission that distinguishes these diseases from the non-communicable.

If diseases are communicable, then they present in an epidemic or endemic form, while if non-communicable as acute or chronic, as follows:

Communicable:

- epidemic (e.g. measles);
- endemic (e.g. malaria).

Non-communicable:

- acute (e.g. accidents);
- chronic (e.g. coronary heart disease).

All these can occur at the same time and in the same place, but communicable diseases are more common in developing countries and non-communicable in the developed world.

Epidemic diseases devastate whole populations, as when measles ravaged Fiji, killing adults as well as children. Populations then have to start again from the survivors to recover their former strength. These are essentially young and growing populations. With endemic diseases, it is children who are particularly vulnerable, so there is a high birth rate to compensate. With so many young people in the population, chronic non-communicable diseases are uncommon, but as people live longer, such diseases become more frequent. Chronic non-communicable diseases, therefore, are a problem of older aged populations as seen in the Western world.

This division between the developed and developing world is purely artificial as far as diseases are concerned. When the plague, or black death as it was known, spread across Europe, it caused as much devastation as when communicable diseases were introduced to newly discovered nations by Western explorers. The population started again from the survivors as it has had to do in the developing countries. Just over a 100 years ago, measles was as serious a cause of childhood death in large European cities as it is in countries today without well-organized vaccination programmes. A tropical environment is more favourable to many diseases than the cooler temperate regions, but even here, tropical diseases like malaria were once common in Europe. There is nothing new or different about these artificially divided parts of the world except for the resources that each is able to devote to the improvement of its population's health. Communicable diseases could be reduced to manageable proportions if sufficient resources, both in financial and educational terms, could be spent on them and much of the reason why certain diseases (as illustrated in Table 1.1) are more common than others is due to poverty.

The difference between communicable and non-communicable diseases was quite clear-cut. When it was an organism that was transmitted, the disease was communicable; otherwise the disease was classified as non-communicable. However, this strict boundary is becoming less well-defined as new suspect organisms are discovered or diseases, by their very nature, suggest a communicable origin. Various cancers are good examples; the link between hepatitis B virus (Section 14.13) and hepatocellular cancer is well established and is now being prevented by routine vaccination. Epstein–Barr virus (EBV) seems to be a pathogenic factor in Burkitt's lymphoma, but there is also a causal relationship with malaria; so controlling malaria (Section 15.6) in Africa and Papua New Guinea, where this tumour is found, could have a double benefit. The EBV might also have a causal effect in non-Hodgkin's lymphoma and nasopharyngeal cancer. Kaposi's sarcoma may well be transmitted by the sexual route as shown by the number of people with it who acquire human immunodeficiency virus (HIV) infection via sexual transmission, compared with those becoming infected from blood transmission, in which case the tumour occurs only rarely. The trematode worms *Schistosoma haematobium* (Chapter 11) and *Opisthorcerchis sinensis* (Section 9.5) are causative factors in bladder cancer and cholangiocarcinoma, respectively. As a result, their control as communicable diseases will also reduce cancer incidence. *Helicobacter pylori*, an organism that thrives in gastric secretions, is probably a causative factor in gastric cancer. The commonest cancer with a communicable cause is cancer of the cervix, which is due to infection with the human papilloma virus (Section 14.11). Prevention of this infection by vaccination, now under trial, offers the greatest hope of reducing this important cause of female mortality.

Equally intriguing is the possibility that atheroma has an infective cause or association. With arteriosclerosis being largely responsible for coronary heart disease (CHD) and a major killer in Western countries, the possibility of preventing an infective causal agent is attractive. *Chlamydia pneumoniae* has been found within atheroma lesions, but not normal arteries, while cytomegalovirus is able to infect the smooth muscle cells of arterial walls. The association of *H. pylori* and CHD now seems unlikely, but herpes virus 1 could induce an endothelial cell response. The cause will probably be found to be multi-factorial, but perhaps in the course of time, nearly all diseases will be shown to have a transmissible factor in their causation. Even road accidents, for which there does not seem to be a necessity to look for a predisposing cause as in a communicable disease, might be made more likely to occur due to infection with toxoplasmosis (Section 17.5).

The key to any communicable disease is to think of it in terms of *agent, transmission, host* and *environment*. These components are illustrated in Fig. 1.1, which will be used as a framework in the description of this section. There needs to be a causative agent, which requires a means of transmission from one host to another, but the outcome of infection will be influenced by the environment in which the disease is transmitted.

1.2 The Agent

The agent can be an organism (virus, bacteria, rickettsia, protozoan, helminth, fungus or arthropod), a physical or a chemical agent (toxin or poison). If the agent is an organism, it needs to *multiply* and find a means of *transmission* and *survival*.

Table 1.1. The burden of communicable diseases in the world. Data from *The World Health Report 2002,* World Health Organization, Geneva.

Disease	DALYs[a] ('000s)		Mortality ('000s)	
	Total	Females	Total	Females
Lower respiratory infections	90,748	42,846	3,871	1,856
HIV/acquired immunodeficiency syndrome (AIDS)	88,429	42,973	2,866	1,338
Diarrhoeal disease	62,451	30,818	2,001	966
Malaria	42,280	22,256	1,124	592
Tuberculosis	36,040	13,411	1,644	569
Measles	26,495	13,260	745	372
Pertussis	12,464	6,240	285	142
Tetanus	8,960	4,497	282	141
Meningitis	6,420	2,961	173	77
Lymphatic filariasis	5,644	1,327	0	0
Syphilis	5,400	2,416	167	70
Trachoma	3,997	2,915	0	0
Chlamydia (STI)	3,494	3,199	8	8
Gonorrhoea	3,320	1,883	2	2
Leishmaniasis	2,357	946	59	24
Hookworm	1,825	893	4	2
Upper respiratory infections	1,815	881	70	35
Schistosomiasis	1,760	678	15	5
Hepatitis B	1,684	605	81	28
Trichuriasis	1,649	800	2	1
Trypanosomiasis (African)	1,598	568	50	18
Otitis media	1,474	719	6	3
Ascariasis	1,181	577	4	2
Onchocerciasis	987	416	0	0
Hepatitis C	844	313	46	17
Japanese encephalitis	767	400	15	8
Dengue	653	366	21	11
Chagas' disease	649	316	13	6
Diphtheria	185	89	5	3
Leprosy	177	79	4	2
Poliomyelitis	164	80	1	0
Total	415,911	199,728	13,594	6,298

[a]DALY, disability-adjusted life year.
The DALY is a calculation of the morbidity and mortality of the particular disease averaged out over the expected life of a person. It reflects the prevalence of the disease and the disability it produces. For example, a common disease such as lymphatic filariasis will have a high DALY because of the large number infected and the disability caused, although nobody dies from the disease.

1.2.1 Multiplication

Two methods of multiplication occur, *sexual* and *asexual* reproduction, which have different advantages. In asexual reproduction, a succession of exact or almost exact replicas are produced, so that any natural selection will act on batches or strains, rather than on individuals. By contrast, sexual reproduction offers great scope for variety, both within the cells of the single organism and from one organism to another. This means that natural selection acts on

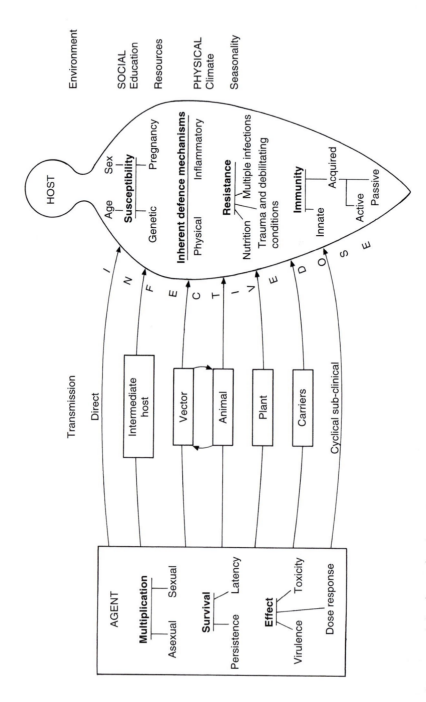

Fig. 1.1. Agent, transmission, host and environment.

individuals and variations of vigour and adaptability occur.

There are different consequences of these methods of reproduction. With asexual organisms, the strain of the organism is either successful or unsuccessful in invading the host, whereas in sexual organisms, certain individuals may succeed while others may not. In continuing its existence, only one organism of the asexual parasite requires to be transmitted, whereas in the case of the sexual parasite, both male and female adults must meet before reproduction can take place. Some parasites seem to be at a tremendous disadvantage, e.g. the filarial worm *Wuchereria bancrofti*, where both male and female individuals go through long migrations in the body to find an individual of the opposite sex, but despite all these problems, they are one of the most successful of all parasites.

Whether the organism reproduces sexually or asexually is relevant in treatment and control. If a treatment is successful in destroying an asexually reproducing organism, then it will also be successful against all the other individuals, unless a mutation occurs, which will also confer resistance to the treatment for all others of that strain. In contrast, sexual reproduction produces individuals of different vigour meaning that some individuals will succumb to treatment, while others will not. However, having two sexes can be a disadvantage for the organism in that methods of control can be devised to attack only one of the sexes or prevent them from meeting.

1.2.2 Survival

Agents survive by finding a suitable host within a certain period of time. They have been able to improve their chances of finding a new host or prolonging this period by a number of different methods.

Reservoirs and parasite adaptability A reservoir is a storage place for water, but serves as an appropriate term to describe a suitable place for storing agents of infection. Reser-

voirs are, therefore, the final host if several intermediaries are used.

The relationship between the parasite and the host is one of continual challenge, or what has been termed a 'biological arms race'. When the parasite first attacks a new species, the host attempts to eliminate it, resulting in a severe reaction. In the course of time, adaptation can occur so that the reaction of the host diminishes and the adaptability of the parasite increases. The parasite is able to live in the host with few ill effects (e.g. *Trichuris trichiura*), forming an established population, continuing with minimal reaction from the host. The host then acts as a reservoir from which parasites attack new hosts of the same species or attempt to colonize different species. Reservoirs can be humans, animals, vectors or the inanimate environment (e.g. soil, water). However, it is always in the parasite's interest to improve its reproductive capability. If a new mutation arises, which is beneficial to this end, then the mutation will be selected, generally to the host's disadvantage so that virulence can increase as well as decrease.

The adaptability of parasites to their human hosts might even have advantages for us. *Ascaris, Trichuris* and the hookworms secrete substances to reduce the host immune response, which inadvertently are absorbed by the gut lining and help reduce allergy such as that due to hay fever. Our more hygienic surroundings, by decreasing these parasites, may be responsible for the increase in allergic diseases such as asthma in the developed countries. It is a strange irony to actually introduce these parasites to combat allergic reactions.

Persistence Another mechanism used by parasites to survive is the development of special stages that resist destruction in an adverse environment. Examples are the cysts of protozoa, e.g. *Entamoeba histolytica* and the eggs of nematodes, e.g. *Ascaris*. Bacteria can persist in the environment by the development of spores as with anthrax and tetanus bacilli (Fig. 1.2).

Latency A developmental stage in the environment that is not infective to a new host is called latency. This allows the parasite time for suitable conditions to develop before changing into the infective form. *Ascaris*, the hookworms and *Strongyloides* exhibit latency.

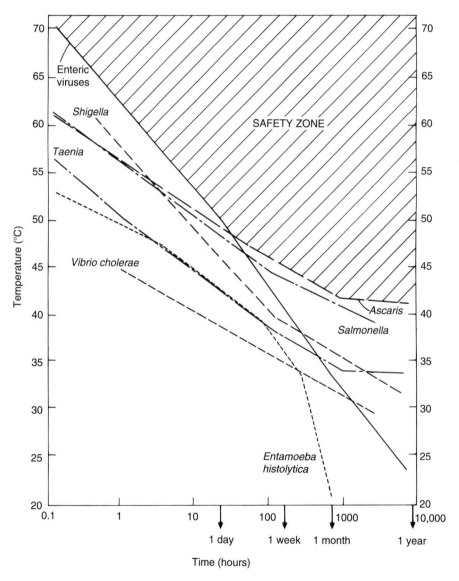

Fig. 1.2. Persistence of pathogens in excreta. The lines represent conservative upper boundaries for pathogen death – that is, estimates of the time – temperature combinations required for pathogen inactivation. Organisms can survive for long periods at low temperatures, so a composting process must be maintained at a temperature above 43°C for at least a month to effectively kill all pathogens likely to be found in human excreta. From Feachem, R.G., Bradley, D.J., Garelick, H. and Mara D.D. (1983) *Sanitation and Disease: Health Aspects of Excreta and Wastewater Management.* World Bank, Washington, DC, p. 79. Reprinted by permission of John Wiley & Sons Ltd.

1.2.3 The effect of the agent

If enough agents survive to infect a new host, they will produce illness, the severity of which is determined by its toxicity and virulence.

Infectious agents produce a toxic reaction due to the foreign proteins they consist of or produce in their respiratory or reproductive process (e.g. malaria). Sometimes the organism produces very little toxicity or it can be out of all proportions to the insignificant primary infection (e.g. tetanus).

Some organisms produce toxins when they grow in food, causing illness at a distance (e.g. *Clostridium botulinum*). Toxic chemicals can also contaminate food (e.g. adulterated cooking oil) producing an illness that has all the appearances of an epidemic produced by a living organism.

Some agents have a very marked effect on their host, while others a mild one. A good example is influenza. In the so-called Spanish flu of 1918, it is estimated that 50 million people were killed worldwide, while subsequent epidemics of influenza have caused mainly mild infections, with mortality only in the young or the aged. As an infection progresses in a community, virulence can increase or decrease due to its passage through several individuals. Generally, virulence decreases, passage through many experimental animals being a method used in developing vaccines.

1.2.4 Excreted load and infective dose

The number of organisms excreted can vary considerably due to the type of infection or the stage of the disease. In diseases such as cholera, there may be vast numbers of organisms excreted (10^6–10^{12} vibrios/g of faeces), whereas in hookworm infection, the number of eggs may be comparatively few. In *Schistosoma mansoni*, asymptomatic children excrete the largest number of eggs, whereas the adult exhibiting severe manifestations may be almost non-infectious. In the otherwise harmless typhoid carrier, a bout of diarrhoea can cause the passage of a sufficient number of organisms to initiate an epidemic.

For each infectious agent, a minimum number of organisms – the infective dose – is required to overcome the defences of the host and cause the disease. A large dose of organisms may be required, such as with *Vibrio cholerae* or very few, as with *E. histolytica*. In most infections, once this number is surpassed, the severity of the disease is the same whether a few or large number of organisms are introduced, while in others, there is a correlation between dose and severity of illness. Estimates of doses have been attempted in cholera and typhoid using healthy volunteers, but variables such as host susceptibility prevent any degree of precision. An example is food poisoning where the severity of the illness is determined by the quantity of the infected food item that is consumed. On the beneficial side, a low dose of organisms may produce no symptoms of disease, but may be sufficient to induce immunity. Poliomyelitis is one of the many examples.

Infections with a low infective dose (e.g. enteric viruses and *E. histolytica*) can spread by person-to-person contact. This means that the provision of a safe water supply or sanitation will have little or no effect. At the other extreme are organisms like typhoid and cholera, when a high infective dose (of the order of 10^6 organisms/ml of water) is required to produce the disease. Improving water quality and the reduction of pathogens in the sewage will be beneficial to the community.

1.3 Transmission

Communicable diseases fall into a number of transmission patterns as illustrated in Fig. 1.3.

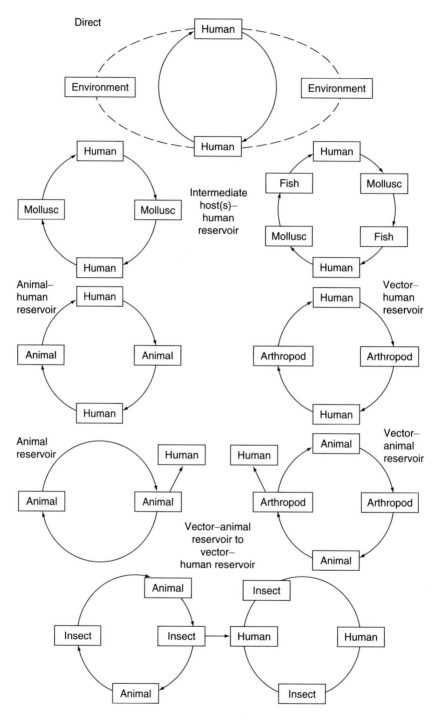

Fig. 1.3. Transmission cycles.

1.3.1 Direct

Direct transmission includes person-to-person contact as from dirty fingers or via food and water in the diarrhoeal diseases. Direct transmission also occurs through droplet infection in the respiratory diseases. Autoinfection can occur where humans contaminate themselves directly from their external orifices. Examples are transmission of *Enterobius* from anal scratching or infection of skin abrasions with bacteria from nose-picking.

1.3.2 Human reservoir with intermediate host

The adults of schistosomiasis live in humans, but for transmission to another human, the parasite must undergo developmental stages in a snail as intermediate host. In *Opisthorchis*, *Paragonimus* and *Diphyllobothrium*, more than one kind of intermediate host is required.

1.3.3 Animal as intermediate host or reservoir

Animals can either be intermediate hosts as with *Taenia saginata* and *Taenia solium* where cysticerci must develop in the animal muscle before they infect humans or they can be reservoirs such as in Chagas' disease. The infection is maintained in a wild rodent reservoir, where the foraging dog becomes infected, bringing infection into the home of a vulnerable human.

1.3.4 Vector

A vector carries the infection from one host to another either as part of the transmission process, such as a mosquito, or it can be mechanical, for example, through the housefly, which inadvertently transmits organisms to the host on its feet and mouth parts. All vectors of importance are either insects, mosquitoes, flies, fleas, lice, etc. or arachnids, ticks and mites. Infection may occur due to the feeding of the arthropod or as a result of its habits. The cycles of transmission are:

- direct insect to human as in malaria;
- insect to animal with humans entering the cycle as an abnormal host (e.g. bubonic plague);
- insect to animal including humans, from whom it is transmitted to other humans by the same or another insect vector (e.g. yellow fever and East African sleeping sickness).

(Snails, especially in descriptions of schistosomiasis, are often called vectors, but they do not carry the infection from one host to another and act only as intermediate hosts.)

1.3.5 Zoonosis

In the classification by transmission cycle, diseases fall into two main groups: the diseases where only humans are involved and those in which there is an animal reservoir or intermediate host. These are *zoonoses*, which are infections that are naturally transmitted between vertebrate animals and humans. They can be grouped according to the intimacy of the animal to the human being:

- *domestic*, animals that live in close proximity to man (e.g. pets and farm animals);
- *synanthropic*, animals that live in close association with man, but are not invited (e.g. rats);
- *exoanthropic*, animals that are not in close association with man (e.g. monkeys).

The importance of this type of classification is that it indicates the *focality* of the disease. As domestic animals are universally distributed, domestic zoonotic diseases are cosmopolitan, whereas at the other extreme, in an exanthropic zoonosis, such as scrub typhus or jungle yellow fever, it is quite possible for humans to live in the same locality, but separately from the disease area. Humans have no part in the disease cycle, but come into contact with it only when they accidentally enter the affected place (focus).

In zoonoses, the animal is all-important in control. In some diseases, such as the beef and pork tapeworms, good hygienic practice and inspection of the animal carcass may be all that is required to interrupt transmission. At the other extreme, a disease such as yellow fever can never be eradicated from the population even if every man, woman and child were immunized because the reservoir of disease remains in the monkey population. In a zoonosis, the animal reservoir is of prime importance and only by studying the ecology of the animal population can any rational attempt be made to control it.

1.3.6 Plants

Vegetable material that is eaten by the host can serve as a method of transmission. This can either be a specific plant, such as water calthrop on which the cercariae of *Fasciolopsis buski* encyst, or non-specific, such as any salad vegetable that might be carrying cysts of *E. histolytica*.

1.3.7 Carriers and sub-clinical transmission

Diseases in which there is an animal reservoir, intermediate host or vector are complex and difficult to control, but even in the simplified transmission cycle of direct spread from human-to-human, complications occur with the *carrier* state. A carrier is a person who can transmit the infective agent, but is not manifesting the disease. There are several types of carriers:

- asymptomatic carriers who remain well throughout the infection;
- incubating or prodromal carriers who are infectious, but unaware that they are in the early stages of the disease;
- convalescent carriers who continue to be infectious after the clinical disease has passed.

The carrier state can either be *transient* or *chronic*.

The important features of carriers are as follows:

1. The number of carriers may be far greater than the number of those who are sick.
2. Carriers are not manifest so they and others are unaware that they can transmit the disease.
3. As carriers are not sick, they are not restricted and, therefore, disseminate the disease widely.
4. Chronic carriers may produce repeated outbreaks over a considerable period of time.

Identification of carriers is a singularly difficult and generally unsuccessful exercise. If the carrier is asymptomatic, the organism is often in such reduced numbers or excreted at such infrequent intervals that routine culture techniques will not detect them. The investigation has to be repeated many times and is probably only successful at specific instances, for example, during a minor diarrhoeal episode in a suspected typhoid carrier. A further difficulty is that clinically unaffected people object to having investigations performed on them, making the coverage incomplete. Examples of diseases in which the carrier state is important are typhoid, amoebiasis, poliomyelitis, meningococcal meningitis, diphtheria and hepatitis B. Cholera can produce more carriers than those that are sick. More on carriers will be found in the sections dealing with each of these diseases.

In some diseases, the carrier state appears to be prolonged or is perpetuated when there are, in fact, no carriers. This may be due to *cyclical sub-clinical transmission* when infection is transmitted within a family or throughout a community, without the subjects being aware of any particular symptoms. One member of a family passes on the disease to another and becomes free of it him/herself. It is then passed on to other family members and eventually back again so that it is maintained in a sub-clinical cycle. When someone who is susceptible to the disease accidentally enters this cycle or the organism is more widely disseminated, then a clinical outbreak occurs. This is a mechanism by which poliomyelitis is maintained in the community.

1.4 Host Factors

If the agent is transmitted to a new host, its successful invasion and persistence will depend upon a number of host factors.

1.4.1 Susceptibility

Genetic Certain diseases can only affect animals and when they are transmitted to man, they are not able to establish themselves. An example is *Plasmodium berghei*, the rodent malaria parasite, which cannot produce disease in man although closely related to the human malaria parasite. However, some newly emergent diseases have succeeded in crossing this genetic barrier, such as HIV and severe acute respiratory syndrome (SARS).

Genetic disposition also determines the host's response to infecting organisms. Mycobacteria are common in the environment, but only certain people develop tuberculosis or leprosy. The type of disease (e.g. tuberculoid or lepromatous leprosy), is also determined by the genetic make-up.

Age During the course of life, different diseases affect particular age groups. The childhood diseases of measles, chickenpox and diphtheria are found at one end of the lifespan, with the degenerative diseases and neoplasms predominating at the other.

Sex The same advantages that parasites derive from having two sexes, producing many individuals of different vigour, also benefit humans, and it is thought that evading parasites might be one of the main reasons why mammals evolved with two sexes. However, one or other sex might more commonly succumb to illness, such

as poliomyelitis and goitre, which are more commonly found in females than males. Occupation can determine which sex is more likely to be involved, such as in East Africa where males, who hunt and collect honey in tsetse fly infested forest, are more likely to contract sleeping sickness. Social habits may also be a determinant, such as the custom of the Fore people in Papua New Guinea, where the women eat the brains of the recently dead, making kuru predominantly a disease of women.

Pregnancy When a woman is pregnant, her physiological mechanisms are altered and she becomes more susceptible to infections. Chickenpox is a severe disease in pregnancy and malaria attacks the pregnant woman as though she had little acquired immunity. The pregnant woman contracting Lassa fever is more likely to die from the illness.

1.4.2 Inherent defence mechanisms

Any infecting organism must be able to overcome the body's *inherent defence mechanisms*. These can either be:

- *physical*, such as the skin, mucus-secreting membranes or acidity of the stomach; or
- *inflammatory*, the localized reaction, which includes increased blood flow, the attraction of phagocytes and isolation of the site of inoculation.

1.4.3 Resistance

The person's susceptibility and defence mechanisms may be altered by the *resistance* of the individual. This may be lowered by the following:

1. *Nutrition*. Where the nutritional status is decreased, the susceptibility to a disease is increased, or the clinical illness is more severe.

2. *Trauma and debilitating conditions.*
Poliomyelitis may be a mild or inapparent
infection, but if associated with trauma,
such as an intramuscular injection, then
paralytic disease can result. The appearance
of shingles or fungal infections in debilitated people is often seen.

3. *Multiple infections.* The presence of one
disease may make it easier for other
infecting organisms. Secondary respiratory
infections commonly occur in measles.
Yaws has been noticed to increase and
spread more rapidly following an outbreak
of chickenpox.

1.4.4 Immunity

Experience of previous infection by a host
can lead to the development of *immunity*.
This can either be *cellular*, conferred by
T-lymphocyte sensitization or *humoral*,
from B-lymphocyte response. Immunity
can either be *acquired* or *passive*.

Acquired (both cellular and humoral) immunity follows an infection or vaccination
of attenuated (live or dead) organisms. This
will induce the body to develop an immune
response in a number of diseases. Immunity
is most completely developed against the
viral infections and may be permanent.
With protozoal infections (e.g. malaria), it
is only maintained by repeated attacks of
the organism.

Passive (humoral only) immunity is the
transfer of antibodies from a mother to her
child via the placenta. Passive immunity is
short lived, as in the protection of the young
infant against measles for the first 6 months
of life. Passive immunity can also be introduced (e.g. in rabies immune serum).

1.5 The Environment

The transmission cycle used by the agent to
reach the host takes place within an environment that determines the success and
severity of the infection. Environmental

factors are subtle, diffuse and wide-ranging.
A few of the more important ones are mentioned in this section. These will be divided
into the social environment and the physical
environment.

1.5.1 The social environment

Education Sufficient knowledge is available
about most of the communicable diseases
for them to be prevented, if only people
were taught how. Education is a complex
process; it is not just teaching people, but
they must understand to such an extent that
they are able to modify their lives. This is
not a sudden process; changes made by one
generation are used as the starting point for
improvements or modifications in the
following. Change is always opposed and
steps that seem easy to the educated may
be insurmountable for the uneducated.
Also, education is not just the adding of
new knowledge, but the rational appraisal
of traditional beliefs and customs.

An improvement in the level of education and understanding was probably the
most important reason why endemic communicable diseases largely disappeared
from the developed world. As education
improved, there was a demand for better
living standards. Good water and proper
sewage disposal were provided, personal
hygiene became a normal rather than an abnormal practice and cleanliness was sanc-
tioned as a desirable attribute. All these
changes occurred before the advent of antibiotics. The decline of tuberculosis in England and Wales (Fig. 13.3) is a classic
example of how the incidence of a major
communicable disease decreased as living
standards rose.

Resources and economics The lack of resources leads to *poverty*, which reduces the
ability to combat disease. The term 'resources' relates to everything that people
need to carry on their livelihood. Perhaps
the most important resource is land, which
is used by the family for living on
and growing crops. Alternatively, this land

can be used to produce commodities that can be sold as part of a manufacturing process. As the society develops, education or the ability to perform a service becomes a resource.

Resources are required to enact the preventive methods or raise standards that have come to be demanded by education. In the simplest terms, food is required to build up body processes and prevent malnutrition. But with a little extra money, a water supply can be built or a better house constructed.

Resources, education and *disease* are inextricably linked. Diseases are best prevented by educating people to overcome them, but resources are required by the educated to achieve this. Greater resources allow increased education and improved education leads to better utilization of resources. Both these factors help in reducing the incidence of communicable diseases.

Making the optimum use of resources and balancing what is needed with what is available is the province of health economics. The sick need treatment, but there may be several alternatives available and the cheapest one producing the desired effect will be the most appropriate for the health service of the country. The World Health Organization (WHO) essential drugs programme has helped to limit unnecessary expenditure. Health economics involves assessing the actual needs of the community, which are expressed as felt needs and translated into demands, but financial restrictions will limit what can be supplied. Health services will need to make choices between implementation of one scheme and another, such as a mass drug administration (MDA) programme or improved curative services, basing their choices on cost-effectiveness and cost–benefit analysis. In cost-effectiveness, programmes that yield the greatest health improvement for the available resources such as a vaccination programme are chosen, whereas in cost–benefit analysis, the outputs of different projects are measured and emphasis given to the one producing the greatest benefit per unit of cost. Although cost–benefit analysis is the more desirable for long-term planning,

measuring the benefit of a health intervention is difficult to do.

A development of these methods involves the concept of marginal costs, which is best illustrated using the three different strategies of a vaccination programme: (i) fixed units; (ii) mobile clinics; and (iii) outreach programmes. Using fixed units (clinics and hospitals), the largest number of children will be reached for the least cost, but to obtain higher coverage it will cost more per child by this method (building more clinics) than by adding an outreach programme to the existing clinics. To contact the remaining children (at the margin of an outreach programme), it will be cheaper to use mobile clinics. So each strategy has its value and it is more cost-effective to use them in this stratified fashion. Another example of the economics of vaccination will be found in Section 3.2.8.

Communities and movements People gather to form communities, constructing some form of habitation in which to live. The type of structure they live in can play an important role in the diseases they succumb to. In South America, the Reduviidae bugs that transmit Chagas' disease live in the mud walls of houses, so replacing these with more permanent materials can prevent the disease. Conversely, if a fire is lit within the house for cooking and heating, the smoke-filled interior leads to an increase in acute respiratory infections, one of the most common of all health problems.

The attraction of cities has resulted in one of the largest demographic changes in recent times. For the majority of the population that lived in rural areas, urban areas now have become the commonest place of residence in tropical countries. Slums have developed in which the diseases of poverty thrive and the imbalance of the sexes has led to an increase in sexually transmitted infections (STIs). At the other extreme is the nomad continually moving from place to place, making it difficult to provide maternal and child health (MCH) services, with the result that children are not vaccinated, making them vulnerable to many childhood infections.

People have to move to get to their place of work, attend school, visit the clinic or for many other reasons, but all such movements incur a health risk. The woman collecting water may make herself more vulnerable to contracting a diarrhoeal disease, by drinking water from a polluted source, while the tsetse fly vectors of Gambiense sleeping sickness favour biting people at water-gathering places. The mother carrying her baby to market with her makes it more liable to contact measles and whooping cough at a younger and more vulnerable age. Fishermen, with their greater contact with water, are more likely to contract schistosomiasis.

Local migrations from one country to a neighbouring country for trade or visiting relatives can pose a risk to the health of individuals or families. In much of Southeast Asia, malaria is more intense along the borders between countries, so that crossing to the next country and staying for a few days has been found to increase the chance of contracting malaria by as much as sixfold. Following trading routes was the way by which classical cholera was taken to East Africa in the 19th century and repeated with El Tor cholera in the 20th century. Schistosomiasis was carried to the Americas and Arabia along with the slaves who were forcibly taken to these parts of the world; a continuing vengeance for the evils inflicted on them.

Travel to another country permanently to seek employment or escape from civil conflict is a particularly vulnerable time for the individual and the family. Refugees, in particular, need extra help, but sometimes this can be misplaced and the situation made worse. During the Cambodian crisis, water containers were provided to households in refugee camps along the Thai border, but these proved to be excellent breeding places for *Aedes* mosquitoes, with the result that there were large outbreaks of dengue. In Tanzania, refugees were settled in a large uninhabited forest area, which was infested with tsetse flies, so soon cases of sleeping sickness began to appear. Refugee health has become a subject in its own right and communicable diseases are one of the many troubles that these unfortunate people suffer from.

As with refugee health, a new speciality has developed around the health of travellers. The phenomenal increase in air travel has brought the risk of contracting a communicable disease in a foreign country to all kinds of people. Over 2000 cases of malaria are imported to England and Wales every year, making it more important than many of the indigenous health problems. HIV infection in European countries has changed from being predominantly in the homosexual community to an increasing problem in the heterosexual, mainly due to infections contracted overseas. Problems also travel in the other direction when students from malaria-infected areas come to temperate countries to study, losing their acquired immunity and rendering them liable to contract serious malaria when they return home.

1.5.2 The physical environment

Topography The nature of the physical surroundings can influence the diseases that are found there. In much of Asia, a complex interaction termed 'forest fringe malaria' describes the greater likelihood of developing malaria at the forest margin. The man enters the forest to fell timber, often illegally, while the woman goes there to collect firewood, bringing them into range of mosquitoes that live within the forest cover. A similar cycle of transmission occurs with yellow fever as illustrated in Fig. 16.3. Destruction of primary forest, to be replaced by secondary growth, makes ideal conditions for the development of 'mite islands', which are important in scrub typhus (Section 16.2).

Human activity not only destroys the natural balance of nature, but also often changes the landscape to make it more suitable for the transmission of communicable diseases. The growing of rice in paddy fields provides suitable conditions for *Culex* mosquitoes that transmit Japanese encephalitis and *Anopheles sinensis*, the vector of malaria in much of China. The construction of dams and irrigation canals has encouraged the proliferation of intermediate host snails of schistosomiasis. However, the *Simulium* fly that transmits onchocerciasis breeds in fast-flowing oxygenated streams that are often destroyed when dams are built, depriving them of their breeding place. All major construction projects should, therefore, have a health evaluation to determine how the health risk can be minimized.

Climate can be divided into different components of *temperature, rainfall* (humidity) and less importantly, *wind*. These attributes of the climate have a marked influence on where diseases are found and the ways in which they are to be controlled.

Temperature varies by distance from the equator, altitude, prevailing winds and the size of land masses. A number of diseases are found only in the tropics, which is the main area for communicable diseases. Temperature decreases with altitude so that malaria will be found at the lower hot altitudes, while respiratory diseases are common in the colder hills. At the fringe of the mosquitoes' range, exceptional conditions of temperature and humidity can produce epidemic malaria.

Temperature not only affects the presence or absence of disease, but also often regulates the extent. The malaria parasite has a shorter developmental cycle as the temperature rises, thereby permitting an increased rate of transmission. Many insect vectors have a more rapid development in the tropics, making them difficult to control. The life cycle of a number of parasites are directly related to temperature.

Rainfall is perhaps the most essential element in human livelihood. Rainfall must be sufficient and regular (Fig. 1.4) allowing people to plant crops and ensure that they come to fruition. An irregular rainfall can be as disastrous as a low rainfall, leading to failed crops, malnutrition and a reduction of resistance to infection.

Rainfall also has a direct effect on certain diseases. Moderate rainfall creates fresh breeding sites for *Anopheles* mosquitoes, but excessive rain can wash out larvae and cause a reduction in the number of mosquitoes. Some diseases, such as trachoma, favour dry arid regions.

Wind produces local alterations to the weather. A major wind system is the monsoon, which brings rainfall to the Indian sub-continent and Southeast Asia. In West Africa, the hot dry Harmattan blows down from the Sahara, reducing humidity and increasing dust. It is these secondary effects on rainfall and temperature that determine the disease patterns.

The winds are appreciated by man to improve his living conditions in the warm moist areas of the world and avoided in the hot dry zones. However, excess wind in hurricane areas or the localized tornado cause destruction and loss of life (Fig. 1.5). Natural disasters disrupt the normal pattern of life, destroy water supplies and provide ideal conditions for epidemics to occur.

Seasonality Temperature and rainfall together determine the best time to grow crops and the seasonal patterns of a number of diseases. In areas of almost constant rain, there is very little seasonal variation, but in the drier regions, seasonality can be quite marked. These areas are illustrated in Fig. 1.4.

The pattern of life determined by seasonality can be generalized as follows:

- Food stores are low or absent during the rains as it is the longest time since the harvest.
- During the rains, people are required to work their hardest when they have the least amount of food.
- The rains bring seasonal illnesses, especially diarrhoea and malaria, which debilitate just when complete fitness is required.
- The time of the rains often coincides with late pregnancy for the woman, conception having taken place during harvest. Since all members of the family are required to work in the fields and much of the burden of cultivating falls on the woman, the

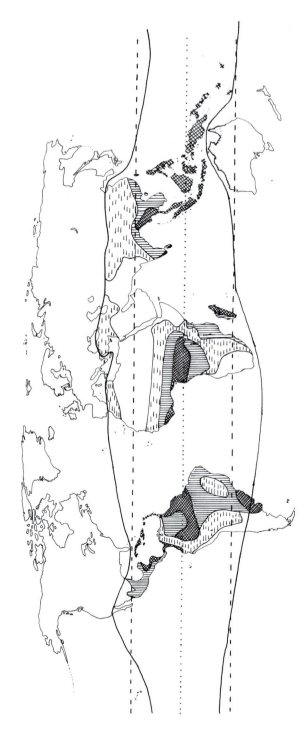

Fig. 1.4. The tropics – rainfall and seasonality. - - -, The tropics, Cancer to Capricorn; ——, developing country zone. Seasonality within the tropical region: ▓, rainfall in every season; ▤ heavy seasonal rainfall; ▨ variable seasonal rainfall; ☐, arid.

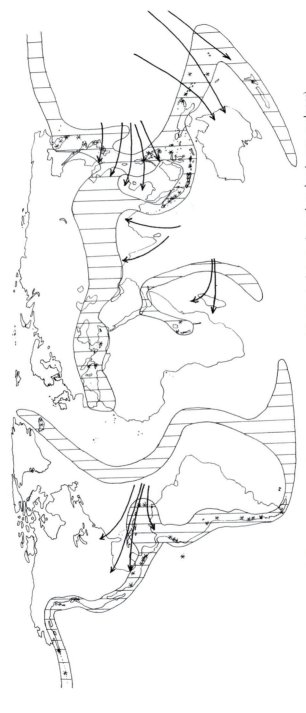

Fig. 1.5. Natural disaster zones. ▦, earthquake areas; *, active volcanoes; ←, revolving tropical storms (tornadoes, hurricanes, cyclones).

increased strain threatens her pregnancy, while her physical reserves are stretched even further.

- Once harvest comes, then body weight is restored, excess crops are stored or sold and some respite taken before the cycle repeats itself.

This pattern leads to the following observations:

1. Attendance for treatment at medical institutions and admission to hospital often follow a cyclical pattern. This is illustrated in Fig. 1.6 where it will be seen that the reporting of ill health is least during the dry months and increases with the rains.

2. Knowledge of the seasonality of a disease can be used in health planning, the deployment of manpower, the ordering of supplies, the best time to take preventive action, etc.

3. Many illnesses show a marked seasonal pattern. Mosquitoes require water to breed, so rainfall will determine a seasonal pattern for many of the vector-borne diseases. The massive contamination of rivers caused by the first rains washing in accumulated pol-

lutants from the many dry months, makes this a period of diarrhoeal diseases. The seasonality of cholera, allows a warning system to be implemented and prevention initiated (see Section 8.6).

4. A different pattern of seasonal diseases occurs with the viral infections, where measles (see Fig. 1.7) serves as a good example. As measles confers life-long immunity, the only way that sufficient susceptibles can accumulate for another epidemic to occur is by immigration or reproduction. If the birth rate is high, a critical number of susceptibles will soon be produced and annual epidemics will occur. If the birth rate is low, then the interval may be every 2–3 years.

5. Knowledge of the seasonality of a disease allows planned preventive services. If a mobile or mass vaccination campaign is used to combat measles, then timing it in the few months before an expected epidemic is the most cost-effective. In Tanzania, measles outbreaks often occur in the rainy season (Fig. 1.7), a time of shortages, malnutrition and difficult communications – the worst possible time to have to do emergency vaccination to contain the epidemic. Just a

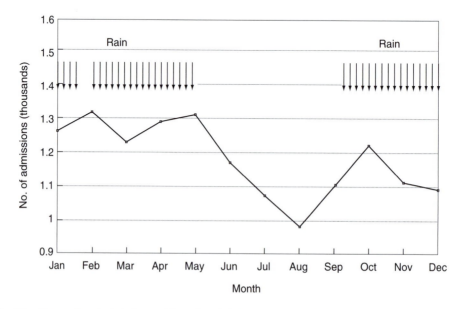

Fig. 1.6. Seasonality of admissions to Mbeya hospital, Tanzania, 1980–1983.

few months before, there was little ill health, nutritional status was high, road conditions good and medical staff were at their slackest. This would have been the best time to ensure that every child was vaccinated.

1.5.3 Climate change due to global warming

The increase in carbon dioxide and other pollutants in the atmosphere due to the burning of fossil fuels (coal, petrol, etc.) has led to an increase in global temperature. Although the temperature increase is comparatively small, it has begun to have a major effect on the climate, with a disruption of weather systems and a raising of the sea level. This has been most marked on a system of currents off the west coast of South America known as the El Niño southern oscillation. Climatic systems are reversed or severely disrupted, with heavy rains and flooding when no rain is normally expected and drought conditions when there should normally be rain. Countries in South America, Southeast Asia and Oceania are the most affected, but its effects are felt all over the world. Even without El Niño,

there has been an increase in the frequency and severity of storms in many parts of the world.

Increase in temperature has the potential to expand the range of infections that are normally constrained by temperature, for example, malaria. This has led to speculation that malaria could become a problem in the developed countries of Europe and North America where it occurred in former times. However, this is unlikely as good preventive measures are able to keep the disease from spreading even if the malarial mosquito re-establishes itself. A good example is Australia where much of the country lies within the tropical region, the main malaria vector *Anopheles farauti* (the same as Papua New Guinea and Solomon Islands) is present, yet control methods have eradicated the parasite and continued surveillance has prevented it from being re-introduced.

A more serious problem is in areas of highlands within tropical countries such as East Africa and South America. At a certain altitude where the lower temperature prevents the mosquito and parasite from developing, malaria is not found, but

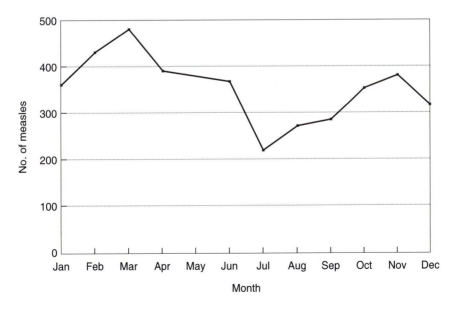

Fig. 1.7. Mean monthly measles cases, 1977–1981, Mbeya region, Tanzania.

evidence from Ethiopia and Kenya has shown that this level is already rising. Malaria is now found at higher altitudes with the rate of ascent linked to the rise in temperature. There is also a greater risk of epidemic malaria with the wider fluctuations of temperature that have resulted and the number of people who have no immunity. Other diseases transmitted by mosquitoes like dengue and Japanese encephalitis, and other arboviruses, such as Rift Valley fever, are likely to increase.

Effects will be most felt at the extremes of the world, i.e. the tropics and the Arctic and Antarctic regions. If ocean levels rise, then small island nations will be threatened by a reduction in land area on which to live and grow their crops and salinity will intrude into freshwater aquifers. Thirteen of the 20 major conurbations are at sea level and the population at risk from storm surges could rise from 45 to 90 million people. Countries at greatest risk are Bangladesh, China, Egypt and the small island nations of the Pacific, Caribbean and Indian Oceans. At the other extreme, a rise in temperature could damage the permafrost, upsetting the balance of nature and the livelihood of the indigenous people who live in these parts of the world. The increase in carbon dioxide will result in preferential conditions for tree growth and the development of forests, which would be beneficial in the long run, but the animals that live in these lands might not be able to adjust to the rate of change and become extinct.

While most of the concern of increase in disease due to global warming has been expressed in the Western world, it is more likely that most of the effects will be concentrated in the poorer regions of the world, with an increase in vector-borne and diarrhoeal diseases, malnutrition and natural disasters.

1.5.4 Medical geography

Features such as topography, climate and altitude are more commonly the province of geography than medicine, but their value is appreciated and epidemiologists are making more use of geographical tools to help them understand the distribution and spread of disease. The classic tool is the map and many examples will be found in several sections of this book where maps are used. A development of mapping is Geographical Information Systems (GIS) using the wealth of data collected by orbiting satellites. These map the surface of the world at frequent intervals so that comparisons can be made over time. Features known to be important in disease transmission, such as the distribution of populations or the breeding places of disease vectors can be identified from satellite images and predictions made without having to laboriously follow-up these features on the ground. Examples are the movement of people into the Amazon jungle where yellow fever is endemic and detailed study of a small area for mosquito-related features, such as rice-paddy, which can then be looked for in satellite images for the whole country. GIS is at the forefront of monitoring changes that are resulting from global climatic change.

2

Communicable Disease Theory

———————————

The previous chapter attempted to unify communicable diseases into basic units, the *agent*, a route of *transmission* to a *host* and the way the *environment* influences the outcome. Generalizations have been made in attempting to limit and clarify all the alternatives and variations that are possible. Developing principles, not discovering exceptions, has been the objective. A stage is now reached where interactions between these various elements can be suggested and tried. The approach can either be intuitive, a method used with reasonable success in earlier attempts at explaining disease dynamics, or analytical, where the precision, ease of modification and extrapolation are considerably greater.

2.1 Force of Infection

In a communicable disease, the number of new cases occurring in a period of time is dependent on the number of infectious persons within a susceptible population and the degree of contact between them. Persons, whether infectious or susceptible, and a period of time are all quantifiable factors, but the degree of contact can depend upon very many variables (some of which have been covered above). The factors,

such as proximity (density) of populations, carriers, reservoirs, climate and seasonality, will have separate effects. To single these out and ascribe values to them will involve considerable, and generally unnecessary, complexity. In some disease patterns, certain factors have sufficient influence that they require to be given values, but for the time being, it is best to consider these altogether as a *force of infection*. This can be summarized as:

The force of infection

= Number of infectious individuals
   × Transmission rate

Therefore:

Number of newly infected individuals
= Force of infection
   × Number of susceptible individuals in
   the population

If the susceptible population is sufficiently large to maintain a permanent pool of susceptibles (as would happen in a disease where there is little or no immunity) and the force of infection is constant, then newly infected individuals will continue to be produced, while infectious individuals remain in the population. One healthy carrier might continue to infect a large number of individuals over a long period of time, or a brief devastating epidemic, with a short period of infectiousness, may infect a large number of people over a short period of time. Parasitic infections, such as hookworm, would be an example of the former and measles, an example of the latter. Of course, measles produces immunity, which will alter the size of the susceptible population.

The proportion of susceptible individuals can be reduced by mortality, immunity or emigration, or increased by birth or immigration. After a certain period of time, a sufficient number of non-immune persons would have entered the population for a new *epidemic* of the disease to occur.

2.2 Epidemic Theory

Epidemics can occur unexpectedly, as when a new disease enters a community, or can occur regularly at certain times of the year, as in epidemics of measles. Epidemic contrasts with *endemic,* which means the continuous presence of an infection in the community and is described by *incidence* and *prevalence* measurements. This section will cover epidemics and how they are measured.

Epidemic means an excess of cases in the community from that normally expected, or the appearance of a new infection. The point at which an endemic disease becomes epidemic depends on the usual presence of the disease and its rate. With

an unusual disease, a few cases could be an epidemic, whereas with a common disease (e.g. gastroenteritis), an epidemic occurs when the usual rate of the disease is substantially exceeded. Criteria can be set so that when the number of cases exceeds this level the *epidemic threshold* is crossed. The epidemic threshold can either be the upper limit of cases expected at that particular time, an excess mortality, or a combination of both the number of cases and the mortality.

Characteristics of an epidemic (Fig. 2.1) are as follows:

1. *Latent period*, the time interval from initial infection until start of infectiousness.
2. *Incubation period*, the time interval from initial infection until the onset of clinical disease. The incubation period varies from disease to disease and for a particular disease has a *range*. This range extends from a *minimum* incubation period to a *maximum* incubation period (see Chapter 19).
3. *Period of communicability*, the period during which an individual is infectious. The infectious period can start before the disease process commences (e.g. hepatitis) or after (e.g. sleeping sickness). In some diseases, such as diphtheria and streptococcal infections, infectiousness starts from the date of first exposure.

Various factors modify the incubation period so that if it is plotted on a time-based graph, it is found to rise rapidly to a peak and then tail off over a longer period (Fig. 2.2). The infecting dose, the portal of

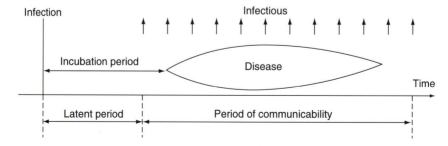

Fig. 2.1.   Parameters of an infection (see text for definitions).

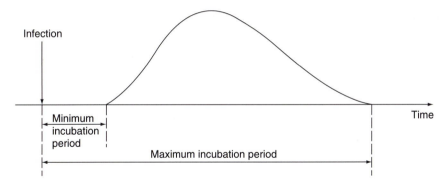

Fig. 2.2.   Distribution curve of incubation times (the epidemic curve).

entry, immune response of the host and a number of other factors modify the normal distribution to extend the tail of the graph. By using a log-time scale, this skewed curve can be converted to a normal distribution and the mean incubation period measured.

An epidemic can either be a *common source* epidemic or *propagated source* epidemic (Fig. 2.3).

- Common source epidemics can further be divided into a *point source* epidemic resulting from a single exposure, such as a food poisoning episode, or an *extended* epidemic resulting from repeated multiple exposures over a period of time (e.g. a contaminated well).

- In a propagated source epidemic, the agent is spread through serial transfer

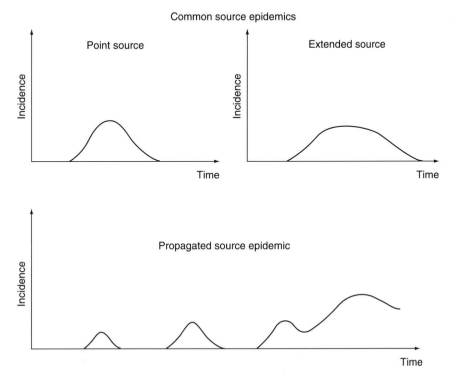

Fig. 2.3.   Epidemic types.

from host to host. With a disease having a reasonably long incubation period, the initial peaks will be separated by the median incubation periods. Chickenpox (varicella) can start as an epidemic in one school; then mingling children will lead to transfer to another school, leading to a series of propagated epidemics.

2.2.1 Investigation of a common source epidemic

In the investigation of any outbreak of a disease, the basic approach is to gather information on the following:

1. *Persons*: age, sex, occupation, ethnic group, etc. comparing the number infected with the population at risk.
2. *Place*: country, district, town, village, household and relationship to geographical features such as roads, rivers, forests, etc. conveniently marked on a map.
3. *Time*: annual, monthly (seasonal), daily and hourly (nocturnal/diurnal). The number of cases occurring within each time-period is plotted on a graph. These aspects will be covered in greater detail later.

In a *point source* epidemic, the number of cases of the disease occurring each day are plotted on a graph to produce an epidemic curve. The earliest cases will be those with the minimum incubation period and the last of the cases are those with the maximum incubation period if all were infected at a single point in time, as illustrated in Fig. 2.4.

Three factors describe a point source epidemic:

- the epidemic curve;
- the incubation period of the disease;
- the time of infection.

If only two of these factors are known, then the third can be deduced. From the epidemic curve, the median (or geometric mean) of the incubation periods is determined. If the disease is known from its clinical features, then the incubation period will also be known (Chapter 19). Therefore, by measuring this known incubation period back in time from the median incubation period on the curve or the minimum incubation period from the beginning of the curve, the time of infection can be calculated. The source now localized to a restricted period of time can be more easily investigated.

If the disease is unknown, but there is evidence of the time of infection (e.g.

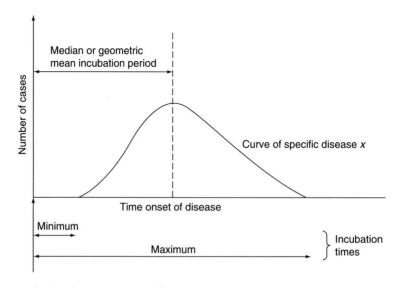

Fig. 2.4.   Investigation of a point source epidemic.

a particular event in time that brought all the cases together or linked them by a common phenomenon), then the incubation period can be calculated and a disease (or aetiological agent producing a disease) with this incubation period can be suspected. This method was used to work out the incubation period for the first epidemic of Ebola haemorrhagic fever, as there were a large number of fatal cases that occurred in one hospital at the same time.

In an *extended source* epidemic, the time of infection can be deduced by measuring back in time from the first case on the rising epidemic curve to the maximum and minimum incubation periods of the diagnosed disease. Search within this defined period of time can elucidate the source.

Epidemics are suitably described by expressing them in *attack rates*. In a common source epidemic, the *overall attack rate* is used:

Overall attack rate

$$= \frac{\text{Number of individuals affected during an epidemic}}{\text{Number (of susceptibles) exposed to the risk}}$$

In a new infection, everyone will be at risk (e.g. with the SARS virus), but as the infection spreads, persons will become immune and are therefore no longer at risk. Where an epidemic occurs at regular intervals (e.g. measles), only those people who have not met the infection before or have not been vaccinated will be at risk.

2.2.2 Investigation of propagated source epidemics

With a propagated source epidemic, phases of infection occur at regular intervals. The time-period between these phases is called the *serial interval* (Fig. 2.5). Features of the epidemic are measured in the same way as a common source epidemic, while an estimate of time of recurrence is given by the serial interval. After several propagated epidemics, cases remaining from the previous epidemic will merge with the next so that the regular serial pattern will be lost.

Contagiousness or the probability that an exposure will lead to a transmission is measured by:

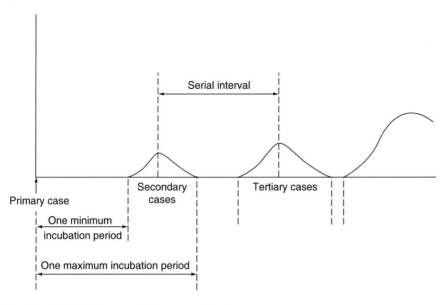

Fig. 2.5. Investigation of a propagated source epidemic.

Secondary attack rate

= Number of cases within the period of one minimum and one maximum incubation period (secondary cases) from the primary case

divided by Number (of susceptibles) exposed to the risk

An example is smallpox, which had a high secondary attack rate and was therefore very contagious. Since smallpox was eradicated and people are no longer vaccinated, the level of immunity has waned and there is the fear that a very similar disease, monkeypox, could now increase and be a threat. However, it has a lower secondary attack rate; so we can rest assured that this is unlikely to happen (see also Section 18.2).

2.2.3 Dynamics of epidemics

The increase in cases in an epidemic has given rise to a measure called the *basic reproductive rate*. This measures the average number of subsequent cases of an infection from a single case in an unlimited, wholly susceptible population. For example, if one case gave rise to two and these two to four, etc., as illustrated in Fig. 2.6, the basic reproductive rate would be 2. This is the most extreme situation. In reality, the epidemic is modified by immunity or the population limited by people having already become infected; therefore, such a rapid increase does not occur. If the basic reproductive rate is less than 1, as illustrated in Fig. 2.7, the epidemic will not take off. The importance of this concept is in control, whereby if the basic reproductive rate can be reduced below 1, then the disease will die out.

The basic reproductive rate has been used in mathematical models of disease, particularly for malaria and filariasis.

2.2.4 Population size

As mentioned above, the continuation of an epidemic is determined by the number of susceptibles remaining in the population.

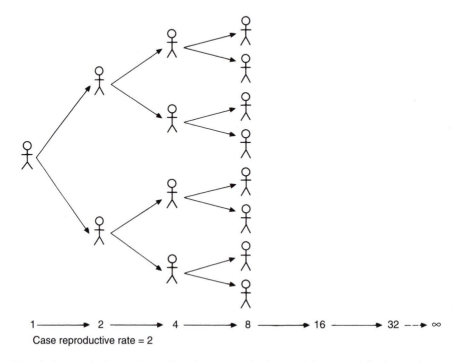

1 → 2 → 4 → 8 → 16 → 32 --→ ∞

Case reproductive rate = 2

Fig. 2.6. Basic reproductive rate increasing – i.e. >1. Maximal transmission: every infection produces a new case.

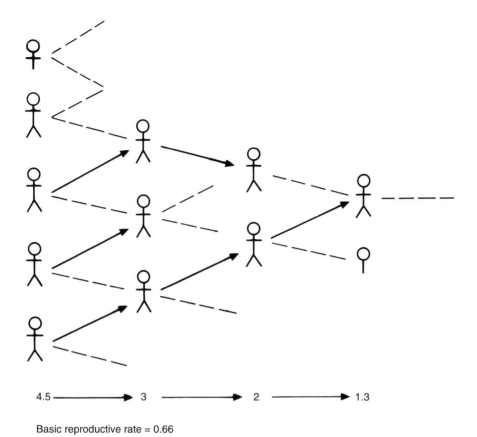

4.5 ⟶ 3 ⟶ 2 ⟶ 1.3

Basic reproductive rate = 0.66

Fig. 2.7. Basic reproductive rate decreasing – i.e. <1. Unsustained transmission: each transmission gives rise to less than one new case and the infection dies out.

Once an individual has experienced an episode of the disease (whether manifest or not), he or she may develop immunity (either temporary or permanent) or die. When a certain number of individuals have developed immunity then there are insufficient susceptibles and the infection dies out. This collective permanent immunity (as occuring in viral infections) is called the *herd immunity*. After a period of time, depending on the size of the population, this herd immunity becomes diluted by new individuals born (or by immigration) and a new epidemic can take place. This is called the *critical population* (the theoretical minimum host population size required to maintain an infecting agent). It depends upon the infectious agent, the demographic structure and the conditions (hygiene, etc.) of the host population. In third world countries with their high birth rates the critical population is less than that in developed countries. Examples of the critical human population size are for measles 500,000 and for varicella 10,000.

If the population is less than the critical size, then regular epidemics will occur at intervals related to the population size. An example is given in Fig. 12.2 of a measles epidemic, which occurred regularly every 3 years in a well-defined community. These regular epidemics can be analysed in the same way as a propagated source epidemic, from which it has been shown that the smaller the community, the longer is the interval between epidemics.

An extension of the concept of herd immunity shows that not everyone in a population needs to be vaccinated to prevent an epidemic. On the same principle as calculating the critical population, the *critical rate of vaccination coverage* can also be worked out. In other words, the population that will need to be successfully vaccinated to reduce the population at risk below the epidemic threshold. It can be similarly shown that even if this target is not reached, then the epidemic will be put off until a future date when the susceptible unvaccinated children will have grown older and therefore be able to cope with the infection better. This is illustrated in Fig. 12.2.

2.2.5 Investigating food- and water-borne epidemics

Other epidemiological techniques are useful for investigating food- and water-borne epidemics, particularly case–control and cohort study methods.

Case–control studies An example of the use of a case–control study in a cholera investigation is given where fish were suspected to contain the aetiological agent. In this community, people preferred to eat fish marinated, but uncooked. Cases were interviewed as to whether they ate raw fish and compared with a similar group who had not had the disease. The results are set out in a two-by-two table: there was a significant finding $\chi^2 = 50.47$; $P < 0.001$.

	Cases	Controls	Total
Ate raw fish	31	8	39
Did not eat raw fish	3	60	63
Total	34	68	102

A reasonable estimate of the *relative risk* can be arrived at (as the incidence rates are not known) from the two-by-two table, using the odds ratio, *ad/cb*:

Suspected cause	Cases	Controls
Present	a	b
Absent	c	d

In the example above, the relative risk of contracting cholera after eating raw fish is

$$\frac{31 \times 60}{3 \times 8} = 77.5.$$

Cohort studies A cohort is a group of people all exposed to the same aetiological agent. By following this group over time, the risk of developing disease can be measured. A modification of the technique can be used in outbreak investigation, particularly food poisoning. This compares the attack rate in the persons exposed to the factor with the attack rate in those not exposed to the factor. In a food poisoning outbreak, where various foods are suspected, then the attack rates in those eating and not eating the range of foods can be compared. This is best illustrated by using an example as shown in Table 2.1. The relative risk for each food item is calculated as above and the results set down in a table. Most of the relative risk values are about 1, but there is over four times the risk of becoming ill if you ate fish, so the investigator would suspect fish as being the most likely cause.

2.3 Endemicity

An endemic disease implies that there is a constant rate of infection occurring in the community. As new individuals are born, they become infected, are cured (including self-cure), retain the infection for life or become immune. Prevalence rates will measure the level of endemicity as it applies to the community. Incidence rates will measure change in the level of infection over a period of time.

While it is useful to compare prevalence from one community to another, on more

Table 2.1. Food-specific attack rates and the relative risks of eating different foods (meal eaten by 152 persons).

Food item	Ate			Did not eat			Relative risk
	Sick	Well	Attack rate (%)	Sick	Well	Attack rate (%)	
Rice	115	28	80.4	45	4	55.5	1.4
Potatoes	111	31	78.2	9	1	90.0	0.9
Fish	93	22	80.9	17	30	18.9	4.3
Beans	101	29	77.7	16	6	72.7	1.1
Coconut	86	22	79.6	24	20	54.5	1.5
Bananas	109	32	77.3	10	1	90.9	0.8

careful investigation, it will be found that within a community, prevalence rates can also vary. These areas of increased prevalence within a community are called foci. Two types of foci occur:

- *host focality*, where some individuals have more severe infection than others, e.g. worm load in schistosomiasis;
- *geographical focality*, where certain localities have a higher prevalence rate than others. Malaria exhibits geographical focality.

These concepts are important in control strategy. When a control method is applied equally to a community, then the overall decrease in disease will leave the foci to maintain infection. However, if the foci are identified and treated, then the infectious source is contained (Fig. 2.8).

Incidence rates show change in the endemicity either upwards, downwards or remaining the same. A decreasing incidence will indicate that the disease may be dying out, especially if control measures have been used. Incidence rates often show a seasonal pattern (Fig. 1.7) and threshold levels that take into account this seasonal variation can be set to give early warning of the disease becoming epidemic.

(a) (b)

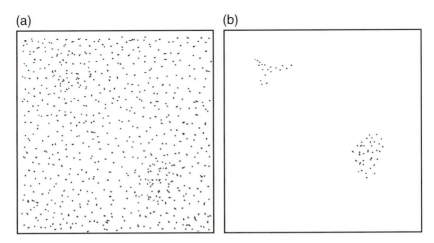

Fig. 2.8. The focality of endemic disease. (a) A universally homogenous prevalence rate is measured in an area. (b) Once control measures have been implemented, foci of persistent transmission are revealed.

2.4 Quantitative Dynamics

Estimates of the magnitude of the infectious process, or the degree of control likely to be achieved, can be calculated. As an introduction to quantitative dynamics, examples of helminth infections are used.

2.4.1 Hookworm

Consider a family of five people with four out of the five infected with hookworms, producing on average some 4000 eggs/g of faeces. Approximately 200 g of faeces are voided by the average person each day, so the four people are excreting $4 \times 4000 \times 200 = 3.2 \times 10^6$ eggs/day. If each of these eggs results in a viable larva, then the potential for infection would be astronomical.

If the head of the household is now persuaded to install a latrine and he encourages his family to use it, then hopefully there should be no further contamination of the surroundings and infection will decrease as the worms die off. Unfortunately, his youngest child does not understand how to use a latrine and despite being taken to it by his mother, half of the stools are still deposited indiscriminately around the neighbourhood. This results in $100(g) \times 4000$ (eggs) $= 4 \times 10^5$ eggs deposited, which

means that the potential for infecting the rest of the family has hardly altered. (This is a simplistic example implying that the eggs will still be concentrated where infection is most likely to occur.)

2.4.2 Schistosomiasis

An idealized situation is illustrated in Fig. 2.9. Ten people with schistosomiasis are all potential polluters of a body of water. Each gram of faeces might contain 80 eggs, but if only half of them reach the water, then there are still 40×200 (an average stool specimen is 200 g) $= 8 \times 10^3$ eggs per person or 8×10^4 eggs from all ten people, reaching the water every day. The miracidium that hatches from the egg needs to find a host snail to complete its development. Snails can reproduce rapidly so that one snail can produce a colony in 40 days and be infective in 60 days. The numbers of cercariae liberated from a snail are immense, but because they need to find a human host within 24 h (generally less), few are successful. The ten people entering the water at the other side of the picture could all become infected, but in reality, only a proportion are likely to be so.

When control is considered, there is the choice of preventing pollution of the

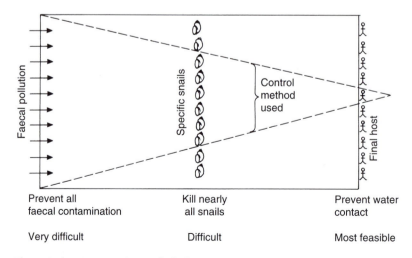

| Prevent all faecal contamination | Kill nearly all snails | Prevent water contact |
| Very difficult | Difficult | Most feasible |

Fig. 2.9. Theoretical environmental control of schistosomiasis.

water, destroying the snails or preventing water contact. (There is also mass treatment of the population which will reduce the total egg load, but for the present argument, it will not be discussed here.) If latrines were provided and nine out of the ten people used them, there would still be 8×10^3 eggs from the tenth person going into the water, sufficient to maintain almost the same level of snail infections. If all the snails were destroyed except a few, then within 60 days, the situation would return to what it was before. However, if any one of the ten people could be prevented from making contact with the water, then his/ her freedom from infection would be absolute.

Of course, the situation is never as clear-cut as this, but the illustration is made to show that a sanitation or molluscicide programme needs to be virtually perfect, whereas prevention from water contact can provide complete protection to the individual. This is a simplified example, but a more realistic situation can be simulated by the use of mathematical models.

Mathematical models will not be covered in any more detail here, but examples will be found in measles (Fig. 12.1), malaria (Section 15.6 and Fig. 15.7) and lymphatic filariasis (Fig. 15.10). They are especially useful in determining control strategy, which is the subject of the next few chapters.

3

Control Principles and Methods

3.1 Control Principles

Control can be directed either at the agent, the route of transmission, the host or the environment. Sometimes it is necessary to use several control strategies. The general methods of control are summarized in Fig. 3.1.

3.1.1 The agent

Destruction of the agent can be by specific treatment, using drugs that kill the agent *in vivo*, or if it is outside the body, by the use of antiseptics, sterilization, incineration or radiation.

3.1.2 Transmission

When the agent is attempting to travel to a host, it is at its most vulnerable position; therefore, many methods of control have been developed to interrupt transmission.

Quarantine or isolation Keeping the agent at a sufficient distance and for a sufficient length of time away from the host until it dies or becomes inactive can be effective in preventing transmission. Quarantine or isol-

ation can be used for animals as well as humans. The former is more effective because animals can be forcibly restrained. Because it is difficult to quarantine humans, it is not widely practised as a method of control, except where the disease is very infectious or the patient can be restrained easily (e.g. in hospital, Lassa fever).

Contacts People who might have become infected because of their close proximity to a case are called contacts. They can be isolated, given prophylactic treatment or kept under surveillance.

Environmental health Methods of personal hygiene, water supplies and sanitation are particularly effective against all agents transmitted by the faecal–oral route whether by direct transmission or complex parasitic cycles involving intermediate hosts.

Animals Whether they act as reservoirs or intermediate host animals can be controlled by *destruction* or *vaccination* (e.g. against rabies). If animals are to be eaten, their carcasses can be *inspected* to make sure that they are free of parasitic stages. The excretions or tissues of an animal can be infectious; so protective clothing and gloves should be worn when handling animals.

© R. Webber 2005. *Communicable Disease Epidemiology and Control,* 2nd edition (Roger Webber)

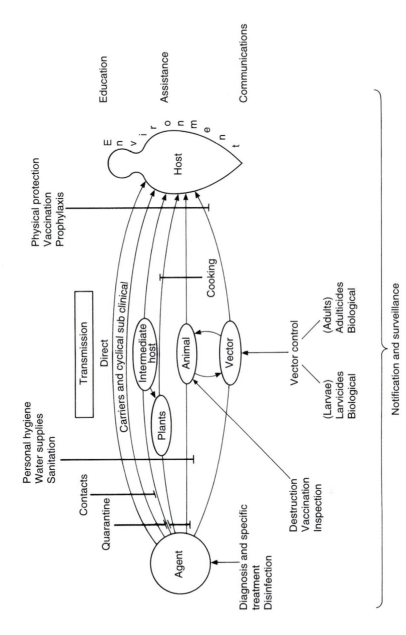

Fig. 3.1. Control principles.

Cooking Proper cooking renders plant and animal produce safe for consumption, although some toxins are heat-resistant. Food should be prepared hygienically before cooking and stored properly afterwards.

Vector control is one of the most highly developed methods of interrupting transmission because the parasite utilizes a vulnerable stage for development and transport. Attack on vectors can either be on their larval stage by using *larvicides* and methods of biological control, or while they are adults with *adulticides.*

3.1.3 Host

The host can be protected by physical methods (mosquito nets, clothing, housing, etc.), by vaccination against specific diseases or by taking regular prophylaxis.

3.1.4 Environment

The environment of the host can be improved by education, assistance (agricultural advice, house building, subsidies, loans, etc.), and improvement of communications (to market his produce, reach health facilities, attend school, etc.). In the course of time, these will be the most effective methods of preventing continuation of the transmission cycle.

3.2 Control Methods – Vaccination

3.2.1 Vaccines

The newborn baby carries antibodies transmitted from its mother across the placenta and from early breast-feeding, protecting it at a very vulnerable stage in life. The effects of these antibodies wear off after 6 weeks to 6 months so that the baby starts making its own from natural or artificial infections that it acquires.

Artificial infection is given by vaccination, or rather the objective is to administer the antigenic substances produced by the disease organisms in a vaccine without the host developing the disease. Vaccine can be given, but immunity does not always result due to poor administration, the vaccine no longer being potent, or the host not developing an immune response. Therefore, the term vaccination is mostly used in this book to indicate the administration of vaccine rather than immunization, which can be misunderstood as immunity has been given.

The immune system of the full-term newborn is capable of producing antibodies and mobilizing cellular defenses. Bacillus Calmette-Guérin (BCG) and polio can be given shortly after birth and killed antigen vaccines are also effective from the first month of life. Some live vaccines like measles do not provide protection if given early because of circulating maternal antibodies.

Vaccines can be of four different kinds:

1. *Live attenuated organisms* give the body an actual infection, inducing antibody production. This is the best kind of vaccine as it generates maximal response from a single dose and as a consequence, immunity is long-lasting. The danger with live attenuated vaccines is that the organisms could revert to the virulent strain. Examples are measles and oral polio, which are attenuated virus infections, and BCG, which is an attenuated bacterium.
2. *Killed organisms* are used when it is not possible to produce a live attenuated strain. Immunity does not develop so well and the vaccine has to be repeated to induce the body defence mechanisms to increase their response. An example is pertussis (whooping cough).
3. *Active components* can be separated from organisms and vaccines made from these organisms. Good immunity is produced, but they are expensive to manufacture. An example is hepatitis B vaccine, which is a recombinant DNA or plasma-derived vaccine.

4. *Toxoids* are detoxified bacterial exotoxins and are an important way of producing antibodies to bacterial toxins. They do not prevent the infection, but counteract the dangerous effects of the toxin. Like killed organisms, several doses have to be given to induce a sufficient antibody response and booster doses repeated from time to time to maintain the level. Diphtheria and tetanus toxoid are two vaccines in this category.

3.2.2 Vaccine schedules

The type of vaccine and the age of risk of developing the target disease determine the optimum time and schedule for administering each vaccine. The characteristics of the principal vaccine-preventable diseases (included in the Expanded Programme of Immunization (EPI) programme in most developing countries) are as follows:

Tetanus can enter the neonate through an infected umbilical cord, producing a high mortality. Protection is by immunizing pregnant women with tetanus toxoid. This protection is short lived and the child should be given tetanus toxoid early in infancy as the combined vaccine diphtheria, tetanus and pertussis (DTP). Toxoid is also given to adults as a course of three vaccinations to prevent tetanus, or if not so protected, when there is a wound, which could possibly be infected with *Clostridium tetani*. The World Health Organization (WHO) policy is to vaccinate all women of childbearing age with a lifetime total of five doses of tetanus toxoid.

Whooping cough (pertussis) is a serious disease of young children, often with a fatal outcome in infants less than 6 months old. Vaccination must start before this time, preferably at 1 month or soon after, to produce a sufficient level of antibodies.

Diphtheria is a dangerous disease at any age, so it is preferable to start protection

early. Diphtheria, pertussis and tetanus are normally combined in a triple vaccine (DTP) given at monthly intervals in early childhood after the first month of age. If resources permit, a booster dose should be given at 18 months to 4 years of age. Adults should have booster doses of adult vaccine (Td) every 10 years.

Poliomyelitis infection is induced by three different strains of virus. The oral polio vaccine (OPV) contains all three attenuated strains of the virus, but the gut may not be infected by three strains at the same time and so three doses are required to ensure protection. In developing countries where wild poliovirus is circulating, a first dose is given as soon after birth as possible, followed by three other doses at the same time as DTP. In the WHO global eradication programme mass vaccination, regardless of previous vaccination, all children under 5 years (two doses at an interval of 4 weeks) are vaccinated, followed by 'mopping up' in areas of low coverage or where continuing transmission is identified. Endemic polio is now only found in Africa and Southeast Asia. Inactivated polio vaccine (IPV) is favoured in many developed countries, but is more expensive and produces less herd immunity. As the reservoir of wild virus is being eliminated, IPV is the preferred vaccine as there is no risk of reversion of the vaccine to a pathogenic form.

Haemophilus influenzae *type b* is an important cause of meningitis and pneumonia in children under 6 years of age, particularly those 4–18 months and a vaccine given before this age gives a high degree of protection. The vaccine is a conjugate known as Hib and has the advantage of inducing antibody response and immunological memory in infants as well as reducing nasopharyngeal carriage of the organism, thereby reducing transmission. It is given at the same time as DTP.

Measles is one of the most important causes of childhood death and disability in the tropics. It reaches maximal prevalence by the end of the first year of life, but many children already would have been infected by 6–12 months. Maternal antibodies do not diminish sufficiently until 6 months for the attenuated virus to be effective, so the optimal time for vaccination is 9 months in developing countries. Prolonged immunity is obtained if vaccine is given later (at 12–15 months) so this is a preferable time in developed countries or those in which there is a low prevalence. A second measles vaccination should be given at 4–5 years or on school entry (see Section 12.2).

Rubella The objective of giving rubella vaccination is to reduce congenital rubella syndrome (CRS), which occurs if a woman becomes infected just before or in the first 20 weeks of pregnancy. If the vaccination programme is efficient, then a strategy to eliminate rubella by giving a combined measles and rubella (MR) or measles, mumps and rubella (MMR) vaccination to all children 9–12 months old can be started. If the objective is to reduce CRS, then all adolescent girls and women of childbearing age should be vaccinated (see Section 12.3).

Mumps An infection of the salivary glands, mumps can cause orchitis and meningitis and more rarely encephalitis. Vaccination is conveniently combined with MR vaccines and given at 9–12 months of age in developing countries or 12–15 months in developed countries, with a second dose at 4–5 years or at school entry (see Section 12.4).

Tuberculosis The maximum age risk of tuberculosis depends on the prevalence of active infection in the community. Where there are many open cases, even small children are at risk, but in a society where most cases are in older people and individuals do not contact many others until they start work in young adulthood, the period of greatest risk is adolescence. In developing countries, vaccination is given at birth, whereas in developed countries, BCG is given when the child starts school or selectively to risk groups such as immigrants from

high-risk countries. BCG should not be given to pregnant women or those with symptomatic HIV infection. However, even in countries where there is a high level of HIV and tuberculosis, BCG should be given to all infants at birth, as it is unlikely that they would have developed symptoms of HIV infection by this time.

Hepatitis B leads to chronic liver disease, especially cirrhosis, which is a predisposing cause of primary liver cell cancer. The prevalence of hepatitis B is as high as 8% in many parts of the world, but if the vaccine is administered before infection, the disease and carrier state are prevented. WHO recommends that hepatitis B vaccine be included in the routine childhood vaccination schedule. It is most conveniently administered in three doses at the same time as DTP, but in countries with a high carrier state, an additional dose at birth is recommended. This will probably only be necessary for a comparatively short period of time because once hepatitis B vaccine becomes widely used, the carrier state will rapidly decline. In developed countries where the incidence is much lower, the vaccine is given in adolescence or to those at risk, but will probably be incorporated into the routine vaccination programme at some stage.

Combinations and schedules Different vaccines can be combined (e.g. DTP), or can be given together (e.g. DTP and polio). A sufficient interval must be left between doses to allow time for the antibody response to take place, 1 month normally being sufficient. All these factors and the national characteristics of a country will determine the vaccination schedule to be followed. A suggested regime is as follows:

Before birth	Tetanus toxoid to all women of childbearing age with at least two doses in the first pregnancy and one in the second.
Birth	BCG. OPV in endemic areas and hepatitis B vaccine in areas of high prevalence

1–2 months	DTP plus OPV plus hepatitis B plus Hib
2–3 months	DTP plus OPV plus hepatitis B plus Hib
3–6 months	DTP plus OPV plus hepatitis B plus Hib
9–15 months	MMR (see Sections 12.2, 12.3 and 12.4); OPV if not given at birth
4–5 years or school entry	MMR

DTP and OPV can be given even if the child has a mild illness. Measles vaccine can also be given if the child is having a mild illness as it does not have any effect for several days, by which time the minor illness would have been cured. Vaccination should always be given to the malnourished child, who is at particular risk from infection. Protective response is good except in cases of severe kwashiorkor. (Further information can be found on individual vaccines under the various diseases.)

3.2.3 Operational factors

In planning vaccination programmes, cultural, logistic and other operational factors largely determine the coverage. Some of these are:

1. The strongest motivation to attend MCH clinics is immediately after the child has been born; the shorter the interval between birth and vaccination, the more likely they are to be brought by their mothers.
2. A range of ages, days and combinations should be available so that the time of attendance is always the right time for vaccination. If a mother is told to bring her child back at a set time or at a particular age of the child, then she probably will not bother.
3. Admission to hospital is an ideal opportunity to check whether the vaccination schedule is up to date. Measles vaccination is particularly important as many children contract serious measles when admitted to hospital for another complaint.

4. A primary course need never be repeated, even if the booster dose is long delayed.
5. An interrupted course can be resumed whenever feasible without starting from the beginning again.
6. If the interval between doses ends up as being longer than planned, the immunological effect will not be reduced. The only disadvantage of long drawn out schedules is that the individual is not rapidly protected.

3.2.4 The cold chain

The cold chain is a descriptive term for the whole sequence of links that must be maintained in transporting the vaccine in a viable condition from the manufacturer to the person to be vaccinated. Vaccines will only survive when they are maintained at the correct temperature. There are certain limits when the vaccine can be allowed to depart from the optimal temperature, but the range and time are very short and vaccines rapidly lose their potency. To vaccinate with non-potent vaccine is not only a waste of time and money, but also brings discredit to the vaccination programme.

Some vaccines are stored at freezing temperature (poliomyelitis, BCG and measles), while others are at the standard refrigerator temperature of 4–8°C (DTP and tetanus). If stored at the wrong temperature, the vaccine will be destroyed. The two elements of the cold chain are speed of transport and maintenance of a steady temperature; hence the fastest means of getting a vaccine from one place to another is used. A temperature-sensitive strip that changes colour if the batch becomes too warm during the period of transport accompanies most vaccines. The viability of the vaccine can then be checked and the problem link in the cold chain detected.

Cold boxes are very well insulated containers lined with freezer packs in which vaccines can be transported or stored for up to 7 days. They are valuable for mobile vaccination teams, but for the individual vaccinator, a hand-held vacuum flask will store vaccines for 1–2 days, depending on the outside temperature.

Certain vaccines, such as measles and BCG, are sensitive to light and need to be protected while they are being diluted, stored and administered to a person. Special dark glass syringes can be obtained, but covering with a cloth is just as efficient. Many potent vaccines are destroyed by being drawn up into syringes that are still warm from the sterilizing process, a sad end to a long cold chain.

3.2.5 Mobile and static clinics

Vaccination can be from static and/or mobile clinics. Their various advantages and disadvantages are given in the following table:

	Static	Mobile
Coverage	Limited to 10 km radius	Large areas
Availability	Always	Occasional
Transport	Not required	Required
Costs	High capital, low recurrent costs	Moderate capital, high recurrent costs
Vaccine supplies	Often erratic	Good

A static clinic responsible for providing primary care services (including delivery) for both the mother and the child is the most effective. A child stands a greater chance of receiving all its vaccines from a static health unit. However, as distance from the clinic increases, the probability of a mother bringing her child to the clinic decreases for every kilometer to be walked. Coverage is best closest to the clinic and decreases further away, with often large gaps between clinics as shown in Fig. 3.2. It is in the inadequately covered areas between the static clinics that an epidemic is likely to occur. Outreach services or mobile clinics then become valuable in vaccinating the in-between areas. For the

economics of static and mobile vaccination clinics, see Section 1.5.1.

Mobile clinics are easier to organize where only one dose of vaccine is required (e.g. measles) and have a special place in mass campaigns.

3.2.6 Seasonality and vaccination campaigns

Many infections follow a seasonal pattern with sufficient regularity that peaks of incidence can be forecast. If the pattern is known, the epidemic can be prevented by carrying out mass vaccination before it is expected (see Fig. 1.7).

3.2.7 Ring vaccination

If an epidemic is spreading, it can be contained by vaccinating everyone in a ring around the site of the epidemic. Villages should be chosen where cases have not yet been reported and an attempt made to vaccinate as many people as possible. If the ring is too close to the epidemic, then the disease might have already affected some people outside the defensive ring and then another will need to be started even further away.

3.2.8 Economies of vaccination

Vaccination coverage is often poor because of constraints put on staff by the cost of vaccines. Vaccines should be supplied in small dose quantities so that a vial can be opened even if there is only one child to be vaccinated. Spare vaccine can often be used up on other children attending the health centre for other reasons. The cost of vaccination is not just the price of the actual vial of vaccine, but includes the whole cold chain and the salary of the vaccinator. To have a vaccinator sitting around not vaccinating because there are not enough children to warrant opening a vial is a false economy.

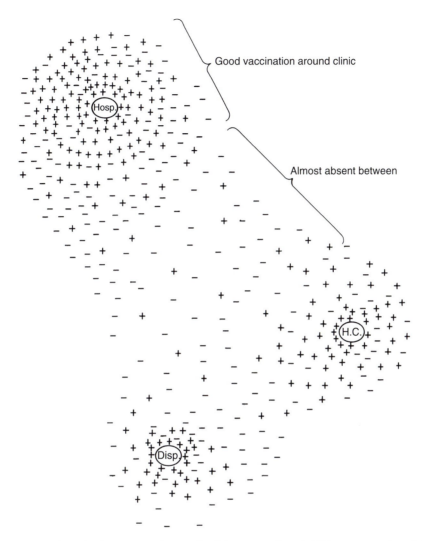

Fig. 3.2. Unequal vaccination coverage from static clinics. +, vaccinated child; −, non-vaccinated child; Hosp., hospital; H.C., health centre; Disp., dispensary.

Proportional costs have been calculated as follows:

Capital	12–15%	Transport	20%
Salaries	45%	Vaccine	5%
Training	2–3%	Others	12–16%

3.2.9 Vaccine efficacy

Vaccine efficacy (VE) is calculated by:

$$VE = \frac{(AR\ in\ unvaccinated - AR\ in\ vaccinated)}{AR\ in\ unvaccinated} \times 100\%$$

where AR is the attack rate (discussed in Section 2.2.1). The VE indicates the maximum achievable level, but poor vaccination technique or storage can reduce this. Also, the more people who are vaccinated, the greater the number of apparent vaccine failures. If the above equation is rewritten to express the percentage of cases vaccinated (PCV) in terms of the percentage of the population vaccinated (PPV) and VE, then:

$$PCV = \frac{PPV - (PPV \times VE)}{1 - (PPV \times VE)}$$

By knowing two of these variables, the third can be calculated. Figure 3.3 shows three curves generated from the equation, each for a different VE. These curves predict the theoretical proportion of cases with a vaccine history. For example, if a measles epidemic is observed in a population with homogeneous measles exposure where 90% of the individuals are vaccinated (PPV=90%) with a 90% effective vaccine (VE=90%), the expected percentage of measles cases with a history of being vaccinated would be 47% (PCV=47%: Example A). However, if only 50% were vaccinated, then 9% of the cases would have been found to be vaccinated (Example B). This is not to say that there is anything wrong with the vaccination programme, but explains why there may appear to be an unexpected number of vaccinated population amongst the cases.

3.3 Environmental Control Methods

Many diseases result from contamination of the environment by faecal matter with transmission by the direct route (e.g. by fingers), or via food and water. The mechanisms are schematically illustrated in Fig. 3.4. The various control methods available are as follows:

- personal and domestic hygiene;
- proper preparation, cooking and storage of food;
- use of water supplies;
- proper disposal of excreta and waste;
- miscellaneous methods including meat inspection and hygiene.

Classifying the water- and sanitation-related diseases into well-defined categories allows

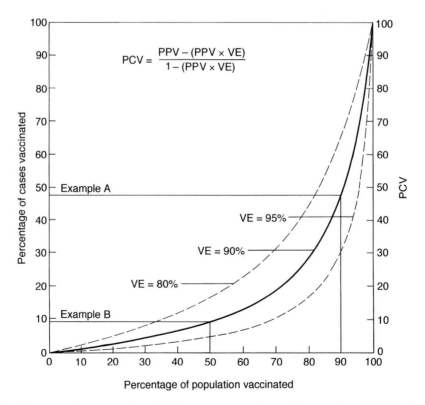

Fig. 3.3. Percentage of cases vaccinated (PCV) per percentage of population vaccinated (PPV), for three values of vaccine efficacy (VE). Reproduced by permission from *Weekly Epidemiological Record 7*, 20 February 1981. World Health Organization, Geneva.

rational control methods to be applied (Table 3.1). The potential impact of control methods is seen in Table 3.2.

3.3.1 Personal hygiene

Personal hygiene is the understanding by the individuals of how infections can be transmitted to them or others by unclean habits, and using appropriate methods to avoid them. Infection can be avoided by preventing bad habits (e.g. promiscuous defecation) or introducing good habits (e.g. handwashing before eating). Infections that can be reduced by personal hygiene are shown in Table 3.3.

Category 1 diseases are reduced by washing of the body and clothing with water, which is best heated and with the addition of soap if available. Categories 2

and 3 diseases are reduced by rigorous hand-washing after defecation and before eating.

Personal hygiene is closely related to the availability of water in sufficient quantity. Water quality is of less importance. Washing is improved by using warm water and soap. Soap reduces surface tension and emulsifies oils, allowing bacteria to be more easily removed. However, large quantities of water can still be effective in the absence of soap.

3.3.2 Protection of foods

Food-transmitted infections can spread either through contamination or by a specific intermediate host. Flies indirectly contaminate food. Protection of the food we eat can be by the following:

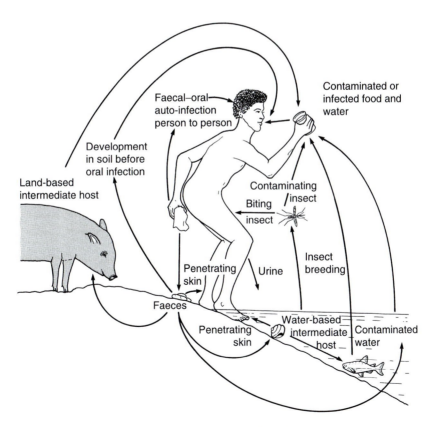

Fig. 3.4. Routes of transmission of the water- and sanitation-related diseases.

Table 3.1. A classification of water- and excreta-related diseases.

Category	Characteristics	Examples	Transmission	Control measures
1. Water-washed disease	Diseases of poor hygiene	Skin diseases, eye diseases, louse-borne typhus	Person-to-person (and autoinfection)	Personal hygiene Increase water quantity
2. Faecal–oral diseases	(a) Low infective dose	*Enterobius*, amoebiasis, enteric viruses	Person-to-person (and autoinfection)	Personal hygiene Increase water quantity
	(b) High infective dose. Able to multiply outside host	Diarrhoeal diseases, cholera, typhoid, hepatitis A	Contamination of food or water	Excreta disposal Cook food Improve water quality
3. Soil-mediated diseases (helminths)	(a) Development in soil	*Ascaris*, hookworm, *Strongyloides*	Larvae penetrate skin or swallowed	Personal hygiene Excreta disposal
	(b) Development in animal (cow or pig) intermediate host	*Taenia* spp.	Cysts in meat	Meat inspection Cook food
4. Water-based diseases	Helminths requiring intermediate hosts			
	(a) Copepods	Guinea worm	Ingested in water	Improve water quality
	(b) Snails only	Schistosomiasis	Penetrates skin	Reduce water contact
	(c) Two intermediate hosts	*Fasciolopsis, Opisthorchis, Paragonimus, Diphyllobothrium*	Eating uncooked specific foods	Excreta disposal Cook food
5. Water- and excreta-related insect vectors	(a) Breeding in water or sewage	Malaria, filariasis, arboviruses	Mosquitoes	Drain breeding sites Maintain water supplies and sanitation
	(b) Breeding or biting near water	Onchocerciasis, trypanosomiasis	*Simulium* Tsetse fly	Water supply at site of use
	(c) Breeding in excreta	Diarrhoeal diseases	Housefly	Excreta disposal

Modified from Bradley, D.J. (1978) In: Feachem, R.G. *et al.* (eds) *Water, Wastes and Health in Hot Climates*. Reproduced by permission of John Wiley & Sons Ltd, Chichester.

- inspection of raw produce;
- packaging and avoiding contamination;
- suitable storage conditions and time-limits;
- washing and correct preparation;
- adequate and even cooking;
- preventing contamination of cooked foods;
- eating cooked foods immediately.

Infections that can be reduced by the proper protection of food are shown in Table 3.4.

Table 3.2. The potential impact of environmental control methods (compare with Table 3.1).

	Disease category	Personal hygiene	Cooking of foods	Water supplies	Sanitation	Miscellaneous
1.	Water-washed diseases	+++	−	++	+	−
2.	Faecal–oral diseases	+++	+	++	+	−
3.	Soil-mediated diseases	++	+++	−	+++	Meat inspection
4.	Water-based diseases	−	+++	++	+	Reduce water contact
5.	Water- and excreta-related insect vectors	−	−	±±	±±	Protection from insects

+++, Very effective; ++, moderately effective; +, effective; −, not effective; ±, can be either effective or not effective.

Table 3.3. Infections that can be reduced by personal hygiene.

Category	Infection
1	Skin sepsis and ulcers
1	Conjunctivitis
1	Trachoma
1	Scabies
1	Yaws
1	Leprosy
1	Tinea
1	Louse-borne fevers
1	Flea-borne infections (including plague)
2	Enteric viruses (including hepatitis A and polio)
2	*Enterobius*
2	Amoebiasis
2	*Trichuris*
2	*Giardia*
2	*Shigella*
2	Typhoid
2	Other Salmonellae
2	*Campylobacter*
2	Non-specific diarrhoeal diseases
2	Cholera
2	Leptospirosis
3a	*Ascaris*

Category 2 infections contaminate food before or after cooking. Flies are often involved. Even if contamination has occurred, correct storage and the disposal of cooked foods after a limited time can prevent sufficient multiplication of bacteria to reach an infective dose.

Categories 3b and 4c (Table 3.4) require specific intermediate hosts in their transmission, so their destruction or proper cooking is an effective means of control. Cooking needs to be at a sufficiently high temperature to kill off the intermediate stages and procedures, such as roasting on a spit or cooking meat 'under done', do not provide high enough temperatures inside the meat. Meat inspection can be effective in *Taenia* infection (3b).

3.3.3 Water supplies

Contaminated water can be the vehicle of transmission of a number of disease-producing organisms. Water is also important in diseases of poor hygiene as a medium for intermediate hosts and as a breeding place for vectors of disease.

The infections and possible improvements that may occur as a result of installing a water supply are shown in Table 3.5.

The provision of water There are four aspects of water supply, which can help to control disease transmission:

• improve water quantity;
• improve water quality;
• reduce water contact by bringing water to site of use;
• prevent spillage by proper maintenance of supplies and drainage.

It will be noticed how this is the normal process in the supply of water. The first objective is to provide water in sufficient quantity, which is followed by improving its quality and finally a piped system is constructed. If this is the pattern followed, then similarly it can be anticipated that the first group of diseases to be reduced will be the water-washed and faecal–oral, then the

water-borne etc. However, water supplies need to be maintained and when they break down, the disease can be expected to return.

In rural water supplies where chlorine treatment of the water is costly, difficult to maintain or inappropriate, then a different standard to that in large centralized supplies may be acceptable. This should not be considered unsatisfactory as the provision of a properly constructed water supply is an improvement on what was used before. Also quality is closely related to quantity. By providing a greater volume of water at a more accessible site, quality will usually be improved.

Health aspects are the concern of the medical worker, whereas the villager looks upon water as a basic necessity. His, or rather her (as women are nearly always the carriers of water), major concerns will be quite different. These are the following:

• availability of water at a more convenient place (preferably in the village);
• a continuous and reliable supply;
• additional water for crops and domestic animals.

Table 3.4. Reduction of infection by food protection.

Category	Infection	Type of food	Possible reduction
2	Enteric viruses (including hepatitis A and polio)	All	+
2	*Hymenolepis*	All	+
2	Amoebiasis	All	+
2	*Trichuris*	All	+
2	*Giardia*	All	+
2	*Shigella*	All, especially dairy produce	++
2	Typhoid	All, especially dairy produce	++
2	Salmonellae	All, especially dairy produce	++
2	*Campylobacter*	All, especially dairy produce	++
2	Non-specific diarrhoeal diseases	All, plus fly contamination	++
2	Cholera	Marine animals, salad	++
2	Leptospirosis	Rat-contaminated foods	++
2	Brucellosis	Milk produce	++
3a	*Ascaris*	All	+
3b	*Taenia*	Cow or pig meat	+++
4b	*Trichinella*	Pig	+++
4c	*Fasciolopsis*	Salad	+++
4c	*Opisthorchis*	Fish (fresh water)	+++
4c	*Paragonimus*	Crustacea (fresh water)	+++
4c	*Diphyllobothrium*	Fish (fresh water)	+++

Refer to footnote of Table 3.2 for the description of +++, ++ and +.

Table 3.5. Expected improvements when installing a water supply.

Category	Infection	Water improvement required	Possible reduction (%)
1	Skin sepsis and ulcers	Increase water quantity	50
1	Conjunctivitis	Increase water quantity	70
1	Trachoma	Increase water quantity	60
1	Scabies	Increase water quantity	80
1	Yaws	Increase water quantity	70
1	Leprosy	Increase water quantity	50
1	Tinea	Increase water quantity	50
1	Louse-borne fevers	Increase water quantity	40
1	Flea-borne diseases (including plague)	Increase water quantity	40
2	Enteric viruses (including hepatitis A and polio)	Increase water quantity	10?
2	*Enterobius*	Increase water quantity	20
2	*Hymenolepis*	Increase water quantity	20
2	Amoebiasis	Increase water quantity	50
2	*Trichuris*	Increase water quantity	20
2	*Giardia*	Increase water quantity	30
2	*Shigella*	Improve water quality	50
2	Typhoid	Improve water quality	80
2	Other Salmonellae	Improve water quality	50
2	*Campylobacter*	Improve water quality	50
2	Non-specific diarrhoeal diseases	Improve water quality	50
2	Cholera	Improve water quality	90
2	Leptospirosis	Improve water quality	80
3a	*Ascaris*	Increase water quantity	40
3a	Hydatid	Increase water quantity	40
3a	*Toxocara*	Increase water quantity	40
3a	Toxoplasmosis	Increase water quantity	40
4a	Guinea worm	Reduce water contact	100
4b	Schistosomiasis	Reduce water contact	60
5a	Malaria	Water piped to site of use and maintenance of water supplies	10
5a	Filariasis		10
5a	Arboviruses		10?
5b	Onchocerciasis	Water piped to site of use	20?
5b	Gambian trypanosomiasis		80

From Bradley, D.J. (1978) In: Feachem, R.G. *et al.* (eds) *Water, Wastes and Health in Hot Climates.* Reproduced by permission of John Wiley & Sons. Ltd, Chichester.

It is a combination of these health and social factors that needs to be used in deciding the appropriateness and benefits of water supplies.

Economic and planning criteria Everybody wants the best possible water supply they can get, but resources are limited so it will be many years before everyone has the supply they desire. Decisions have to be made as to which sections of the com-munity should be served, when they should receive their supply and the level of availability. There are many alternative strategies that may be, or inadvertently will be, used. They might include the following:

- priority of an area on health grounds;
- priority to an area of water scarcity;
- encouragement of development to an area of high potential;

- priority to communities that can contribute in money and labour;
- first come, first served;
- political favouritism.

Other alternatives in the nature of the supply can also be considered:

- supplying a large number of people with the simplest of supplies;
- restricting supplies to certain demonstration areas with a high standard;
- start with the most available natural water sources;
- plan a major project, such as a dam, followed by extension of supply in subsequent years.

This will depend on how much the country, region, district or village is prepared to pay for the price of water. Savings can be made by the following: (i) economies of scale; (ii) standardizing the equipment; and (iii) self-help labour.

The initial water master plan is best formulated by skilled engineers, but its execution can be by a purpose-trained technician, utilizing community effort. The plan needs to take account of health, engineering, political and community demands.

Water capacity and use In selecting a suitable source, the amount of water it produces and its regularity need to be known. If a spring or stream does not flow all the year round, then it is not suitable unless a dam is also built. Measurements of water flow should be made at the end of the dry season and the people asked if the source has ever dried up. A temporary dam can be constructed and the rate of filling a measured bucket estimates the flow. Wells can be mechanically pumped out and the fall noted for a given flow of water. Rainwater catchment is derived from the simple formula:

1 mm of rainfall on 1 m² of the roof in plan will give 0.8 l of water.

As an example, if the roof plan area is 10 m × 5 m and the average annual rainfall

is 650 mm, then $10 \times 5 \times 650 \times 0.8 = 26{,}000$ l/year or 71 l/day, on average.

The demand for water will be determined by the availability, the number of people and the use to which it is put. Availability is the most crucial factor as water that has to be carried some distance will be used much more sparingly than when there is a tap inside the house. Average figures taken from a number of studies are as follows:

Rural supply	20 l/person/day
Standpipe	40 l/person/day
Single tap in the home	80 l/person/day
Multiple taps with bath, W.C., etc.	200–300 l/person/day

At least 50% extra capacity is allowed for future growth of the community and expansion of the supply. A water source is chosen where the expected demand on the supply will never be exceeded, even in the driest time of the year. If this is not possible, then some form of storage will be required. Water use during the night is far less than during the day, so a poor supply can be boosted by providing a storage tank that fills at night. In areas of wide seasonal variation, more extensive storage facilities may be required, such as a dam, to save the rainfall in the few wet months.

Choice of water supply Choosing a water source will depend upon the following:

- proximity to user;
- reliability;
- quantity of water;
- quality of water;
- technical feasibility;
- resources available;
- social desirability or taboo;
- maintenance.

The alternative choices are illustrated in Figs 3.5 and 3.6. Rainwater naturally seeps through the earth until it finds an impervious layer (such as clay) on which it collects. When this impervious layer comes to the

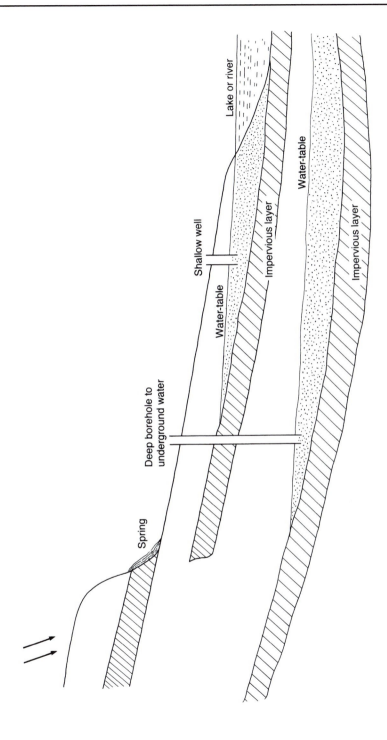

Fig. 3.5. Sources of water.

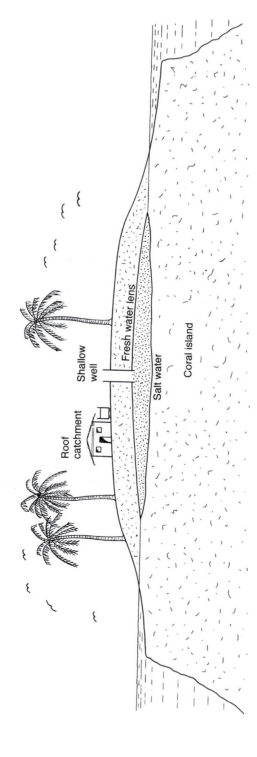

Fig. 3.6. Water catchment and the fresh water lens of coral islands.

surface, water runs out of the ground as a spring. It can also form the bed of a river or in an enclosed area, a lake. This groundwater can be tapped by a shallow well. At a much deeper level, a second impervious layer can trap a large quantity of water. A deep well or bore hole is required to reach this source of water. Island populations (Fig. 3.6) have particular problems in obtaining water and are generally left with only two alternatives. Provided they have suitable roofing material (e.g. corrugated iron), rainwater can be collected and stored in a tank. The other alternative is to sink a well to tap the freshwater lens. Due to a fortunate quality of coral rock, it acts like a large sponge, holding fresh water that has percolated through, floating on the denser sea water. Provided the well is sunk just far enough and not pumped out too hard, freshwater can be obtained. The different water sources are summarized in Table 3.6.

Wells are often a good supply, as long as contamination can be prevented and have the advantage that they can be sited close to houses. This can be achieved by sealing them and having a pump fitted, but this will require maintenance. Deep wells and bore holes need special equipment for their construction and complex pumps to lift water from these depths. They are mainly applicable in areas of severe water shortage such as deserts. Lakes and rivers provide conveni-

ent, but poor quality water. Other sources should be used if possible, but if there is no alternative, then some form of water treatment, such as filtration and storage, should be incorporated. A constant spring that never dries up is a very suitable source, as it is comparatively free from contamination and can normally be led to an outlet without requiring pumping. Maintenance costs will, therefore, be low, so greater capital expenditure can be allowed for protecting the spring and piping its water to the village.

Rainwater catchment is an underutilized source of pure water, either as a main method or as subsidiary (for drinking water). So much good water runs to waste off large expanses of roof that have already been paid for in the construction of the building. This water can be tapped for good use. With the additional cost of guttering and a tank, a family can have a good, safe source of water inside or very close to their house. Storage tanks can either be close to the roof or large concrete structures built underground. Their main danger is that if water is allowed to collect in poorly maintained gutters or uncovered tanks, then mosquitoes can breed there.

The ideal is to find a source that has both constant quantity and good quality, but where the latter is not available, then it can be improved by simple methods, such as the three-pot system (Fig. 3.7).

Table 3.6. Sources of water, their advantages and disadvantages.

	Spring	Shallow well	Bore hole	River	Lake	Catchment
Proximity	Distant	Near	Intermediate	Near	Near	Near
Reliability	Good	Variable	Good	Unreliable	Good	Unreliable
Quantity	Good	Moderate	Good	Variable	Good	Poor
Quality	Good	Moderate	Good	Poor	Poor	Good
Technology	Easy	Moderate	Difficult	Easy[a]	Easy[a]	Moderate
Cost	Low	Moderate	High	Low[a]	Low[a]	Moderate to high
Community preference	High	Moderate	Moderate	Low	Low	Moderate
Maintenance	Low	Moderate	High	Low	Low	Moderate

[a]These assessments are for taking water by hand from the river or lake. If a pump and supply system are used, then the technology is difficult and the cost high.

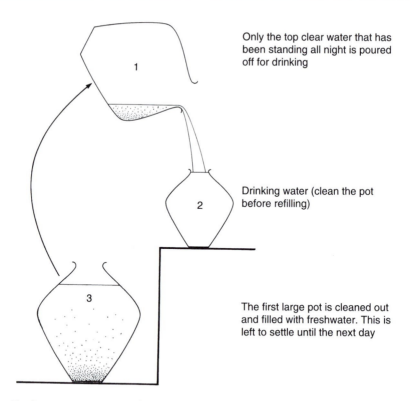

Only the top clear water that has
been standing all night is poured
off for drinking

Drinking water (clean the pot
before refilling)

The first large pot is cleaned out
and filled with freshwater. This is
left to settle until the next day

Fig. 3.7. The three-pot system – a simple means of improving water quality.

3.3.4 Sanitation

With food and water supplies, the emphasis is on the prevention of contamination, but with sanitation, it is reducing the source of the contamination. Social habits concerned with excreta disposal are often strongly held and unless these are approached in a sensible manner, any new system will fail. Sanitation is not just the provision of latrines, but a complex and inter-related subject involving people, water supplies and all other aspects of environmental health.

Health factors As shown in Table 3.1, the main impact of sanitation is on groups 2, 3a, 4c and 5c. The installation of sanitation may produce a reduction in the infections shown in Table 3.7.

The provision of sanitation When providing sanitation, there is a sharp contrast with water supplies. Everybody wants a water supply, but nobody wants to change his or her defecation practice. This is quite simple to explain in that substances taken into the body can be understood as a direct cause of illness, whereas excreting something from the body cannot. Defecation is a necessary, but private business and is not a matter for discussion. There are also social reasons that are set by religious, racial or cultural practice. These may dictate where and where not to defecate, will probably separate the sexes and define particular anal-cleansing practices. With all these patterns and customs that have been taught since childhood, any change becomes a long and difficult process. If a family can see the benefits of a latrine, then they will install and look after it; the health authority can then assist in technical specifications and subsidize costs. Any attempt to impose systems or even build them free of charge will cause resentment or non-use.

Like water, sanitation has to be paid for, but here costs are even less accepted by the population. People are only prepared to pay for the minimum possible in getting rid of their excreta. Only in urban areas will it be considered necessary to pay for the removal of excrement; in rural areas, there is sufficient space. A subsidizing scheme then becomes the main way in which sanitation can be improved. For instance, in pit latrine construction, villagers will need to dig their own hole, but might be sold a bag of cement at a reduced price or be provided with a squatting slab free of charge.

Cost is related to convenience, which is why people are prepared to pay for improved systems, their willingness to pay usually having nothing to do with health. A good pit latrine can be as effective in disease control as a conventional water-carried sewage system, the only difference being that the former is outside the house, while the latter carries excreta from within the house. The cost of this convenience is typically ten times that of a pit latrine.

In choosing the most appropriate excreta disposal system, the emphasis should be on simplicity. Only when a simpler method becomes outmoded because of rising standards and expectations will a more sophisticated system become appropriate. A simple incremental process, as illustrated in Fig. 3.8, can be planned. The first stage is to bury excreta, which will lead on to using a pit latrine. If pit latrines are already accepted by the community, then demonstrating the advantages of improved pit latrines will be the next step. The type of facility will also be determined by the availability of water. As mentioned in Section 3.3.3, the provision of water should precede any sanitation programme as

Table 3.7. The expected improvements from the installation of sanitation.

Category	Infection	Through reduced contamination of	Possible reduction
1	Trachoma	The environment; flies (group 5c)	+
2	Enteric viruses (including hepatitis A)	Vegetables	+
2	*Hymenolepis*	Food and water	+
2	Amoebiasis	Vegetables	++
2	*Trichuris*	Food and water	+
2	*Giardia*	Food and water	+
2	*Shigella*	Food and water	++
2	Typhoid	Food and water	++
2	Other Salmonellae	Food and water	++
2	*Campylobacter*	Food and water	++
2	Non-specific diarrhoeal diseases	Food and water	++
2	Cholera	Food and water	++
3a	*Ascaris*	Soil	+++
3a	Hookworm	Soil	+++
3a	*Strongyloides*	Soil	+++
3b	*Taenia*	Soil	+++
4b	Schistosomiasis	Water	+
4c	*Fasciolopsis*	Water	+
4c	*Opisthorchis*	Water	+
4c	*Paragonimus*	Water	+
4c	*Diphyllobothrium*	Water	+
5	Housefly-transmitted diseases	The environment; flies	±±[a]
5	Filariasis	Water and *Culex quinquefasciatus* breeding	+

[a]Sanitation, if not properly built or maintained, can be as responsible for increasing the fly nuisance as well as decreasing it. Refer to footnote of Table 3.2 for the description of +++, ++, + and ±.

personal hygiene can only be taught if there is water at hand to wash with. The quantity and proximity of this water will then determine the type of sanitary system that can be used. In the second part of Fig. 3.8, the incremental progression of a water-utilizing sanitary system is shown. A pour–flush latrine can be installed where water is obtained from a village standpipe, but with a septic tank or sewerage, a water-flushing system requires in-house water connections.

Siting and contamination The unit must be sited so that it does not contaminate the environment in such a way as to threaten the health of others. With a pit latrine, bacterial pollution can travel downwards for a distance of up to 2 m. If the contamination reaches the water table, it will flow horizontally for up to 10 m. This means that any latrine should be sited at least this distance away from a water supply, such as a well. The latrine should also be placed downhill to the well, although excessive pumping will draw water into the well from all directions, including possibly from a latrine. If a latrine is built less than 10 m from a river or stream, it can pollute it, as the water table will be flowing towards the stream. Latrines in this situation can be potent sources of pollution if the river is used for drinking water. Pollution of the soil is a complex subject and the rough rule of 10 m distance between a latrine and source of drinking water is given as a guide. Contamination is dependent upon the following:

- the velocity of groundwater flow (should be less than 10 m in 10 days);
- the composition of the soil (not fissured, e.g. as in limestone).

Expert advice should be obtained before embarking on a latrine programme.

In a sealed system such as a septic tank or an aquaprivy, contamination of the soil will not take place unless there is a crack in the structure. However, the effluent is highly charged with pathogens and must be disposed of properly. Running it into a storm drain, as often happens, is a bad practice and poses considerable threat of infection. The easiest solution is to lead it into a soakaway, but precautions similar to a latrine need to be taken.

3.4 Vector Control

Parasites are transmitted from one host to another by vectors, often utilizing the stage in the vector to undergo multiplication or development. In some parasites (e.g. malaria) the vector is the definitive host, whereas in others such as *Wuchereria bancrofti*, it is the intermediate host. Whichever part the vector plays, it is a vital one for the parasite and it cannot continue if the vector is destroyed or reduced to sufficiently low numbers. The time of changing from one host to another is a precarious time for the parasite and considerable loss may occur. Malaria gametocyte development must coincide with a mosquito taking a blood meal and both male and female gametocytes are required for fertilization and maturation to take place in the insect's stomach. *W. bancrofti* suffers considerable parasite loss during the vector stage. The vector, therefore, does not have to be completely destroyed, but must be kept at levels too low for transmission to take place. So vector control means vector reduction and not vector eradication.

3.4.1 Mosquito control

The various ways in which mosquitoes can be controlled are as follows:

- adulticides;
- repellents;
- personal protection;
- larvicides;
- biological control;
- environmental modification.

These are all illustrated in Fig. 3.9.

Adulticides Killing the adult mosquito can either be done while it is flying using a

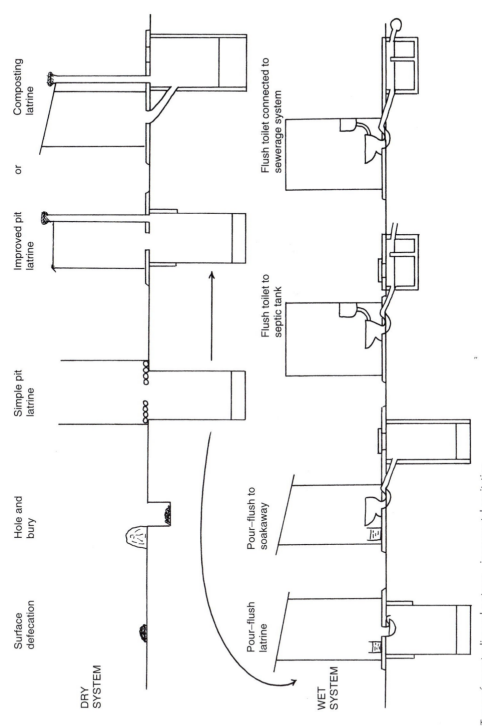

Fig. 3.8. Types of excreta disposal systems – incremental sanitation.

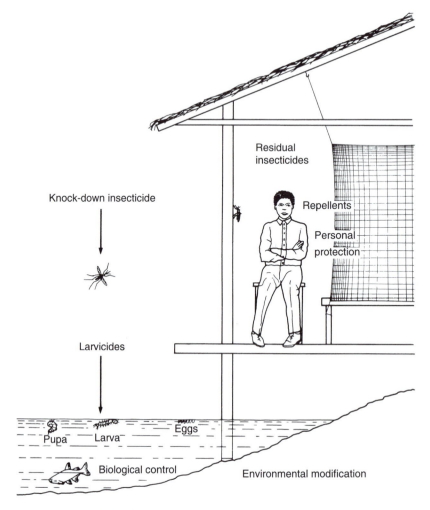

Fig. 3.9. Mosquito control methods.

knock-down spray or when it is resting with a residual insecticide. Knock-down insecticides will kill adult mosquitoes at the time of application only, whereas residual insecticides continue to have a lethal effect for a considerable period of time.

KNOCK-DOWN INSECTICIDES are used to control epidemics of vector-transmitted disease where an explosive increase in the number of flying adults is responsible. They have been used in malaria epidemics, but have perhaps their greatest value in dengue and the control of arbovirus infections. They are used as space sprays (aerosols) in the house, for mosquito survey counts and for disin-

fecting aircraft. Knock-down sprays commonly contain pyrethrum, derived from a species of chrysanthemum grown in highland areas of East Africa. They can be dispersed in aerosols, smoke generators (fogging) or ultra-low volume (ULV) aerial sprays.

RESIDUAL INSECTICIDES Residual spraying is the main method for control of mosquito-transmitted disease because the insecticide continues to remain active for 6 months or more. By careful organization, repeated applications made at regular intervals can maintain a continuing killing effect. Ideally they should be sprayed just before the start of the main transmission season, especially in areas where malaria is seasonal.

Residual insecticides act on the resting mosquito. Mosquitoes need to rest after they have taken a blood meal and generally choose the nearest place, which is the wall of the victim's house. If the wall has been sprayed with residual insecticide, then the mosquito will absorb a lethal dose through its legs while it is resting. The insecticide can either be sprayed as an emulsion or wettable powder, as few of the insecticides commonly used go into solution with a cheap and easily obtainable medium such as water. Emulsions are best on non-absorbent surfaces, while wettable powders are suitable for mud, leaf or other poor quality walls. The wettable medium (generally water) soaks into the wall and leaves the powder on the surface. Some of the insecticide is taken into the porous surface, but this gradually comes out, maintaining a steady concentration. Once residual insecticide has been sprayed on a wall, then it must not be washed or painted.

Residual insecticide sprayed on a surface depends upon a number of factors:

• the proportion of active insecticide in the preparation;
• the amount of insecticide mixed with the fluid medium;
• mixing, before and during application;
• the distance from the surface that is sprayed;
• the speed of application.

These are all specified for a particular insecticide and sprayers must be trained to ensure that the right concentration is delivered. A measured area of plaster can be scraped and the insecticide content analysed.

Residual spraying is carried out by a team of sprayers with manually operated spray apparatus covering a village at a time. Houses are emptied and pets and domestic animals restrained at a suitable place some distance away (as they are sensitive to insecticides). Any insects, beetles and lizards that are killed should be swept up and disposed of before the domestic animals are allowed back into the houses. This takes a considerable amount of organization with a strict schedule of notification, followed by spraying. The supervisor answers any questions, ensures that the work is done and arranges logistic support. If residual spraying is not adequately explained to people, then organizational resistance will develop. The target is to spray every dwelling house whether permanently or temporarily occupied.

Deterrents and repellents can be either smokes or applications to the body in the form of creams and solutions. They do not kill the insect, but deter it from biting.

Mosquito coils or heated pads have a combined deterrent and repellent action. They are made with small quantities of pyrethroids in a slow burning base, but other insecticides can be added to enhance the activity. Used in a still atmosphere, they can be most effective. If they do not prevent all the bites, they reduce the number, which is important in filariasis transmission. They reduce the probability of being bitten by an infective mosquito carrying any disease.

The most commonly used repellent is diethyltoluamide (DEET), which can be applied to the person, clothing, tents and mosquito nets. The solutions can either be dissolved in methylated spirit or emulsified with water and applied to the surface. It is not absorbed by synthetic fabrics and a cotton or wool base is essential if it is to remain for some time. Four weeks of activity is given if continuously exposed, but if the garments (such as a shawl or leg bands) are kept in a polythene bag, then repellent action can continue for 3–6 months. Precaution should be taken while applying DEET to the skin as some individuals are sensitive, while neurological toxicity can be produced in children. Natural repellents made from eucalyptus oil are preferable for application to the person.

Mosquito nets and personal protection Personal protection is a valuable precaution in reducing the number of mosquito bites.

Clothing that covers the arms and legs especially if combined with a repellent can protect an individual most effectively. With the appearance of widespread insecticide resistance, greater reliance must now be placed on personal protection.

The use of mosquito nets is a well-tried method of personal protection. Mosquito nets are fitted to the bed and the edges tucked under the mattress. A knock-down spray applied prior to retiring will prevent any mosquitoes entering the net when the occupant goes to bed. Young children should be placed under nets before it gets dark. If the custom is to sleep on a mat on the floor rather than a bed, then mosquito nets can still be used. The sale of subsidized mosquito nets can be an effective method of malaria control, if they are subsequently treated with an insecticide.

Mosquito nets are treated with synthetic pyrethroids, such as permethrin, deltamethrin, lambda-cyhalothrin or alpha-cypermethrin. They deter mosquitoes from entering should the net be torn or kill it if it touches the net. Nylon nets are better than cotton because they absorb less solution and are stronger, but this has to be offset by their greater cost. Additional advantages of treated nets are that they provide some protection to other people sleeping in the same room. They also kill fleas, lice, bed bugs and cockroaches and even if rolled up will still provide some protection. A modification of this method is to treat curtains that are used to cover doors, windows or any opening. These methods are used in community malaria control programmes.

Nets are treated by soaking them in a solution of the insecticide when new or after they have been washed. The amount of insecticide is $200\,mg/m^2$ permethrin, $25\,mg/m^2$ deltamethrin or $10\,mg/m^2$ lambda-cyhalothrin, calculated by measuring the area of the net. Some treated net programmes are using standard sized nets, all of which are made of the same material, to avoid having to measure each one, but a rough approximation can be made by weighing each net. Once nets have been treated, they should not be washed again until just before re-treatment (normally every year) as this decreases the effectiveness of the insecticide.

Some people suffer from nasal congestion when sleeping under a net that has recently been treated with deltamethrin or lambda-cyhalothrin and it is probably better to put it to one side for the first 2 days if either of these insecticides has been used. Otherwise they are perfectly safe and no long-term effects have been recorded.

One of the problems of treating mosquito nets is that they need to be retreated at annual or 6-monthly intervals, so a recent innovation has been long-lasting insecticidal nets (LLIN) where the insecticide is impregnated into the fibre of the net before it is woven. Such nets are effective for 4 years or more and, therefore, are being actively promoted for malaria control.

A less satisfactory alternative is to screen the whole house, but this is expensive and a torn area will destroy the whole effect. Air conditioning, by providing a sealed room, generally prevents mosquitoes from entering. Even so, it is preferable to use a knock-down spray in the evening to prevent any mosquitoes that may have entered. The cost of these methods is considerably higher than using treated mosquito nets.

Larvicides Substances that block the breathing apparatus of mosquito larvae and destroy the surface tension (so they sink to the bottom) or poison them are known as larvicides. Kerosene spread on water covers the siphon of the larvae so that it dies from asphyxiation. High-spreading oils have been developed, which inactivate the force of surface tension that larvae use to float on the surface. Insecticides sprayed on collections of water will kill larvae as well as many other organisms (including fish), are expensive and generally objected to by the public and hence are rarely used as larvicides. Such preparations as temephos (Abate), with its very low toxicity, are a notable exception.

Larvicides are not efficient methods of mosquito control, their main use being in urban and periurban areas, especially against culicine vectors. Drains and gutters can be sprayed and temephos added to water containers and septic tanks. Surface sprays must be renewed at regular intervals.

To control *Culex quinquefasciatus*, the main vector of urban filariasis, which breeds in latrines or soakaways, expanded poly-styrene beads can be placed in the pit. The beads float on the surface of the water so larvae are dislodged and prevented from breathing, while the function of the latrine or soakaway is not disrupted. The polystyr-ene is manufactured as fine granules and when placed in boiling water, it expands into beads.

Biological control The term biological con-trol is used to describe the natural method of reducing vectors. Various natural agents that have been tried include predators such as larvivorous fish, microbial organisms (e.g. *Bacillus thuringiensis* and *B. sphaeri-cus*) or modification of the insect itself. Male insects can be sterilized by radiation or with chemosterilants and then released into the environment. If these sterile males compete successfully with the unsterilized males, then the females will not be fertilized. Un-fortunately, this technique requires the preparation and release of a sufficient number of males to outnumber those in the natural habitat, which is generally imprac-tical. An alternative technique is to breed mosquitoes that are refractory to the target disease. This can either be through genetic manipulation or by introduction of a closely related natural species. Species replace-ment, as the method is called, offers some promise because similar, but competitive species can be obtained from different parts of the world.

The problem with any biological method is that nature requires a balance. If a predator destroys all its food supply, then it will die. As a result, an equilibrium is reached where the number of predators and those they prey on remain in sufficient numbers for both to exist. Biological control is, therefore, more an aid rather than a definitive method.

Environmental modification In some situ-ations, it is possible to modify the environ-ment to make it unsuitable for the vector. This can include simple methods such as burying tin cans or cutting holes in old tyres to drain water, to clearing vast tracks of forest for tsetse fly control. Any method of environmental modification on a large scale must carefully consider other systems that may be damaged. Clearing large areas of forest can affect the water retention of the soil and deforesting river banks can lead to severe erosion. On the other hand, filling-in or draining a swamp can provide extra land. Eucalyptus trees, which absorb large amounts of water from the soil, can be planted and at a later time, their wood can be used.

Specific methods of environmental modification, such as for trypanosomiasis, will be found under the particular disease, while the emphasis here will be on mosquito control. One of the most successful methods for reducing surface water and preventing breeding places is the construction of sub-surface drains. This should be within the ability of most health personnel. The system of drains should follow the contours (Fig. 3.10) and be at least 1.5 m below the surface. The gradient needs to be between 1 in 400 and 1 in 30. Various materials can be used for constructing the drains, such as stones, bamboo or poles laid length-wise in the bottom of the drain. An-other method of environmental control is to use a siphon, which flushes out mosquito larvae, or a simple dam as shown in Fig. 3.11.

3.4.2 Insecticides

Insecticides for vector control include the following:

1. *Poisons* (e.g. Paris Green, which was used extensively as a larvicide). *Anopheles gambiae* was eradicated from Upper Egypt by this preparation. In view of the resistance to insecticides that has developed, it could be reconsidered.

2. *Fumigants* (e.g. hydrogen cyanide, methyl bromide and ethyl formate) can

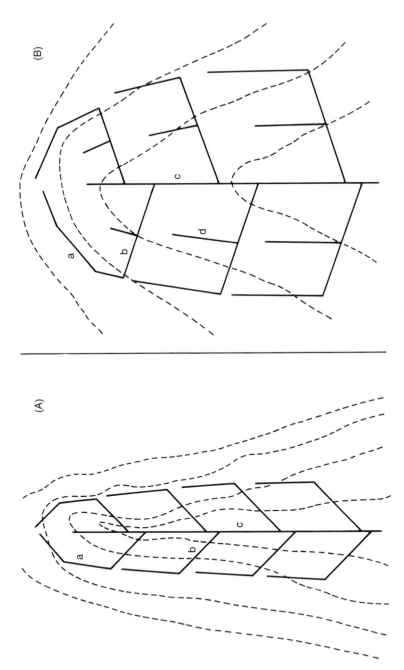

Fig. 3.10. Contour drains in a (A) narrow ravine and (B) wide ravine. (From Davey, T.H. and Lightbody, W.P.H. (1987) *The Control of Diseases in the Tropics.*)

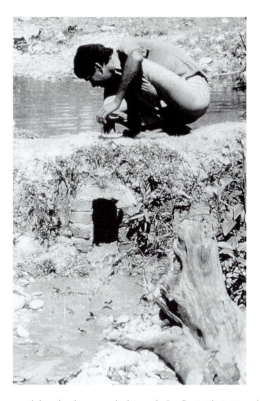

Fig. 3.11. A locally constructed dam for the control of *Anopheles fluviatilis* in Nepal. Every 3 days, the bung is removed and the head of water rushing down the stream is sufficient to dislodge developing mosquitoes.

be used on grain or clothing to destroy infestations.

3. *Knock-down* (e.g. pyrethrum, bioresmethrin and bioallethrin).

4. *Residual,* which are sub-divided into organophosphates, carbamates and pyrethroids. (Organochlorines, 4,4'-dichlorodiphenyl-1,1,1-trichloroethane (DDT), benzene hexachloride (BHC) and dieldrin, which were widely used originally, are no longer available due to their toxic and long-lasting effects on the environment.)

Organophosphates Organophosphates, such as malathion and fenthion, are volatile substances that require frequent application. They act by inhibiting cholinesterase at the nerve junctions and, therefore, can produce temporary paralysis (and respiratory failure) in humans as well as insects. They do not have a long residual action or persist in the environment. Chlorpyrifos (Dursban) and temephos (Abate) are low-toxic compounds widely used as larvicides.

Carbamates Carbamates act in a similar manner to the organophosphates except that they compete with acetylcholinesterase rather than combining with it, making their effects more easily reversed and thereby conferring an advantage to humans. Examples are propoxur and carbaryl.

Pyrethroids Pyrethrum is a naturally occurring insecticide, obtained from a species of chrysanthemum, that has been synthesized to produce a range of more active forms with good residual ability. These are stable substances with low mammalian toxicity and are widely used both for agricultural and medical control. Examples are permethrin, deltamethrin and lambda-cyhalothrin, which are particularly valuable for treating mosquito nets.

3.4.3 Resistance

When an insecticide is being chosen for a control programme, the vector must be tested against various strengths of the insecticide to determine the discriminatory dose (this is when 99.9% mortality of the sample occurs). These tests need to be repeated from time to time during the course of the programme to determine whether the vector remains sensitive. If there are technical reasons why this cannot be done, then resistance will probably only be noticed by an increase in number of insects or cases of the disease. This might, however, indicate deficiencies in the spraying programme and these should first be ruled out. Correct application of insecticide can be measured as mentioned above, while a simple field test for suspected resistance can be performed by placing a few of the insects in a glass jar held against the sprayed surface for a minute. If they are not all killed, then resistance should be suspected and entomological assistance obtained.

Resistance may be partial or complete. If partial, then increasing the concentration of insecticide may be sufficient to control the vector. Unfortunately, complete resistance is soon likely to develop. Resistance is a genetic character and resistant strains are selected out under pressure of insecticides. Initially resistance to one insecticide occurred, but subsequently cross-resistance has developed making several insecticides ineffective. Some species now have multiple resistance. Biological control or trying a completely different strategy may be effective.

3.4.4 Ectoparasite control

Ectoparasites live on the outside of the body, such as fleas, lice, bedbugs, mites and ticks. They are responsible for transmitting a number of diseases covered in Chapter 16. There are various control methods:

- personal hygiene;
- reduction of interpersonal contact from overcrowding and clothes sharing;
- regular and effective washing of clothes and bedding;
- repellents;
- improved house construction;
- insecticides.

Ectoparasites favour dirty dark places, whether they are searching for a suitable habitat on a person or a vantage place in the house from which to mount an attack. Fleas and lice are not removed by washing, but the continued use of warm water and soap considerably deters them. If this is combined with washing of clothes, then fleas can rapidly be controlled. Where possible, clothes and bedding should be boiled or at least subjected to very hot water as fleas are not affected by cold water. Some communities practice head shaving to control lice, while short hair makes them easier to control.

Fleas and lice favour overcrowded conditions, such as those occuring during wars, famines or refugee camps. Efforts should be instituted to reduce overcrowding, but where this is impossible, washing and laundry facilities should at least be provided. Wearing of other people's clothes or sharing combs are common methods of transferring ectoparasites in tropical areas.

Repellents have been used successfully in areas where infection is likely. Impregnated socks and trousers can be effective when passing through micro-habitats of scrub typhus or wild rodent plague. Ticks, bedbugs and reduviids are repulsed by repellents.

Bedbugs, ticks and reduviid bugs live in cracks in the walls of poorly constructed houses, coming out at night to attack sleeping persons. Improving house construction or applying a layer of unbroken plaster to a wall discourages these arthropods permanently. Bed nets can protect the individual from being bitten.

Insecticides are especially useful in epidemic conditions. Dusting clothing, using a puffer to supply the insecticide up trouser legs and skirts and down collars and sleeves, can quickly reduce the number of ectoparasites in concentrations of people. Insecticide solutions can be applied to the hair to kill off head lice or to clothing if repellents are not available. Rat burrows and runs should be dusted with insecticides to kill off plague-carrying fleas before rat catching. Benzyl benzoate or BHC is effective against scabies mites.

3.5 Treatment and Mass Drug Administration

Treatment of the sick is not only a humanitarian action, but reduces the length of illness and, therefore, the period of communicability, thereby aiding control. However, where treatment is incomplete, it can actually prolong the period of communicability, encourage the development of carriers or worst of all, resistant organisms. Case finding and treatment is the main method of control for leprosy (Section 12.6) and tuberculosis (Section 13.1), but careful follow-up is essential to ensure that treatment is taken for the whole period. Rapid diagnosis and treatment is particularly important in acute respiratory infections (Section 13.2) and meningitis (Sections 13.6 and 13.7). The development of effective single dose therapy for the treatment of the sexually transmitted infections (STIs, Chapter 14) has been one of the great challenges of chemotherapy, but the 'power of the needle' has also been the means of transmission of several communicable diseases. In many societies, having an injection (irrespective of what is given) is seen as the panacea of all ills, but unfortunately improperly sterilized needles (including intravenous infusions) have been responsible for much of the transmission of HIV infection and hepatitis B.

Mass drug administration (MDA) is used as a method of control of filariasis (Sections 15.7 and 15.8). However, an MDA needs to cover the entire population in the infected area and the full dose of treatment seen to be swallowed. This becomes an administrative exercise requiring a large number of assistants to ensure that the drug has been properly taken. One of the most successful campaigns, in the Pacific Island of Samoa, used women's groups who are a very well-organized segment of society, with the result that the coverage was over 90%. Generally, such organizations are not available resulting in a lower coverage rate.

Mass treatment is also used in the control of trachoma (Section 7.5). Treatments and MDA regimes will be found under the relevant diseases in Chapters 7–18.

3.6 Other Control Methods

The zoonoses often require specific control methods to reduce or eliminate the animal reservoir. Dogs are the major animal source of human disease (Table 17.1) so only those animals which are useful in the society, should be kept, and strays and unwanted dogs should be destroyed. Laws to reduce dog-fouling are reasonably effective in developed countries and could perhaps be applicable to urban areas of some developing countries.

Rats are a serious transmitter of disease, especially plague (Section 16.1), leptospirosis (Section 17.8) and Lassa fever (Section 17.9). Methods of controlling rats will be found in Box 16.1. Other methods of disease control and prevention will be found under the specific diseases.

4

Control Strategy and Organization

The first two chapters covered the elements and theory of communicable diseases and the previous chapter discussed how to interrupt transmission with the various methods of control available. This chapter considers how to put all this information into action when faced by an outbreak, or the application of control methods in an established endemic disease.

4.1 Investigation of an Outbreak

In any communicable disease outbreak, the following sequence of events will need to take place:

- outbreak detection;
- investigation;
- confirmation;
- notification;
- analysis;
- treatment of cases;
- interruption of transmission;
- prevention of recurrence;
- analysis and writing of a report;
- surveillance.

These are not mutually exclusive stages, and although they are in order of action,

several events can be carried out at the same time.

Excess cases, unusual deaths, exceeding the epidemic threshold or an unexpected clustering of cases will be indicators that an outbreak of a new or known epidemic disease is taking place. The cause will need to be identified and an estimate made of the magnitude and distribution of cases. Field investigations are organized and active surveillance set up to find any new cases. The disease can be confirmed by using an agreed case definition, specific laboratory test or sero-epidemiological technique. The disease must be notified as soon as possible, both nationally and possibly internationally (see Chapter 6). Judgement needs to be used in spending time on making an accurate diagnosis, or starting treatment with the information that is available. There will be great pressure to treat cases, which is a necessary humanitarian action, but until transmission is interrupted more cases will occur. Once the disease is under control, methods must be implemented to prevent recurrence. Finally, the outbreak is analysed and written up. A surveillance system is on the look-out for the first indications of the communicable disease starting again. These stages will be considered in more detail.

4.1.1 Identification

The start of an epidemic can be dramatic with a large number of cases being reported or many people dying. However, the cause may well be anticipated, as the agents of most communicable diseases are now known. The person reporting the outbreak will probably have made a provisional diagnosis or it might be anticipated, having been reported in a neighbouring region. It will need to be confirmed by laboratory methods or by careful clinical judgement (e.g. measles). A case definition is a useful tool for ensuring that everybody understands what they are looking for. This can either be very general, such as fever with no obvious cause as in a suspected malaria epidemic, or a more detailed description, such as with the rash and symptoms of measles. In the general case definition, this will indicate that laboratory confirmation is required, as in the example of malaria with a blood slide being taken.

Normally, the confirmation of diagnosis is relatively easy, but several laboratory specimens may be required and restraint exercised in rushing to a diagnosis (e.g. in typhoid). Alternatively, it may be a unique and rare disease in which the aetiology and transmission have not been worked out. If this is the case, expert assistance is sought, while general principles of control are carried out.

Enquiry and search is made to determine the extent of the outbreak, whether there are many more cases, especially in areas where there are no medical facilities. Cases may be hidden or exaggerated to avoid or attract medical attention. Is this the first case or have there been several cases over a period of time? Have the cases come from another administrative area or country, and is there a risk that they might infect other areas? Was notification received and should notification be given?

4.1.2 The epidemiological investigation

Collecting information on the cause and method of transmission utilizes the three pillars of epidemiology – *persons, place* and *time*. Information should be collected from as many angles and from as wide a field as possible. The more pointers there are to a method of transmission, the stronger will be the case.

It will generally not be possible to complete a detailed epidemiological investigation before starting some control methods, for example, if it is diarrhoeal disease, then emergency boiling of drinking water can be started. However, a full investigation must be made and completed, as quite often different factors come to light. A full investigation will help prevent a recurrence.

The method used in an epidemiological search is as follows:

1. Look for a common event that is shared by all the cases.
2. Study exceptions to see if there are rational explanations.
3. Base these findings on the population at risk.
4. Elucidate changes that have occurred in the environment, which may have favoured the outbreak.
5. Make a hypothesis of cause, route of transmission and method of control.

Ideally, information should be collected on every case, but this might be scant or absent in the first few cases. However, it is important to investigate these first cases thoroughly so that the start of the epidemic can be accurately fixed and an epidemic curve drawn (see Chapter 2). If it is a very large epidemic, then it might be preferable to take a sample of cases and study these in detail, but some record of the total number of cases will always be required.

Information on *persons* should be available, and sex and age classification can readily give an indication as to the cause of the epidemic. If it is just children who are involved, then it is a common disease in which adults have obtained immunity such as measles. If there are more cases in one sex than another, then this might indicate a division of duties such as women (who are the main collectors of water) succumbing to cholera in larger numbers than men.

The address of each case should be plotted on a map and a note made of the most affected areas and whether there is any clustering. Look for associations, such as rivers, breeding places of vectors, forests that might harbour reservoir animals, or any other feature that the nature of the disease indicates to be important. If maps are not available, then constructing a simple sketch map might be necessary, especially if it is a very well-defined epidemic. Typhoid cases often occur in communities, so the houses of individual victims will need to be identified on a sketch map of the village or town. Any clustering or association of cases might lead to the carrier from which the epidemic started. Exceptional cases can often provide definitive evidence of an association such as the visit by a person resident in a different area, which subsequently becomes infected.

All calculations, such as the morbidity and mortality rates, must be done on the population at risk. Normally, this is the population of the entire area, district, region or country, but in a very localized epidemic, the population of the village, town or group of villages might give a better estimate. Population figures are available from census data, malaria control programmes and often collected by the village authorities. Otherwise, a sample needs to be taken of the number of occupants in a random number of houses, followed by counting of all the houses in the area and multiplied by the average house occupancy.

There is normally a reason why an epidemic has occurred at a particular period in time. Diarrhoeal diseases often start at the beginning of the rainy season and influenza is more common during winter months. Religious gatherings or other large collections of people provide ideal conditions for the transmission of disease. If there are strong indicators, then these can be used in future surveillance and to initiate preventive action.

A working hypothesis is established as soon as possible so that emergency control action can be commenced, but a detailed investigation must be completed. Search back within the maximum and minimum incubation period from the first case or cases using other indicators gained from person and place data. Laboratory confirmation of cases might give a different pattern from clinical assessment, especially where several medical staff are involved. If available, samples might need to be taken from a suspect cause, such as a food item, or from the environment, such as a river used for drinking water, which will all take time to be analysed. However, a negative result will not necessarily alter the hypothesis; the specimen may have been collected too late or from the wrong place. It is the strength of association of all the different pieces of evidence that should be used to decide on the cause.

4.1.3 Treatment of cases

The priority is to organize the treatment of cases rather than become involved in the clinical management, and concentrating time on investigating the outbreak and instigating control. This should be by:

- setting up emergency treatment centres or arranging transport of cases to hospital;
- mobilization of staff, medicines and equipment according to need;
- formulation of a standard treatment schedule;
- making rules on period of quarantine, management of contacts, prevention of carriers and disposal of the dead.

As the epidemic means a large number of cases of a single disease, once the diagnosis has been made, the treatment of all the cases will be the same. There may be a complicated case that requires special attention, but the priority of the investigating doctor is to interrupt transmission and bring the epidemic to an end. A standard treatment schedule should be devised and all available staff at every level made available to help with treating the cases. Instead of trying to bring all the cases to a hospital, it may be better to set up emergency treatment centres in the proximity of the outbreak. Schools, community centres, religious buildings and warehouses can be utilized for this purpose. Not only does this avoid the problem of transporting cases, but frees the hospital from fresh contamination or disruption.

4.1.4 Interruption of transmission

Once a hypothesis of causation is made from the epidemiological investigation, a method of control is commenced. This can be done in three different phases:

- emergency;
- specific;
- long-term prevention.

If the communicable disease is in epidemic form and threatening a large number of people, then emergency methods must be implemented as soon as possible. These are often non-specific and should commence before the detailed investigation has been finished. As an illustration of these three different strategies, an epidemic of dengue can be used. The emergency method would be a knock-down spray, such as fogging which kills all adult mosquitoes indiscriminately. This will control the immediate problem, but once the number of adult mosquitoes builds up again, the epidemic might recommence. The specific method would be a programme selectively against the *Aedes* mosquito vector by destroying all temporary breeding places and using larvicides in water containers. Long-term prevention would be by permanently altering breeding places, placing mosquito netting over water tanks, repairing broken guttering and all the techniques that are available for removing the mosquito permanently.

4.1.5 Analysis and report

A communicable disease outbreak should be analysed in detail and written down as a report. This will be based on the investigations made, the control methods used and their outcome. The number of cases and deaths are items of information that authorities are particularly interested in. The functions of a report are to:

- inform planning and organizing authorities of what has happened;
- notify other workers who are or might soon be participating in a similar outbreak;
- make a record to be referred to in future outbreaks;
- evaluate actions taken and improvements that should be made;
- provide information for the general public;
- elicit funds for more permanent preventive measures;
- illustrate for teaching purposes;
- be used for the advancement of science if of an original nature.

4.1.6 Outbreak organization and community participation

Outbreaks occur suddenly and often with little warning so there is no time to wait for help to arrive; the doctor, nurse or other health worker must take control. Generally, the temptation is to become so involved in patient management and treatment that no investigation is done. But until the cause of the outbreak is investigated, cases will continue and generally increase in number.

Help in patient care can be obtained from many sources, such as other health workers, public health inspectors, hospital porters, even cleaning staff, but probably the main resource will be relatives. In most societies, relatives will come with the patient and remain with them until they are cured. Care needs to be taken that they do not become patients themselves if it is a highly infectious disease, so instructions on preventive methods will need to be given and enforced.

In many communities, there is a local organization that should be involved at an early stage. This may be official, a village chief or headman; religious, the village priest; or just a respected member of the community such as a school teacher. In some countries, the local organization will have a person responsible for the health of the community or a village health committee. They will be of value in identifying cases, but even more useful in seeing that control measures, such as boiling drinking water, are enforced. They will also have a role in preventing the epidemic from starting up again in the future, such as ensuring that all children are vaccinated.

4.2 Surveillance

Surveillance of communicable diseases is the continuous watching for any changes in known diseases and the monitoring of the environment for any new diseases that may appear.

The key to surveillance is reporting, developed in such a way that a continuous record is kept, not the desperate call of an established epidemic. Surveillance methods are of several kinds and are discussed below.

4.2.1 Routine or passive surveillance

All health facilities collect data in their record keeping, at its simplest being the name, age and sex of the individual and the symptoms or diagnosis of their illness. Considerable use can be made of well-kept records and it is worth doing an analysis of the type of information collected to determine the best system to use with the resources available. Hospital records, while more detailed than in small clinics, will not be representative of the population.

Additional categories can be added to the basic data collected, but care must be taken not to overload the health staff so that an unreasonable amount of their time is taken up with filling in forms. Every additional entry must be tested by a small pilot study to ensure that it is collecting the information required and is within the means of the staff to collect it. If it is too onerous a task, then there will be a tendency to either

not bother to collect the information or even worse, to falsify the data. Even the routine data already collected should be looked at in detail; for example, staff may record the number of patients reporting headaches, which will not be a valuable criterion. Recording fever rather than headache (and taking a blood slide) is far more useful.

Accuracy of data collection can be improved by training, with regular refresher courses so that all staff are taught the same method at the same time. Regular feedback of an analysis of the data will encourage staff to be vigilant in their returns. Comparing one area with another will show up weaknesses, which can then be strengthened. Formulating case definitions encourages a more consistent diagnosis.

Where facilities are available, laboratory confirmation is always desirable. Every fever case in a tropical area should routinely have a blood slide taken, and sputum smears always made from persons with a chronic cough. In special circumstances, having a screening programme can enhance routine investigations. Examples are antibiotic resistance patterns of STIs, *Aedes aegypti* index in dengue-susceptible areas, vaccine coverage in under-fives clinics and rainfall records to measure seasonality.

All data collected must be analysed or there is no point in collecting it in the first place. The well-established criteria of persons, place and time will be the basic model, but special techniques may also be required. Data from one level are sent to the next higher level where they are analysed, and a copy of the analysis sent both to the level above and to those collecting the data in the first place. Special reporting may be required for notifiable diseases. Evaluations need to be made at regular intervals to modify and improve the system.

4.2.2 Active surveillance

Active surveillance is the deliberate search for target data. This has been used particularly in malaria control programmes, where contacts of malaria cases are visited and blood slides taken, as illustrated in Fig. 4.1.

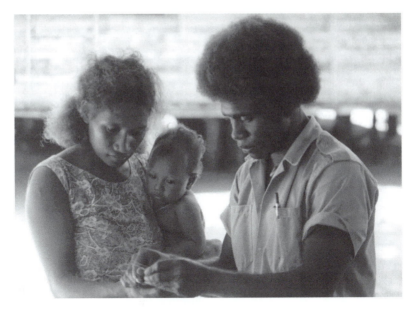

Fig. 4.1. An active case detection (ACD) technician taking a blood slide from a woman suffering from fever in a malaria eradication programme (St Isabel, Solomon Islands)

Another example is a leprosy field worker who visits all the villages in his/her area and examines the population for any signs of early disease. Suspect cases are then sent to clinic or hospital for further tests.

4.2.3 Sentinel health service surveillance

Special health problems involving detailed or laboratory investigation are often best collected by using sentinel health services. These are given extra staff or facilities to enable them to identify the disease. Influenza information is often collected in this way, as it is notoriously difficult to distinguish influenza from the common cold and other causes of a respiratory infection. Several sentinel health centres will then give a reasonable estimate of the problem in the entire area.

4.2.4 Emergency surveillance

Emergency surveillance is set up during an outbreak to monitor special risk areas, such as contacts and bacteria counts, among others. Suspect cases or contacts should be kept under observation. Monitoring of treatment can detect the appearance of resistant organisms or an imbalance in the treatment regime. Utilization of staff and equipment can also be built into an emergency surveillance system.

4.2.5 Serological and virological surveillance

Where laboratory facilities permit, a record of certain diseases can be obtained from serological or virological studies. An example is the use of anonymous testing of blood samples collected at antenatal clinics for HIV and hepatitis B infections. Care must be taken to ensure that the data are representative of the population and are measured continuously.

As the incidence of a parasitic disease declines, it becomes increasingly difficult to detect the parasite and serological surveillance can be of more value. This method has been used in malaria programmes nearing eradication.

4.2.6 Other forms of surveillance

Where all information reaches a single central authority, it is reasonable to assume that it is representative of the entire area from which it is collected. An example would be a public health laboratory, where more complex and standardized results are available.

Other allied disciplines may collect data that is relevant to health, such as veterinary and entomology services. Sleeping sickness is a more widespread and devastating disease in cattle than humans, so outbreaks in cattle are indicators to take precautions in associated human communities. Anthrax and bovine spongiform encephalopathy (BSE) are other examples.

Epidemics may first be reported by persons in authority, such as village leaders, school teachers, priests, etc. Indeed, they can often be relied upon to give continued and reasonably accurate information for the community they serve. It is often one of the functions of a village leader to collect data on births and deaths, which can be valuable in estimating the population.

More information on surveillance can be found in Section 5.3 and under each disease in Chapters 7–17.

4.3 Control and Eradication

A communicable disease can be *controlled* or *eradicated*. By controlling a disease, it is kept at such a minimum level that it no longer poses a health problem. Eradication on the other hand sets out to eliminate the disease completely. The difference between control and eradication can be summarized in the following table.

The attraction of putting the entire health effort, funded by international support into the eradication of a disease requires organization of the very highest order. There have been five global eradication efforts, out of which two were successful, the other two almost successful and the remaining one was not successful. The eradication of smallpox worldwide has been one of public

	Control	Eradication
Objective	Minimal incidence	Complete elimination
Duration	Indefinite	Time-limited
Coverage	Areas of high incidence	Entire area
Method	Effective	Faultless
Reservoir	Animal or environment	Human only
Organization	Good	Perfect
Costs	Moderate for a long time	High for limited period
Complications	Acceptable	Extremely serious
Imported cases	Not important	Very important
Surveillance	Reasonable	Very good

health's greatest triumphs against disease. This was only possible because the vaccine was extremely effective, there was no other reservoir but humans and the organization was very good. Recently, an entirely different kind of disease, Guinea worm, has been eradicated from all countries except one (where there is a civil war) by a programme of 'protected-well' construction. Poliomyelitis has been eliminated from WHO regions of the Americas, Europe and Western Pacific and in 2001 only 600 cases were reported from the rest of the world. The global yaws campaign eradicated yaws from large areas of the world, but it is still endemic in some places and on the increase in others. The tremendous progress of the malaria eradication campaign, followed by an equally impressive resurgence of the disease, has been a devastating setback to the doctrine of eradication. (There have been other localized eradication programmes such as *Anopheles gambiae* from South America.)

With eradication, it is an all-or-none process – if eradication is not complete, then the disease can return to its former levels and all effort has been wasted. In these circumstances, it is preferable to choose the alternative target of control, which will be the method used in the majority of infections.

A new terminology has been introduced by WHO – *elimination*. This uses a special programme and enhanced resources similar to an eradication programme, but accepts that eradication will not necessarily be achieved. Lymphatic filariasis, Chagas' disease, trachoma, maternal and neonatal tetanus have been designated as suitable for elimination programmes.

4.4 Campaigns and General Programmes

Communicable diseases can be controlled by campaigns (called special programmes by WHO) or made a function of the general health services. Special campaigns have the attraction of putting all the effort into one particular disease, often with considerable initial success, but over the long term, breaking down again. Integrating the control method with the general health services often gives a more consistent result. The advantages and disadvantages are as follows:

	Campaigns	General health services
Effectiveness	Initially very good	Only moderate
Continuation	Poor	Moderate
Duration	Short	Long
Staff	Special required	General health workers
Salary	Inflated	Average
Staff problems	No career structure	Addition to routine duties
Cost	High	Low
Integration	Low	High

It is the integration of the campaign into the general health services that destroys the good progress made. There are difficulties of emphasis, staff absorption and resentment by the multi-purpose worker. Campaign workers are often specially recruited for the task, probably from non-medical backgrounds and are paid inflated salaries to offset the time-limited nature of the operation. The general health services are not used to dealing with the special disease and feel they are being given extra work, while still being paid the same. An alternative might be to use the general health services for a brief special effort, which can continue to be maintained in their routine services. An example is a mobilization of the general health services to do a mass vaccination campaign before the start of the rainy season (Section 3.2.6). For the rest of the year, they can continue with the routine vaccination programme.

4.5 Control Organization

During the malaria eradication campaigns, a high level of organizational methodology was developed, which is a useful model for any communicable disease control programme. The four stages are as follows:

- preparatory;
- attack phase;
- consolidation;
- maintenance.

4.5.1 Preparatory

The preparatory stage is perhaps the most important, and time spent on collecting baseline data, trying to forecast problems and assessing the feasibility of the proposal is always time well spent.

Surveys are made of the disease to measure its prevalence over as wide an area as possible. A good sample survey might be sufficient to measure the endemicity, but this will not reveal the foci of infection, which normally cause the most problems. In addition, a surveillance system needs to be established, if there is not one already, to continually collect data on cases as the programme proceeds.

The population will need to be enumerated and it might be justified to spend money on carrying out a census if one has not been done recently. Maps are essential and if suitable ones are not available, then they need to be drawn. They must contain up-to-date village locations, preferably with the population marked on them. Figure 4.2 is an example of a map prepared in this way.

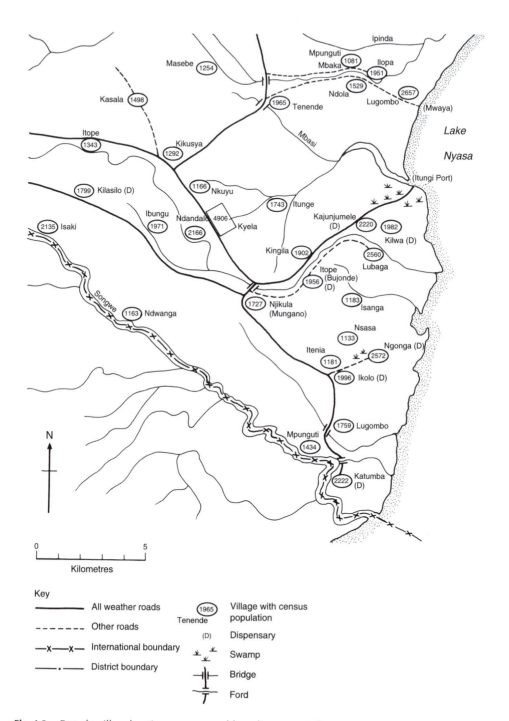

Fig. 4.2. Part of a village location map prepared for a disease control programme.

Every level of society must be committed – from the senior administrative head, through divisional chiefs and influential people, to the established health worker. This will require regular meetings, with the establishment of key contacts. Without the complete and continued cooperation of the people, any special effort is doomed to failure.

Planning of the persons, money and materials (logistics) to be used in the programme is often the easiest part to initiate, but one of the most difficult to maintain. Utilizing existing staff who retain all their usual functions and continue in an established pattern of service is preferable to recruiting special staff, but this should not be at the expense of existing services. If special staff need to be recruited, then conditions of service must be carefully worked out so that no conflict arises with existing staff.

Adequate funding is required, as no disease control programme has remained within estimates; they nearly always cost more than expected. Additions arise that were not foreseen, inflation increases faster than allowed for and the programme takes longer than planned. If adequate finances cannot be secured and the programme has to be abandoned, then the net result is worse than doing nothing in the first place. More serious is the damage done to the existing health services by diverting funds from them.

Included in the preparatory stage is a *pilot programme* to try out the techniques and organization in a limited area. The pilot programme is a scaled down version of the full programme, not a special effort to show what can be done. The area chosen should be fully representative of the larger area to be covered. If there are marked variations, then several pilot studies of differing criteria may be required.

The pilot programme can be for a set period of time, or continued into the full programme after it has been assessed. If there are major difficulties, then the programme should proceed no further, but the whole strategy reworked. If there are minor problems, then these are indicators of major problems in the future.

4.5.2 Attack

In the attack phase, the method that was found to be effective in the pilot programme is extended to the whole area. Alternatively, the area can be covered in sequence, but if this is done, then measures may need to be instituted to prevent re-infection. Time tables and procedures are required to ensure that separate teams cover the area in a regular manner. Realistic targets are set and organization developed to make sure they are kept. The delay in one part will cause the delay of everything else.

During the attack phase, the number of cases found by the passive surveillance services will rapidly diminish, so progress is assessed by making serial surveys. Incidence is more useful than prevalence data; therefore, surveys are conducted at regular intervals in sample areas. However, this can pose a strain on relations with the population that is being sampled and areas of higher prevalence may be missed, so new sample areas may need to be used after a time.

To ensure that all the remaining cases are found, an *active surveillance* system can be established. This involves special workers, each with an assigned area which is visited on a regular basis. Active surveillance is no substitute for passive surveillance, the two should work closely together.

4.5.3 Consolidation

In the consolidation phase, the full apparatus of disease reduction is disbanded and reliance placed on small specialist teams that can rapidly respond to the active surveillance system. If a focus of malaria is found, then focal spraying and radical treatment of cases is implemented. If a yaws or polio case is suspected, then mass treatment or vaccination is given in the surrounding area. The essence of the consolidation phase is speed and efficiency. If rapid remedial action cannot be carried out, then the disease is liable to return.

4.5.4 Maintenance or a continuing level of control

If the target of the programme is to eradicate the disease, then the maintenance phase will be an efficient monitoring system to ensure that any introduced cases are rapidly detected and treated. If it was to reduce the disease to an acceptable level that the amount of funds and staff availability permits, then this might need to be continued indefinitely. A limited control programme may be sufficient to reduce the burden of disease to allow a rise in the standard of living, which in the long term will have the most sustained effect on controlling the disease.

5

Notification and Health Regulations

Due to the serious nature of a disease or the ease by which it is transmitted, some diseases are notifiable. Individual countries will have their own priorities as to which diseases these should be, whereas international agreement specifies certain diseases which must be notified to other countries, generally via the WHO.

5.1 International Health Regulations

International health regulations require that certain diseases be notified. The purpose is to warn other countries and intended travellers to the country of the health risks involved. Assistance can also be requested, once the disease has been notified.

Diseases subject to the International Health Regulations (1969, 1974 and 1992) are as follows:

- plague;
- cholera;
- yellow fever.

Diseases under surveillance by WHO are as follows:

- louse-borne typhus;
- relapsing fever;
- paralytic poliomyelitis;
- malaria;
- influenza;
- human immune deficiency virus (HIV);
- smallpox;
- severe acute respiratory syndrome (SARS).

The initial case is notified by e-mail to www.who.int/csr/alertresponse and subsequent summaries of the number of cases suspected and confirmed are sent at weekly intervals.

The regulations are being revised and instead of the current list of three diseases, this will be replaced by a requirement for all countries 'to notify WHO of all diseases or events of international public health importance'. This will mean that such events, as the first cases of a new infection, such as SARS, must be reported.

In addition, a region (e.g. the South Pacific Commission or Association of Caribbean States), may initiate its own regulations, for example, for the following disease:

- dengue;
- diphtheria;
- typhoid;
- whooping cough;
- scrub typhus.

5.2 National Health Regulations

Countries have their own system of national notification of some diseases, including the following:

- tuberculosis;
- leprosy;
- sleeping sickness.

5.2.1 Notifiable diseases for England and Wales

Very rare infections	Rare infections	Common infections
Anthrax	Leptospirosis	Food poisoning
Leprosy	Yellow fever	Viral hepatitis
Typhus	Cholera	Whooping cough
Relapsing fever	Diphtheria	Tuberculosis
Plague	Poliomyelitis	Malaria
Smallpox	Typhoid fever	Meningitis
Viral	Paratyphoid	Meningococcal
haemorrhagic	fever	septicaemia
fever	Rabies	Ophthalmia
	Tetanus	neonatorum
	Encephalitis	Measles
		Dysentery
		(bacillary and
		amoebic)
		Rubella
		Scarlet fever

5.3 Special Surveillance

The principles of surveillance were mentioned in Section 4.2. A country at particular risk may be advised to set up a surveillance system of international or national importance. Some suggestions are:

- in plague areas, any case of fever, glandular enlargement and death;

- any person or persons dying from diarrhoea;
- any person dying of jaundice in the yellow fever zone (see Fig. 5.1);
- *Aedes aegypti* index;
- severe case of chicken pox or other unusual pox rashes;
- any case of acute flaccid paralysis following a feverish illness;
- severe pneumonia with difficulty in breathing.

Any case coming within one of these categories is reported immediately to the responsible Medical Officer or doctor in charge, who is required to investigate the report.

WHO has set up an international surveillance team to investigate any case of suspected smallpox reported. The suspected case must be isolated and WHO informed immediately. There is also concern about emergent diseases and the strengthening of surveillance systems, so the linking of one country's reporting with another will assist in detecting new diseases before they become a serious problem.

5.4 Vaccination Requirements

The only vaccination now required for international travel is yellow fever for persons who come from or pass through a yellow fever zone (Fig. 5.1).

Cholera vaccination is no longer required by international regulations. A yellow fever vaccination must be recorded on the prescribed form with the signature of the doctor; the batch number and official stamp of the vaccination centre. The vaccination is valid for 10 years, 10 days after the date of the vaccination or revaccination.

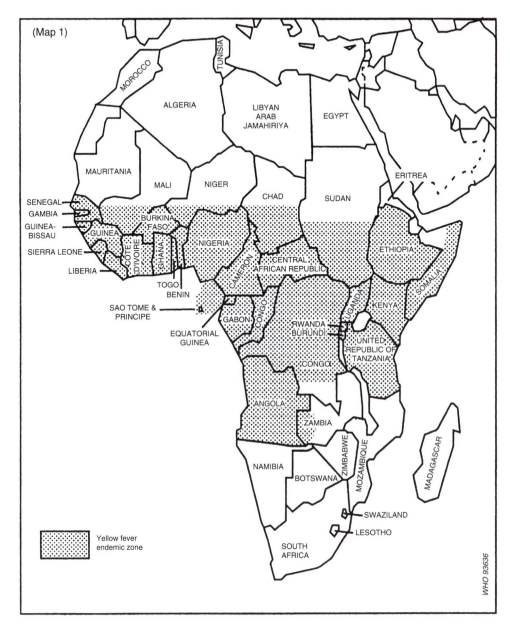

Fig. 5.1. The yellow fever endemic zones in Africa (Map 1) and Central and South America (Map 2, see next page). Yellow fever endemic zones are areas where there is a potential risk of infection on account of the presence of vectors and animal reservoirs. Some countries consider these zones as infected areas and require an international certificate of vaccination against yellow fever from travellers arriving from these areas. (Reproduced, by permission, from WHO (2004) *International Travel and Health, Vaccination Requirements and Health Advice*, World Health Organization, Geneva.)

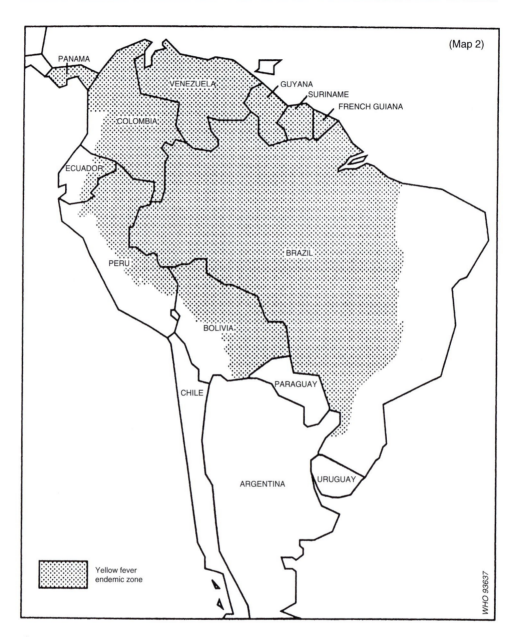

Fig. 5.1. Map 2.

6

Classification of Communicable Diseases

No biological system is perfect and communicable diseases in particular are not readily classified; however, any grouping makes it easier to understand and remember, so the objective of this short chapter is to look at the different ways this can be done.

A disease is a morbid condition of the body (e.g. measles or plague). As the cause of diseases were discovered, they became identified by the causative organism, such as trypanosomiasis or pneumococcal meningitis, but confusion arose because there are two forms of African trypanosomiasis and one of American, while the pneumococcus is an important cause of pneumonia as well as meningitis. This confusion continues. Instead of settling on one system or another, I have tried to list all the communicable diseases by either the disease state or the organism by which they are best identified. For example, in the case of gastroenteritis, one of the commonest causes of diarrhoea in developing countries, it is preferable to separately list the various organisms that can cause it. Where these are particularly distinct, such as rotavirus infection, then they are put into the list. On the other hand, the streptococcus is responsible for such an array of diseases that just to put down streptococcal infection would fail to reveal important diseases such as rheumatic fever or otitis media. With these

provisos, all the communicable diseases are listed in Chapter 19, at the end of the book, rather than here, so quick reference can be made to them.

There are 340 diseases listed in Chapter 19, of which the commonest causative organism is a virus, being responsible for 185 diseases, with arboviruses causing 118 infections. Bacteria and chlamydia account for 66 and the larger parasites for 54 infections, of which the nematodes cause 21 diseases, protozoa 17 and helminths 16. The commonest method of transmission is, therefore, the vector, with the mosquito being incriminated in a staggering 76 infections, ticks in 31, and other or unknown biting insects in 42 of the infections. In methods of control, with vectors being so frequent, vector control is the commonest, which proved useful in 134 of the disease conditions, but simple methods, such as using repellents and sleeping under mosquito nets, are all that are required most of the time. Next comes personal hygiene, invaluable for preventing 90 infections – just washing your hands, not spitting and making an effort to be clean can be remarkably effective. Allied to personal cleanliness is food hygiene, ensuring that food is prepared properly, adequately cooked and stored under safe conditions, accounting for 57 of the preventive methods. Allied to the proper cooking of

© R. Webber 2005. *Communicable Disease Epidemiology and Control,* 2nd edition (Roger Webber)

food is the control of animals either in their farming, slaughter, and the control of domestic pets, this group being responsible for 41 disease preventive actions. Chemotherapy as a method of control is valuable in 40 diseases and vaccination in 35, but several of these are major disease problems, such as tuberculosis, measles and the STIs. The provision of a good water supply will reduce 39 conditions and sanitation another 23, while the control of rats is important in 17 conditions. The social and educational methods appropriate to controlling STIs will be valuable in 20 conditions, while the screening of blood donors will avoid 14 diseases and the proper sterilization of needles, instruments and giving sets could prevent nine diseases.

No attempt is made in the next few chapters to cover all 340 of the diseases listed, but to select only those of worldwide importance, which are major problems in certain parts of the world, or to illustrate a particular disease pattern. Readers might find it useful to refer to the list in Chapter 19 first, before turning to the fuller description in the following pages.

Diseases are normally classified by the causative organism, which has much to recommend it for the clinician and the pathologist, but different organisms can cause similar diseases, such as *Escherichia coli*, a bacteria and *Giardia intestinalis*, a protozoa, both producing diarrhoea in the individual. Control methods are similar; as a result, an epidemiologist will find it preferable to include them in the same group. On the other hand, the closely linked group of viruses that cause hepatitis are very different in their means of transmission – hepatitis A is transmitted by the faecal–oral route and hepatitis B by blood and other body fluids, so it is preferable to separate these two diseases into different categories. Transmission is the key to the epidemiology of communicable diseases. Once the means of transmission is known, it leads to the best method of control, so it is preferable to use this as the method of classification. Based on these criteria, all communicable diseases can be classified into 11 groups as follows:

	Chapter
Water washed diseases	7
Faecal–oral diseases	8
Food-borne diseases	9
Diseases of soil contact	10
Diseases of water contact	11
Skin infections	12
Respiratory diseases and other airborne transmitted infections	13
Diseases transmitted via body fluids	14
Insect-borne diseases	15
Ectoparasite zoonoses	16
Domestic and synanthropic zoonoses	17

Water-washed diseases could be called person-to-person diseases, but many diseases including skin infections and respiratory diseases are also transmitted from one person to another, so a preferable description is to include the main method of control, which is washing. They could also be called diseases of poor hygiene, but since hygiene is involved in the control of very many diseases, to call them this would make this category far too large. Faecal–oral is a very large group and could quite easily incorporate many of the diseases in the chapter on food-borne diseases, but it is easier to consider control methods if a separate chapter is made. There are important diseases that are acquired by contact with either soil or water, which means that methods of control are very specific. Skin infections are obvious in their presentation and most of them are transmitted directly by skin contact but also use other modes of transmission, so it is more convenient to classify them by their most common method of presentation. Instead of putting leprosy in a separate chapter as in the previous edition, because its means of transmission has not been fully worked out, it is included in the chapter on skin infections. The respiratory infections are transmitted by the airborne route, which is also a method of transmission of several other infections that present in different ways. The chapter on diseases transmitted via body fluids is an attempt to bring together common themes in the transmission and control of diseases transmitted via blood, seminal fluid, cervical secretions, saliva and other less common methods of transmission. It includes the STIs, which would warrant a chapter of their own, but other diseases that share many common features, such as hepatitis B and non-venereal syphilis, are better included with them. Insect-borne diseases not only include a large number of health problems, but also some of the most important diseases in the world such as malaria. It is already the largest chapter and could be even bigger, but the combination of ectoparasite transmission (by fleas, lice, etc.) and zoonosis is a very specific one, so a separate chapter has been included for this category. The rest of the zoonoses, where a vector is not included, form the last chapter in the classification.

No classification system is perfect and not every disease fits neatly into the 11 categories. For many diseases, there is more than one means of transmission and these can also be important in developing control methods. However, the categories are sufficiently broad to encompass minor differences. Bringing them together into such a system demonstrates similarities and associations, making it easier to understand the complexities of the many communicable diseases.

The fewer groups there are, the easier it is to remember all of them, sparing the onerous task of learning about each disease in detail. However, if each group is too broad, much of the essential information is also lost, thereby defeating its purpose. For example, Vietnam had classified all its communicable diseases into just four groups, but this was found to lack the precision to work out the best control strategy for each group, so this was replaced by an abbreviated classification, as follows:

1. Person-to-person (skin and eye diseases).
2. Faecal–oral transmission.
3. Soil-contact.
4. Airborne (respiratory infections).
5. Diseases transmitted via body fluids (includes STIs).
6. Vector-borne diseases.
7. Zoonoses.

This simplification was due to the absence of such diseases as schistosomiasis and Guinea worm, which are the only members of the 'diseases of water contact' in the classification above, and several others, which allowed amalgamations. Any country might similarly like to draw up its own classification system based on the important diseases found there.

7
Water-washed Diseases

The simplest disease transmission is by person-to-person contact (see Fig. 1.3). The diseases of poor hygiene arise from direct contact of the skin, conjunctiva or mucous membrane. Alternatively, organisms from the skin or in conjunctival secretions can be transported by an intermediate vehicle. The essential mechanism is contamination due to lack of hygiene.

There are two groups of diseases in this category – skin diseases and eye diseases – and it is convenient to describe them in this order. The skin diseases include infections of scabies and lice and the superficial fungal diseases. Tropical ulcers, for which a means of transmission has still not been defined, are conveniently included here. The eye diseases of significance in public health are trachoma, epidemic haemorrhagic conjunctivitis, epidemic keratoconjunctivitis and ophthalmia neonatorum.

The main method of control of the diseases of poor hygiene is to increase water *quantity*. They are the first category in Table 3.1 called the 'water-washed' diseases. Providing an adequate volume of water for washing encourages personal hygiene.

7.1 Scabies

Organism Infection of the skin is by a mite *Sarcoptes scabiei.*

Clinical features There is a skin rash and intense itching where the mite burrows into the superficial layers of the skin. It favours the wrists and hands, although in heavy infections, it may be found in almost any area of the body, but not the head or face. Due to scratching, the affected skin can become thickened and discoloured leading to a mistaken diagnosis of eczema. Secondary infection is common and glomerulonephritis can occur.

Diagnosis is made from clinical presentation, but skin scrapings can be made and the mite viewed microscopically.

Transmission of scabies is due to close personal contact, permitting the mite to pass from one person to another. It can be transmitted by shared clothing and is potentiated by poor hygiene. Where possible, infected individuals should be prevented from infecting others, for example by keeping children away from school until they are cured of the infections. Careful search should be made for unreported or unrecognized cases in the community. Scabies can be spread amongst adults as a STI. Intractable scabies in adults, not responding to treatment, can indicate HIV infection.

Incubation period 2–6 weeks.

Period of communicability As long as there are viable mites on the individual, up until 1 week after the first course of treatment.

Occurrence and distribution Scabies is found worldwide, but favours the hot, moist tropics and flourishes in conditions of poverty. It mainly occurs in children, but anyone who comes in contact with infected individuals (e.g. mothers and school teachers) can become infected with scabies.

Control and prevention Scabies is a community problem and treatment of an individual is insufficient unless the whole family, school or village is similarly treated. In communities with poor hygiene, the provision of adequate water is the most effective method of controlling the disease. People should be encouraged to wash themselves with soap and water and wash their clothes and bedding. Improving the water supply to provide an adequate quantity of water is the main method of prevention.

Treatment Specific treatment is by benzyl benzoate, but this may need to be accompanied by an antibiotic if there is secondary infection. A 10% emulsion of benzyl benzoate is liberally applied to the whole body and left for 24 h before being washed off. Treatment is repeated after 7 days to kill off larvae that have hatched from eggs. The whole family is treated at the same time, ensuring that only clean clothes and bedding are used. Alternatively crotamiton 10% or sulphur 6% in petrolatum is applied to the entire body for 2–3 days before being washed off. The insecticide permethrin,

used in the control of malaria (Section 16.5.10) or the naturally occurring *Chrysanthemum* from which it is derived, is also effective. Reduction in scabies can be an additional benefit of insecticide-treated mosquito nets, otherwise permethrin can be administered as a 5% cream or 1% lotion. Ivermectin, used in the treatment of filariasis and onchocerciasis (Sections 15.7 and 15.8), can be given systemically as a mass treatment on its own or is a side-benefit of one of these control programmes. If none of the special preparations are available, then repeated applications of oil to the skin can be effective. Any oil usually used by people to rub on the skin, such as coconut oil, can be effective. As the mite lives in a small burrow through which it breathes, to seal-off the opening with a film of oil asphyxiates it. This requires careful and repeated application to the whole body after washing.

Surveillance School teachers should be encouraged to regularly examine school children or do spot checks on any child found to be scratching.

7.2 Lice

Body lice are potential vectors of typhus (Section 16.2) and relapsing fever (Section 16.3), but the main worry of people is personal infestation.

Organism *Pediculus humanus corporis*, the body louse, *P. h. capitis*, the head louse and *P. thirus pubis*, the crab louse. Lice glue their eggs to body hairs (nits) in which they are resistant to treatment until the nymphs hatch.

Clinical features and diagnosis Intense, localized itching at the site of bite will indicate lice, which can be found and identified with a hand lens. If *P. h. corporis* is not on the skin, they will be amongst body hair or in the clothes.

Transmission is by close contact between people, the sharing of clothes, hats and combs. Crab lice are generally transmitted during sexual contact.

Occurrence and distribution Body lice are found worldwide in conditions of poverty or where people are forcibly driven together, such as in refugee camps. They are more common in colder regions of the world or in mountainous parts of the tropics where people huddle together to keep warm. Head lice are found both in the tropics and the colder regions, especially amongst school children.

Incubation period Eggs hatch in 10–14 days.

Period of communicability is as long as there are viable lice on the individual, up until 2 weeks after the first course of treatment. Body and head lice remain alive for up to 1 week on clothing not being worn, and nits for 1 month.

Control and prevention Washing with warm water and soap at frequent intervals is the main method of prevention. Clothes of an infected person should be boiled or insufflated with insecticide powder. The practice of pressing clothes with a hot iron might have originated as a method of controlling lice. Combs should be washed regularly and only used by one person.

Treatment is with 1% permethrin cream rinse, naturally occurring pyrethrins (from *Chrysanthemum*) and oral ivermectin. The treatment should be repeated after 10–14 days to kill any young lice recently hatched from nits. Shaving of heads is a rigorous and effective method of control of head lice, but not of body lice. In epidemic situations, whole communities should be treated irrespective of whether lice have been found or not (Section 16.2). Clothes and bedding can be treated with 1% malathion, 0.5% permethrin, 2% temefos (Abate), 5% iodofenphos, 1% propoxur or 5% carbaryl.

Surveillance Parents or older siblings should carefully search through children's hair, looking for nits, if the child is found to be scratching his/her head. In situations such as refugee camps, people should be encouraged to examine their clothes and those of their children at regular intervals.

7.3 Superficial Fungal Infections (Dermatophytosis)

Organism Fungi of the genus *Trichophyton, Microsporum, Epidermophyton* and *Scytalidium.*

Clinical features Also called tinea, the fungi attack specific sites on the body, the moist skin in the feet or groin, the nails, the scalp or the body. Tinea corporis (often called ring worm) produces well-defined, circular lesions that spread out from the centre causing slight depigmentation as they proceed. Tinea capitis causes areas of baldness, hairs becoming brittle so that they break off. Tinea versicolor produces a blotchy hypopigmentation that can sometimes be misdiagnosed as leprosy. Tinea imbricata is particularly common in Western Pacific Islands, producing serpiginous scaly designs that can cover the whole body.

Diagnosis is clinical, but infected hairs fluoresce in ultraviolet light.

Transmission is by close bodily contact, the sharing of clothes, towels, etc. Dogs, cats and other animals also carry the fungus.

Incubation period 4–14 days.

Period of communicability Fungal material can persist on articles, such as towels and clothing, for considerable periods of time.

Occurrence and distribution Superficial fungal infections are widely distributed throughout the world, being found in developed as well as developing countries. Children are most commonly affected.

Control and prevention Prevention is by washing the body with soap and water, and not sharing clothes, towels, combs, etc. Towels should be boiled.

Treatment Local applications, such as tolnaftate, miconazole, ketoconazole, clotrimazole, econazole, naftifine, terbinafine or ciclopirox, can be used. Acetylsalicylic acid ointment or benzoic acid compound (Whitfields's ointment) are effective if applied regularly for nearly 3 weeks. In resistant cases, griseofulvin, itraconazole or oral terbinafine can be given by mouth for a sufficiently long period to clear all the fungal residue.

Surveillance School children should be examined regularly, especially the head, feet and groins.

7.4 Tropical Ulcers

Tropical ulcers are a common debilitating condition. They cause tissue loss and pain, which temporarily invalids the person, making daily work an agonizing burden. The condition can last for several months and even when it heals, the victim is left with a scar that may lead to contracture. There are two types of tropical ulcers: non-specific or due to a *Mycobacterium*, often called Buruli ulcer. These should both be differentiated from yaws (Section 14.1).

7.4.1 Non-specific tropical ulcers

Organism No specific organism is normally detected, but initial infection is often accompanied by cellulitis, probably caused by a *Streptococcus*.

Transmission Flies are responsible for contaminating small wounds and scratches or occasionally biting insects transmit infecting organisms directly. Scratching of the wound by the host can be a potent method of instilling organisms into the skin.

Clinical features The initial wound becomes red and indurated, with cellulitis spreading to the regional lymph nodes, and systemic fever. An ulcer that refuses to heal then develops at the initial point of infection, producing increasing tissue loss.

Incubation period Uncertain but probably between 1 and 5 days.

Period of communicability Unknown, but probably as long as there are moist lesions.

Occurrence and distribution Tropical ulcers are found in the warm, moist areas of the world, where the temperature and humidity are fairly constant. All ages and both sexes are susceptible.

Control and prevention Tropical ulcers can be prevented by taking scrupulous care over minor cuts and abrasions. As soon as any break in the skin surface occurs, it should be cleaned, an antiseptic applied and covered with a dressing. Where dressings are in short supply, certain kinds of leaves can be used. Flies should be controlled by the provision of sanitation (Section 3.3.4) and the disposal of garbage.

Treatment During the invasive stage, antibiotics should be given both systemically and locally, and the limb rested. Once the ulcer has formed, antibiotics have no effect and a cleaning solution, such as Eusol, should be applied. In coastal areas, soaking the affected limb in seawater is a cost-free method of cleaning out the ulcer. Skin grafting may be necessary.

7.4.2 Buruli ulcer

Organism *Mycobacterium ulcerans* is found in the exudate of the ulcer.

Clinical features There is at first just a small papule surrounded by shiny skin, but this soon breaks down to reveal a large necrotic ulcer with undermined edges. Tissue damage may be extensive involving bone and other structures.

Diagnosis is made on clinical grounds and a stained smear of the exudate.

Transmission The method of transmission has not been elucidated, but there are presumed to be environmental factors due to the relationship with rivers and wetlands. The role of aquatic insects has recently been suggested as *M. ulcerans* has been found in the salivary glands of insects. Focal outbreaks have followed migrations and movements of people, for example due to floods or dam construction. In Australia, koalas and opossums are found naturally infected.

Incubation period Unknown.

Occurrence and distribution Central Africa, Central and South America, Southeast Asia, Australia and New Guinea. Children and women living near rivers or wetlands in a rural region are predominantly affected. There has been a progressive increase in cases and more attention is being paid to working out the transmission and how to control the infection.

Control and prevention Several trials have been made with BCG vaccination and although these showed some early protection, it was not sustained. Health education in areas of high endemicity, with the provision of facilities for treating lesions as soon as they occur, has reduced the period of debility and the severity of the deformities.

Treatment Anti-mycobacterial drugs, such as streptomycin, dapsone, rifampicin or thiambutosine, have been found to be helpful, especially in the early stage, but essentially treatment is surgical with excision of the ulcer and skin grafting.

7.5 Trachoma

A common infectious disease, trachoma is the major cause of blindness in the world.

Organism *Chlamydia trachomatis*, a microorganism that has features both of bacteria and viruses.

Clinical features Commencing as a keratoconjunctivitis, the first sign is *red eye*. There may be irritation and discharge, but it is passed off as a self-limiting infection. A follicular infiltration of the conjunctiva then takes place particularly in the upper lid. Blood vessels grow into the periphery of the eye, forming pannus. Trachoma is often complicated by secondary infection. It is at the late stages of the disease, when it is non-infectious that scarring, particularly of the upper eyelid, turns the eyelashes inwards to rub on the eye, a condition called trichiasis. This constant rubbing of the eyeball, aided by the dryness of the conjunctiva, damages the cornea, leading to scarring and finally blindness.

Diagnosis is usually made on clinical grounds, but can be confirmed by finding the characteristic inclusion bodies in scrapings taken from the conjunctiva.

Transmission Trachoma is a disease of poor sanitary conditions where a combination of close contact and dirty conditions encourages transmission. Within the family unit, transmission is from child-to-child or by flies that are attracted to the discharges around the eyes. These are mainly *Musca sorbens*. Cycles of reinfection and recrudescence continue to damage the eye and lead to blindness at school age. The usual method of wiping away secretions with hands, towels or clothing, which is then used by the adult on other children or themselves, is a typical pattern of transmission.

Incubation period. 5–12 days.

Period of communicability continues as long as active lesions are still present. Once treatment commences, infectivity ceases within 2–3 days although the clinical disease persists.

Occurrence and distribution Trachoma is found mainly in the dry regions of the world (Fig. 7.1), especially Africa, South America and the extensive semi-desert

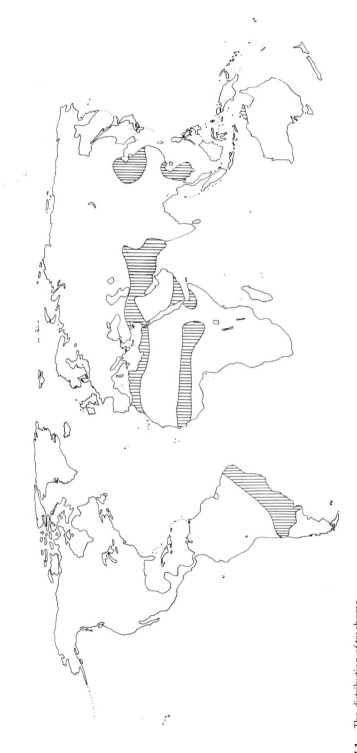

Fig. 7.1. The distribution of trachoma.

regions of Asia. A disease of antiquity, it was first described by the ancient Egyptians.

In endemic areas, 80–90% of children are infected by the age of 3 years. In conditions of improved sanitation, there is a natural cycle lasting until the age of 11 years, with little residual damage. Females develop trachoma and blindness as adults more commonly than males because they are directly concerned with looking after children. The chance of acquiring infection is increased by large families with short birth intervals, as there are more children of a young age living in close proximity.

Control and prevention The use of water to wash away secretions, clean clothes and the surroundings is perhaps the single most effective method. Washing the face often has been shown to reduce the risk of developing trachoma so regular daily face washing should be encouraged. Long-term preventive measures include improved sanitation and the provision of water supplies.

Flies proliferate in rubbish and excrement, reaching their maximum numbers during the dry, sunny period of the year. The damp, moist conditions in open pit latrines may be more important in encouraging fly breeding than non-use of latrines. Any flushing mechanism or improved latrine will discourage flies.

A strategy for a control programme is as follows:

- conduct a survey to find the worst-affected areas;
- give mass treatment;
- conduct health education through schools, stressing regular face washing;
- provide back-up services.

WHO has launched a programme for the global elimination of trachoma by 2020 and given it the acronym of SAFE. This stands for:

- Surgery for trichiasis;
- Antibiotics;
- Facial cleanliness;
- Environmental improvement.

Treatment Mass treatment is preferable, as the majority of the population in an infected area will have trachoma. This is given easily in schools, but is better done at home, where the main transmission takes place. A single dose of azithromycin (20 mg/kg) is better than topical tetracycline and one dose a year may be sufficient to eliminate the blinding propensity of trachoma. Mothers can be taught to regularly treat all children in the household.

Preventing blindness, once scarring and trichiasis have developed, is very easily done by a simple operation that a Medical Assistant can be trained to do. This involves cutting through the scarred conjunctiva of the upper lid and everting it so that the eyelashes no longer rub on the cornea.

Surveillance After the initial survey, follow-up surveys should be conducted at regular intervals. This is most easily done in primary schools.

7.6 Epidemic Haemorrhagic Conjunctivitis

First recognized in Ghana in 1969, epidemic acute haemorrhagic conjunctivitis has caused epidemics in a number of parts of the world, which have given their name to the disease (e.g. Nairobi eye).

Organism Enterovirus 70 is the most important aetiological agent and has been responsible for tens of millions of cases. Coxsackievirus A24 has also been responsible for large outbreaks.

Clinical features The infection starts suddenly, with pain and sub-conjunctival haemorrhages. There is often much swelling and discomfort in the eye; however, it is a self-limiting condition, terminating within 1–2 weeks. In a few cases, there are systemic effects involving the upper respiratory tract or central nervous system (CNS). CNS effects are identical to those of poliomyelitis and residual paralysis can occur.

Diagnosis is clinical once the first few cases of an epidemic have been identified. Laboratory confirmation can be made by isolating the virus from a conjunctival swab.

Transmission is from one person to another from the discharges of infected eyes. Where there are systemic infections, transmission may be by the respiratory route. As with trachoma, intra-familial transmission is common and in situations of poor hygiene and overcrowding, large epidemics can occur.

Incubation period 1–3 days.

Period of communicability 4 days from the start of symptoms.

Occurrence and distribution It occurs in epidemic form infecting a large number of people in the immediate vicinity. Epidemics have been mainly in tropical cities in Africa, Asia, South America, the Caribbean and Pacific Islands.

Control and prevention Careful hand-washing, use of separate towels and sterilization of ophthalmologic instruments are important in preventing transmission. Methods to improve hygiene and reduce overcrowding will prevent major epidemics.

Treatment There is no treatment, so mass administration of eye ointment is not applicable.

Surveillance The first cases of an epidemic should be notified centrally and neighbouring countries warned.

7.6.1 Epidemic keratoconjunctivitis

Organism Adenovirus 5, 8 and 19.

Clinical features Epidemic keratoconjunctivitis is similar to epidemic haemorrhagic conjunctivitis, but a keratitis also develops in some 50% of cases, 7 days after onset. This normally resolves in about 2 weeks, but a minority is left with conjunctival scar-

ring. Upper respiratory symptoms and fever often accompany the eye disease.

Transmission Similar to epidemic haemorrhagic conjunctivitis.

Incubation period 4–12 days.

Period of communicability 14 days from onset of disease.

Occurrence and distribution Epidemics have occurred in Asia, North America and Europe.

Control and prevention are similar to epidemic haemorrhagic conjunctivitis.

Treatment and surveillance As with haemorrhagic conjunctivitis.

7.7 Ophthalmia Neonatorum

Infection of the eye of the newborn infant can lead to blindness.

Organism Neisseria gonorrhoea or C. trachomatis.

Clinical features and transmission If the mother has gonorrhoea or non-gonococcal urethritis (NGU) caused by C. trachomatis (see Sections 14.5 and 14.6), the infant's eyes can become contaminated with infectious discharges as it passes through the birth canal. This leads to conjunctivitis and in gonococcal infection, an important cause of blindness, especially in developing countries.

Diagnosis is made by microscopic examination of maternal vaginal discharges.

Incubation period is 1–5 days in gonococcal infection and 5–12 days with Chlamydia infection.

Period of communicability As long as genital or ocular infection persists.

Occurrence and distribution Infection is found more commonly in sex trade workers and the sexually promiscuous. It is more common in developing countries, where routine testing of expectant mothers is not performed.

Control and prevention Detection and treatment of the initial infection in the mother (see Sections 14.5 and 14.6) is the best strategy. Any vaginal discharge occurring during pregnancy should be examined, cultured and treated.

Treatment At delivery, all babies' eyes should be routinely wiped and a 1% aqueous solution of silver nitrate instilled. Wiping both eyes at delivery alone can reduce the incidence of infection if silver nitrate is not available and should always be practised. A 2.5% solution of povidone—iodine, tetracycline 1% or erythromycin 0.5% eye ointment, can be used as alternatives to silver nitrate.

Surveillance. All vaginal discharges during the antenatal period should be examined and cultured. Where an infant is born with ophthalmia neonatorum (sticky eye), the parents and any sexual contacts should be fully investigated (Section 14.5).

7.8 Other Infections

Many of the faecal–oral diseases covered in Chapter 8 and those due to soil contact in Chapter 10 are due to poor personal hygiene. Streptococcal and staphylococcal infections of the skin (Section 12.6) are also prevented by good personal hygiene. Yaws (14.1), pinta (14.2) and endemic syphilis (14.3) are readily cured by penicillin, but in the long-term, personal hygiene is the best preventive strategy. A full list of diseases prevented by good personal hygiene can be found in Section 3.3.1.

8

Faecal–Oral Diseases

The faecal–oral group of diseases is transmitted by person-to-person contact, through water, food or directly to the mouth. The absence of a proper water supply, rubbish and dirty surroundings with an abundance of flies are the typical situations in which these diseases thrive. The incidence of these diseases can be controlled by: (i) breaking the faecal–oral cycle with personal hygiene; (ii) increase in water quantity; (iii) improvement in water quality; (iv) food hygiene; and (v) the provision of sanitation. The disposal of garbage and the control of flies are also important.

Many of the diseases in this group cause diarrhoea (Table 8.1).

8.1 Gastroenteritis

Gastroenteritis is a common form of diarrhoea that predominantly attacks children. It is endemic in developing countries, but seasonal epidemics occur. Attempts to find a specific organism as a cause are often unsuccessful and not essential, as management and control are the same. Strains of enterotoxigenic, enteropathogenic and enteroaggregative *Escherichia coli* as well as enteric viruses, particularly rotavirus, are the main organisms. *Campylobacter* (Section 9.2) is now a major cause.

Clinical features Profuse, watery diarrhoea with occasional vomiting, but despite the fluid nature of the stools, faecal material is always present. There is never the rice-water stool characteristic of cholera. Water and electrolytes are lost, which in the young child may be sufficient to cause dehydration and ionic imbalance, leading to death. Normally, a self-limiting condition, but in unhygienic surroundings, or where babies' bottles are used, repeated infections occur leading to chronic loss of nutrients and subsequent malnutrition. A serious infection in neonates, mortality decreases with age until in adults, it is just a passing inconvenience (travellers' diarrhoea).

Diagnosis is made on clinical criteria unless laboratory facilities sufficient to identify viral infections are available. Specific DNA probes are likely to be the most appropriate method of identifying causative organisms in developing countries if they can be made cheap enough.

Transmission Epidemics occur in families or groups of children sharing similar surroundings. Infection is often seasonal, for example, the beginning of the rains heralding an outbreak. This would suggest transmission by water and simple control measures, such as boiling of water, can

Table 8.1. Diarrhoeas.

Presentation	Disease	Organism	Characteristics
Acute watery diarrhoea	Salmonellosis, food poisoning	*Salmonella, Staphylococci, B. cereus, C. perfringens, V. parahaemolyticus*	Sudden onset with vomiting in group of people associated by food
	Gastroenteritis (bacterial)	*E. coli* or non-specific	Common, mainly in children, epidemic
	Gastroenteritis (viral)	Rotavirus and other enteroviruses	Occurs in children, often in institutions (hospitals, schools, etc.)
	Cryptosporidiosis	*Cryptosporidium*	
	Cholera	*V. cholerae*	Severe, dehydration, rice-water stools, epidemic
Acute diarrhoea with blood	Bacillary dysentery, Campylobacter	*Shigella* sp., *C. jejuni*	Severe, seasonal, all ages Sporadic, from contaminated food, animal reservoir
Chronic diarrhoea	Giardiasis (Sprue or malabsorption syndromes)	*G. intestinalis*	Mainly children and travellers Adults, mostly males; nutritional deficiencies especially of folic acid
Chronic diarrhoea with *blood*	Amoebiasis	*E. histolytica*	Cooler climates, mainly adults
	Balantidiasis	*B. coli*	Similar to amoebiasis; associated with pigs
	Schistosomiasis	*S. mansoni*	Endemic areas, characteristic eggs in stools

B. (cereus), Bacillus; C. (perfringens), Clostridium; V. (parahaemolyticus), V. (cholerae) Vibrio; E. (coli), Escherichia; C. (jejuni), Campylobacter; G. (lamblia), Giardia; E. (histolytica), Entamoeba; B. (coli), Balantidium; S. (mansoni), Schistosoma. Many other diseases cause diarrhoea (e.g. measles, malaria, tonsillitis).

stop the epidemic. Improperly sterilized babies' bottles or their contents are a common method of infecting the neonate.

Incubation period 12–72 h (generally 48 h).

Period of communicability 8–10 days.

Occurrence and distribution Gastroenteritis is found throughout the world, especially in developing countries and in conditions of poor hygiene. It is particularly common where bottle-feeding has been recently introduced, such as by unscrupulous infant-feed companies. A seasonal distribution suggests contamination of the water supply.

Control and prevention is by the following methods:

- promotion of breast-feeding;
- use of oral rehydration solution (ORS) in the community;
- improvement in water supply and sanitation;
- promoting personal and domestic hygiene;
- vaccination (rotavirus and other vaccines, e.g. measles).

Breast-feeding not only provides a sterile milk formula in the correct proportions (in contrast to the often-contaminated bottle), but also promotes lactobacilli and contains lactoferrins and lysozymes. Promoting breast-feeding and the administration of

ORS solution in the community are the main control strategies. Improvement in water supplies and sanitation, with the promotion of personal hygiene, are long-term measures.

The oral cholera vaccine WC/rBS has been shown to be about 60% effective against enterotoxigenic *E. coli* so might have some place in control although its protective effect in infants is considerably less. Rotavirus vaccine (RRV-TV) has so far been shown to be less effective in developing countries than the developed and several cases of intussusception has resulted in its withdrawal from use in the latter. Preventing other childhood infections by vaccination, especially those associated with gastro-intestinal disease, such as polio and measles, can reduce the severity of gastro-enteritis.

Treatment is by replacement of fluid and electrolytes using ORS in the moderately dehydrated and intravenous replacement in the severely dehydrated.

A suitable ORS is made by dissolving the following constituents in 1 l of water:

Sodium chloride (salt)	3.5 g (Na$^+$ 90 mmol)
Trisodium citrate dihydrate	2.9 g (citrate 10 mmol)
Potassium chloride	1.5 g (K$^+$ 20 mmol, Cl$^-$ 88 mmol)
Glucose anhydrous (dextrose)	20.0 g (glucose 111 mmol)

These ingredients can be obtained separately or in packets of readily prepared mixtures. In the absence of prepared packets, a simpler formulation can be made as shown in Fig. 8.1, which consists of mixing salt and sugar in 1 l of clean water. Potassium is not an essential constituent, but addition of the juice of one orange is useful. Tea leaves also contain potassium, so the mixture can be prepared as tea with the addition of salt and sugar. Teaspoons vary in size and it is dangerous to give too much salt; hence a useful check is for the mother to taste the solution before adminis-

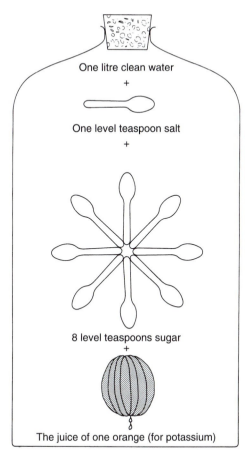

One litre clean water

+

One level teaspoon salt

+

8 level teaspoons sugar

+

The juice of one orange (for potassium)

Fig. 8.1. Preparing a simple oral rehydration solution.

tering it to her child. If it tastes salty, then more water should be added.

A naturally available rehydration solution is the fluid from a green coconut. A 7-month coconut has been found to be the most suitable. Rice-water made from a handful of rice boiled in a saucepan of water until it disappears, plus the appropriate amount of salt for the volume of water, makes a simple rehydration solution. Carrot water can also be used.

If mothers are taught how to make up these solutions, then they can treat their children as soon as they start to get diarrhoea. The mother should use a cup and a spoon and sit with her child giving it small quantities of fluid at frequent intervals. Severe dehydration can usually be prevented by primary care from the mother.

There is no need to use an antibiotic or an antispasmodic, both of which are contra-indicated. Lactobacilli, which inhibit *E. coli*, colonize the gut in the breast-fed infant. In some countries, lactobacilli are administered in yoghurt (curd).

Surveillance In countries with a seasonal rainfall pattern, gastro-enteritis outbreaks often start with the beginning of the rains, so monitoring the weather can provide early warning of an impending outbreak.

8.2 Cryptosporidiosis

Organism *Cryptosporidium parvum* is a protozoan parasite found in poultry, fish, reptiles and mammals, especially cattle, pigs, sheep, dogs and cats, from which the infection can be acquired.

Clinical features Cryptosporidiosis presents as an acute watery diarrhoea associated with abdominal pain. Fever, anorexia, nausea and vomiting can also occur, especially in children. There may be repeat attacks, but these do not normally continue for more than a month. In the immunodeficient, especially those with HIV infection, the disease enters a chronic and progressive course.

Diagnosis is by finding the oocyst in faecal samples. Alternatively, the intestinal stages can be looked for in intestinal biopsy specimens.

Transmission is from person-to-person via the faecal–oral route, from animals or faecal-contaminated water. The oocyst can survive in nature for a considerable period of time. The infecting dose is very low.

Incubation period. 1–12 days. Mean of 7 days.

Period of communicability Up to 6 months in faecal material.

Occurrence and distribution. Cryptosporidiosis has a worldwide distribution, found particularly in conditions of poor hygiene. It is endemic in many developing countries where infection is acquired at an early age. Massive epidemics have occurred in developed countries when the water purification system had failed (such as the 1993 Milwaukee epidemic where there were 500,000 cases). In other areas, it is a disease of animal handlers, homosexuals and institutions. There is a marked seasonality in the northern hemisphere with peaks of disease in spring and autumn.

Control and prevention is by personal hygiene, the provision of sanitation and safe water supplies. Domestic animals and pets can be important sources of infection and therefore precautions should be taken when handling them.

Treatment is with oral rehydration to replace fluid loss (Section 8.1).

Surveillance Animals, particularly cattle and pigs, can be examined for *Cryptosporidium* infection.

8.3 Cholera

Organism. *Vibrio cholerae.* Classical cholera is caused by *V. cholerae* 01, while most of the recent epidemics have been due to the El Tor biotype. *V. cholerae* 0139, which appeared in 1992, is a more virulent serogroup variant of the El Tor biotype.

Clinical features A profound diarrhoea of rapid onset that leads to dehydration and death should be considered as a case of cholera until proved otherwise. The diarrhoea contains no faecal particles, but is watery and flecked with mucus (not cells), the so-called rice-water stools. The passage of large quantities of fluid leads to rapid and extreme dehydration, which can be fatal. Vomiting can also be present in the early stages.

Diagnosis *V. cholerae* can be identified from the diarrhoeal discharge, vomitus or by rectal swab. Its characteristic mobility (it vibrates, hence being called a vibrio) can be seen by dark ground or phase-contrast microscopy and is inhibited by specific antiserum. Confirmation of the diagnosis is made by culture on TCBS sucrose agar. A suitable transport medium is Carey Blair, or alternatively 1% alkaline (pH 8.5) peptone water, which can also be used for water samples.

Transmission Classical cholera is a disease of water transmission, whereas El Tor is by both water and food. Generally, epidemic cholera is transmitted by water and endemic cholera by food. It may appear in a seasonal pattern, often in association with other causes of diarrhoea (Fig. 8.2). It is the endemic nature of El Tor and its persistence in the environment that has been responsible for its prodigious spread.

For every clinical case of El Tor cholera, there can be as many as 100 asymptomatic cases, explaining how epidemics spread from one region to another, but not how infection persists in the environment. Vibrios may be able to persist in an aquatic environment, such as in the mucilaginous covering of water plants or fish, in association with copepods or other zooplankton. An alternative method may be due to continuous person-to-person transmission in a sub-clinical asymptomatic cycle. When a susceptible person enters the cycle or there is an environmental or climatic change, a fresh epidemic starts.

V. cholerae in water are easily destroyed by sunlight, chemical action or competing bacteria. However, where these elements are not present, it can survive in fresh water for some time and in saline water for at least a week. The level of salinity needs to be between 0.01% and 0.1% as is found in estuarine or lagoon water. *V. cholerae* in these saline environments can be taken up by shellfish or fish, which then form an alternative method of infection when eaten uncooked.

The isolation of *V. cholerae* from river water has been perplexing because epidemiological investigations show this source of infection to be important, but bacteriologists have not isolated organisms in sufficient numbers. One possible explanation is the presence of non-agglutinable vibrios (alternatively known as non-cholera vibrios), which are closely related to *V. cholerae* except that they do not agglutinate antisera. These are known to be mutations so that shifts between typical vibrios and non-agglutinable forms may occur. If this is a regular feature in nature, then it could help to explain where cholera goes to (especially the classical form) during interepidemic periods. The appearance of non-01 cholera (vibrio 0139) supports this view.

V. cholerae has been found to remain viable in crude sewage for over a month and in sewage-contaminated soil for up to 10 days, a possible source of infection carried over to rivers or wells. It has been isolated from a number of foodstuffs especially those with a pH between 6 and 8, such as milk produce (e.g. ice cream), sugar solutions, meat extracts or articles of food preserved by salt. Uncooked fish and vegetables, which have been washed or irrigated by sewage effluent, have been responsible for outbreaks.

Direct person-to-person spread or via fomites, such as utensils or drinking straws (in home-brewed alcohol parties), do not appear to be as important as expected. Even for persons attending the death of a cholera victim, it is more likely that infection will result from drinking water or consuming food that has been prepared for the mourning ceremony, rather than from the dead person or their shrouds.

A case of cholera can excrete between 10^7 and 10^9 *V. cholerae* per millilitre of diarrhoeal discharge and since the volume of this discharge may be in excess of 20 l/day, the potential for contamination of the environment is enormous. Clearly, though the severe case is unlikely to be anything but a transitory source, it is the asymptomatic case passing from 10^2 to 10^5 organisms/g of stool in a spasmodic manner that poses the greatest hazard.

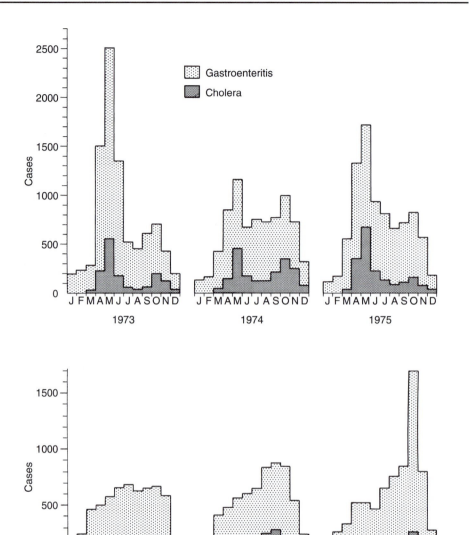

Fig. 8.2. Similar pattern of gastroenteritis and cholera in Calcutta, India (1973–1978). (Reproduced with permission from the Indian Council of Medical Research (1978) *National Institute of Cholera and Enteric Diseases, Annual Report,* Indian Council of Medical Research, Calcutta.)

A high dose of *V. cholerae* is required to infect the healthy subject. Some 10^6–10^8 organisms are needed, but if the person has a decreased gastric acidity, then 10^3 organisms may be sufficient. Lowered gastric acidity is found more commonly than expected and may be related to malnutrition or diet. Cannabis smoking is known to de-press gastric acidity. Blood group O is associated with an increased severity of cholera.

Carriers are of short duration; 70% of cholera cases are free of vibrios at the end of the first week and 98% by the end of the third. Long-term carriers are rare and of no epidemiological importance.

Incubation period 1–5 days.

Period of communicability is until about 5 days after recovery, but prolonged excretion of organisms can continue in some individuals. Antibiotics reduce the period of communicability.

Occurrence and distribution Humans are the only known reservoir, but the persistence of the organism in the environment, in possibly a changing form, as discussed above, may be another source. In endemic areas, cholera is a disease of children (adults having developed immunity in childhood), whereas in its epidemic form, adults are the more usual victims. The disease is associated with poverty and poor hygienic practices.

Classical cholera is restricted to South Asia and caused by *V. cholerae* 01. The El Tor biotype has infected Asia, Africa, Europe, Pacific Islands and South America; the majority of cases are now found in Africa. First isolated from pilgrims to Mecca in the quarantine station of El Tor in West Sinai (now Egypt) in 1906, it differs from the classical variety by producing a soluble haemolysin. It is classified as either Ogawa, Inaba or Hikojima of the classical serotypes. The importance of the El Tor biotype is that it can survive longer in water, is more infectious, can cause mild infections and more frequently produces the carrier state. All these characteristics have assisted in the extensive spread of this organism. The new and more virulent *V. cholerae* 0139 has spread to many parts of Asia and been responsible for epidemics in India, Bangladesh, Myanmar, Thailand and Malaysia.

Control and prevention Control is aimed at the cause. All too often a panic situation develops, foods are banned, vaccination given and quarantine instigated. If cholera is epidemic and preliminary investigations indicate that water is the vehicle of transmission, then the supply should be steril-ized by super-chlorination (adding two to three times the calculated amount of chlorine required for the volume of water) or people should be advised to boil the water they use for drinking. Boiling water is unpopular as it uses vital firewood, monopolizes scarce cooking pots and the water has a flat taste. However, there is no reason why water cannot be boiled at the same time as the meal is cooked and simple clay pots used instead of metal ones. Boiled water can be re-aerated by shaking it up. A not so safe, but easier method is to leave water to stand and then decant off the supernatant. A simple way of doing this is the three-pot system (Fig. 3.7). Chlorine can be added to a well or community water supply, but any vegetable matter in the water will inactivate chlorine and several times the amount calculated may be required.

The banning or restriction of food should only be made on good epidemiological evidence. If fish are properly cooked before being eaten, then they are unlikely to be a source. Disruption of a fish-eating practice may have dire consequences on other aspects of people's health. It is more often the fisherman rather than the fish, or the farmers, rather than their produce that are the purveyors of cholera.

Quarantine is rarely effective, as bribery or evasion of the barricades by the few who might be carrying the infection negates the hardships borne by the many who are not. Giving tetracycline to immediate contacts of cases will reduce the number of asymptomatic carriers, but the widespread distribution of the drug will encourage tetracycline resistance.

The original inactivated *V. cholerae* vaccination gives about 50% protection and only lasts for 6 months. It does not prevent the asymptomatic disease state and can actively encourage the spread of infection and, therefore, is not recommended as a method of control. A new oral vaccine (WC/rBS) consisting of killed whole *V. cholerae* 01 in combination with a recombinant B subunit of cholera toxin confers protection of up to 90% for 6 months and has been found to be effective in preventing cholera in high-risk areas, such as refugee camps and urban slums. Protection was found to last for 3 years in 50% of those vaccinated at the age of 5 years or above. Another oral vaccine (CVD 103-HgR) conferred good protection and was also effective in infants as young as 3 months of age. Either of these vaccines can be used pre-emptively in high-risk areas, epidemic situations and to protect travellers entering areas of high endemicity.

Persons dying from cholera should be buried quickly and the ceremony kept to a minimum. Disinfectants and hand-washing facilities should be provided at treatment centres and when bodies are prepared for burial. Flies should be controlled by disposing or covering all faecal discharges, although they have not been shown to play a significant role in transmission.

Treatment The vibrio binds to the cells and produces an enterotoxin, which activates adenyl cyclase, an intracellular enzyme that initiates a system of fluid and ion transport from the plasma to the intestinal lumen. There is no mucosal damage and increased permeability is unlikely, which explains why glucose and electrolytes can still be absorbed by the mucosa. This allows large quantities of low-protein fluid, bicarbonate and potassium to escape through an essentially undamaged intestine. Management is to correct dehydration in this otherwise self-limiting disease.

Fluid replacement must be rapid and adequate, the most easily available being the first choice. If rehydration can be started as soon as cholera symptoms begin, then oral rehydration will be all that is required. ORSs can either be prepared from ready mixed packets of salts (Section 8.1) or by making a sugar–salt solution (Fig. 8.1). Unfortunately, most cases have already lost a considerable quantity of body fluid on presentation, which means that they will require intravenous infusion. If available, Ringer lactate solution (Hartmann's) contains the nearest approximation of electrolytes to that lost in the diarrhoeal fluid. As a second best option, a mixture of two units of normal saline and one unit of sodium bicarbonate can be used. The patient should be rehydrated intravenously as rapidly as possible, the rehydration substituted by ORS once the patient can swallow. This allows the body mechanisms to regulate electrolytes, as ionic imbalance can rapidly occur with intravenous infusion to which many patients succumb. The body fluid deficit should be restored, followed by maintenance of one and a half times the equivalent amount of bowel loss. Fluid loss can be measured by directing fluid into a bucket placed under the bed. A bed or cholera cot is not essential though and the patient can be nursed on a plastic sheet laid on the ground with the earth hollowed out under the pelvis to take a receptacle to collect the outpouring fluid.

Tetracycline is not essential in treatment, but shortens the duration of the illness and quantity of fluid replacement required. Tetracycline is given in a dose of 500 mg 6-hourly for 3 days or Doxycycline in a single dose of 300 mg. Sensitivity must be monitored as the development of tetracycline resistance will necessitate changing to another antibiotic.

The management of a cholera epidemic requires speed and good organization. Essentially treatment is taken to the people by setting up treatment centres at strategic places in the vicinity of the epidemic. These can be dispensaries, schools, church halls or even tents, supplied with staff and fluids. Cholera patients do not need to be treated in hospital.

Surveillance for cholera is both national and international. An outbreak of cholera must be reported to WHO, providing an advance warning system to neighbouring countries. Nationally, a warning system can be implemented for diarrhoeal diseases where an increase in numbers or persons dying from diarrhoea may indicate an underlying outbreak of cholera (Fig. 8.2). Where cholera exhibits a seasonal pattern, the population and health staff can be placed on the alert when the next season starts.

8.4 Bacillary Dysentery (Shigellosis)

Organism Bacillary dysentery is due to *Shigella* invading the bowel. The species and strains of *Shigella* are numerous. There are four main groups:

- *S. dysenteriae* with 12 serotypes;
- *S. flexneri* with 14 serotypes;
- *S. boydi* with 18 serotypes;
- *S. sonnei* with one serotype.

The most severe are *S. dysenteriae* and the least severe *S. sonnei*, with *S. flexneri* being the most common in endemic areas. Another form of bloody diarrhoea is due to enteroinvasive and enterohaemorrhagic *E. coli*, particularly serotype 0157.

Clinical features Bacillary dysentery presents as an acute diarrhoeal illness with blood in the stools, more acute and severe than amoebic dysentery. In mild infections, blood may be absent with a similar presentation to gastroenteritis. In severe cases, the stools are a mixture of pus and blood, and tenesmus is common. Fever accompanies the illness and nausea or frank vomiting can occur. Severity is determined by the strain of organism and age of the person, with a moderate mortality in the very young and very old.

Diagnosis If bacteriological facilities permit, the organism should be identified, typed and sensitivity determined. A suitable transport medium is Carey Blair. Where this is not possible, a simple epidemiological investigation may provide sufficient information to indicate the mode of transmission.

Transmission is by the faecal–oral route with either food or water as the main vehicle carrying the infection. Bacillary dysentery can occur in small outbreaks amongst families, suggesting food as the mode of transfer. Seasonal epidemics coinciding with the arrival of the rains indicate water-borne spread. Flies can be important in hot dry months when garbage accumulates and massive fly breeding takes place. Only 10–100 organisms are required to produce the disease.

Carriers can be important and sporadic epidemics in institutions might indicate a food handler with unsanitary habits.

Incubation period 1–7 days.

Period of communicability 4 weeks, but may persist for longer in the carrier.

Occurrence and distribution Any outbreak of an acute diarrhoeal disease with blood should be considered to be bacillary dysentery until proved otherwise. Distribution is worldwide with sporadic outbreaks occurring in both the developed and the developing world. Infection is often carried from one area to another or across international boundaries by carriers.

Control and prevention Bacillary dysentery is likely to present as an outbreak; so control will need to be implemented in the manner described in Section 4.1. Generally, it is better to bring treatment to the site of the outbreak, setting up temporary treatment centres, unless the outbreak is a small one and the hospital has sufficient facilities to isolate cases. A seasonal outbreak will suggest that water supplies need to be improved. Search for carriers is generally unsatisfactory and investigation should be restricted to food handlers.

Breast-feeding is protective for babies and infants and should be continued even by the sick mother. Washing hands with soap and water is the most effective method of interrupting transmission.

With widespread antibiotic resistance, *Shigella* infections could be controlled by vaccinating susceptible groups, especially if there is an outbreak in the vicinity. A live oral vaccine of *S. flexneri* (SC602) is currently under trial, while others are in the developmental stage.

Treatment Management is the same as with other diarrhoeas – to replace fluid and

electrolytes lost. ORS is adequate and effective in all cases, but the severely dehydrated
will require intravenous rehydration. There
is a place for antibiotics in the treatment
of bacillary dysentery although sensitivity
must be determined, as resistance is
common. Ampicillin, nalidixic acid,
TMPX–SMX, ciprofloxacin or ofloxocin
can be given as a 5-day course. Antibiotic
treatment should not be relied upon as resistance makes control more difficult and the
disease can relentlessly spread though a
country.

Surveillance is similar to cholera (Section
8.3) with notification of any outbreaks
and monitoring of the weather for seasonal
occurrences.

There are many similarities between
cholera and bacillary dysentery, especially
in the management and control so further
help can be found in Section 8.3.

8.5 Giardia

Organism The small flagellate *Giardia intestinalis* (*lamblia*) is a common commensal of
the human small intestine, but heavy infections can cause diarrhoea.

Clinical features Faeces are loose and greasy
with an unpleasant odour. Bloating and
abdominal distension can occur. Chronic
infections can produce partial villous atro-
phy with a resulting malabsorption syndrome. Giardia is one of the causes of
traveller's diarrhoea.

Diagnosis The characteristic 'face'-shaped
flagellate is occasionally seen in the faeces,
easily detected by its high motility, but the
cysts are more commonly found (Fig. 9.1).
Jejunal biopsy or the duodenal string test
may be performed in the differential diagnosis of the malabsorption syndrome.

Transmission is by person-to-person transfer
of cysts from the faeces of an infected individual or by contamination of food or water.
Infected food handlers are often responsible

for infecting people in restaurants, while a
poorly maintained water supply dissemin-
ates infection more widely. The cysts can
survive for several weeks in fresh water
and are not killed by normal levels of chlorine. An animal reservoir might also be responsible.

Incubation period 3–25 days; mean 7–
10 days.

Period of communicability The organism can
persist in the bowel for many months and
during all of this time the infection can be
transmitted.

Occurrence and distribution The infection is
found worldwide, but is more common in
the tropics and where conditions of hygiene
are poor, ensnaring the unsuspecting traveller with chronic diarrhoea. Heavy infections
occur in children, especially those in institutions or debilitated by other conditions.

Control and prevention Individuals who are
rigorous with their personal hygiene can
largely avoid infection. Drinking water can
be boiled or treated with five to ten drops of
iodine per litre of water. Proper food handling and preparation, especially the washing
of hands is essential, while long-term prevention is through proper sewage disposal
and the protection of water supplies.

Treatment is with tinidazole either as a
single dose of 2 g or 300 mg a day for 7 days.
Metronidazole can also be used.

Surveillance *Giardia* is a common infection
in travellers and a routine stool examination
after travelling to a less-developed area is
advisable.

8.6 Amoebiasis

Organism Amoebiasis is caused by the
protozoan *Entamoeba histolytica*, which
exists in an amoeboid form in the human
large intestine and as a cyst in the environment.

The pathogenic amoeba enters a mucosal fold and feeds on red blood cells (RBCs). Penetrating through the muscularis mucosae, an abscess is formed with vascular necrosis taking place at its base. This leads to tissue disintegration and the development of an ulcer (the so-called flask-shaped ulcer). Active amoebae can be found in the base of an ulcer.

Clinical features Illness presents as acute diarrhoea with frank blood, chronic diarrhoea or as an abscess with no apparent transitional period of diarrhoea. If the amoebic ulcer penetrates a blood vessel, fresh blood is passed in the stool, which is a characteristic feature. Amoebae from the breached circulatory system are carried to various parts of the body, the liver being the commonest. In the liver, an abscess is formed, with the right lobe being the predominant site. Liver damage is a predisposing cause with liver abscess more common in males than females. The expanding abscess can track outwards through the peritoneum, abdominal wall and on to the skin or upwards to form a sub-phrenic abscess or enter the pleural cavity. The most serious site of amoebic abscess development is in the brain. All these features are illustrated on Fig. 8.3.

Symptoms of an abscess are fever, weight loss and localized tenderness. Amoebic pus is characteristically a pale reddish brown colour (without odour) and can be discharged on to the skin from a penetrating ulcer, or coughed up from the lung. In a chronic infection, an amoeboma can be formed, which may be confused with carcinoma.

Diagnosis is made by examining fresh stool specimens within half an hour of their production for motile amoebae with ingested RBCs. Amoebae are occasionally found in amoebic pus, which similarly must be examined as soon as possible as the active forms rapidly die off. The finding of cysts indicates infection, but search must be made of fresh stool or pus for motile amoebae. Liver abscess is diagnosed by X-ray (raised diaphragm) or by ultrasound. The abscess is usually not tapped, unless in differential diagnosis from a bacterial abscess or is about to burst.

Transmission Cysts of *E. histolytica* are formed in the large intestines and passed into the environment in the faeces. They survive in faeces for only a few days, but if they enter water, they remain viable for considerably longer periods. Infection occurs through drinking contaminated water or eating irrigated salad vegetables. Flies can carry cysts for some 5 h. In circumstances of poor hygiene, direct faecal–oral transfer via food, or by utensils, can take place.

Cysts can survive in the cold for considerable periods, but they are killed by a temperature over 43°C, which must be obtained in any composting system where human faeces are used. Non-survival of amoebic cysts is a useful indicator of effective decomposition (see Fig. 1.2).

Incubation period 2–4 weeks.

Period of communicability Cyst passing can continue for many years.

Occurrence and distribution Amoebiasis is a disease of poor hygiene, more commonly found in cooler environments than hot ones. In the tropics, it predominantly occurs in highland areas or where there is a large temperature fluctuation. It is an infection of adult life and if the period of residence in an endemic area is long, there is greater chance of becoming infected.

Control and prevention is by personal hygiene, food hygiene and the proper provision of water and sanitation. Sand filtration, especially if it is combined with alum flocculation, removes cysts from water supplies. A high concentration of chlorine is required to kill cysts (3.5 ppm residual) although they are more sensitive to iodine.

Treatment of all stages of the disease is by metronidazole 2.4 g single dose for 3 days or

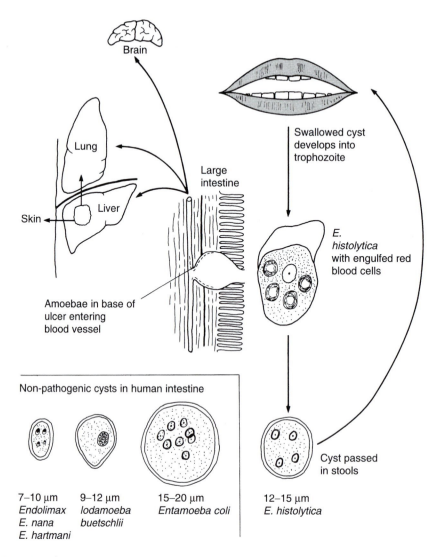

Fig. 8.3. Amoebiasis.

2 g daily for 5 days or by other derivatives of the 5-nitroimidazole group of compounds (tinidazole, ornidazole and nimorazole). Cyst passers can be given diloxanide furoate (Furomate), 500 mg 8-hourly for 10 days.

Surveillance Routine stool specimens should be examined for amoebic cysts. Cysts of *E. histolytica* can be differentiated from other cysts by size and number of nuclei (Fig. 8.3).

8.7 Typhoid

Organism *Salmonella enterica* serovar Typhi.

Clinical features Although transmitted by the faecal–oral route, typhoid manifests mainly as a systemic infection, generally presenting as a fever. The fever starts gradually, increasing in a stepwise fashion over the first 1–2 weeks, with a progressive malaise, disorientation and drowsiness. At the end of the first week, a rash of characteristic rose spots may appear (not seen in black skins).

The stools are normally constipated at first, but may later change to diarrhoea. If the organism localizes in the Peyers patches of the small intestine, ulceration, haemorrhage and perforation may occur.

Diagnosis is difficult and depends upon finding the organism in blood, stool or urine. A blood culture (3–5 ml) taken in the first week is the most satisfactory. Culture from the stools can be obtained if repeated examinations are made from the start of the illness, with a greater likelihood of becoming positive as the illness progresses, provided antibiotics have not been used. Finding the organism from urine, in which it is excreted spasmodically, is more difficult. Where the diagnosis has still not been made and further investigation considered necessary, *S. enterica* can be cultured from the bone marrow or bile (by duodenal string test). Bone marrow culture has the advantage of occasionally being positive even if the patient has received antibiotics. Sewage culture can be used in the investigation of epidemics.

The Widal test on the patient's serum can indicate infection, but a search for *S. enterica* must also be made to confirm the diagnosis. The Widal test has three components, the H (flagella) the O (somatic) and Vi antigens. The H antibody titre can be raised by any *Salmonella* infection and remain raised (giving an estimate of previous exposure), whereas the O antibody indicates recent infection. However, both H and O levels will be raised by a recent typhoid immunization, negating any value of the test. A titre of 1/40 or higher is required. Added weight is given to the diagnosis by making a series of tests and demonstrating a rising titre. The Vi antibody is produced during the acute stage of the disease and persists while the organism is present and, therefore, has a value in detecting the carrier state.

Transmission The main method of transmission is water, contaminated by faecal material from a carrier. These water-borne outbreaks may not always be explosive and where low-grade infection of the water source is taking place, groups of cases, spread over time, may occur.

S. enterica has been found to survive periods of 4 weeks in fresh water, but if the water is stored in bright sunlight (as in a reservoir), then the number of organisms rapidly dies off. It can survive in aerobic conditions with organic nutrient present, as found in contaminated streams. If the stream is polluted with raw sewage, then the organism can survive over 5 weeks and within solid faecal material for considerable periods of time. Seawater is bactericidal, but where a sewage outfall is near a shellfish bed, then the organism is filtered and concentrated providing a potent source of infection if the shellfish are eaten raw.

Milk and dairy products provide ideal culture media and can become infected during handling by a carrier, or rinsing of containers with polluted water. Contaminated ice cream has been responsible for several outbreaks. Pasteurization of milk at 60°C is effective in killing *S. enterica*. Infection of meat products and canned foods is less common, but can occur in the cooling process (if carried out in polluted water).

Flies can transmit the organism from faeces to food, whereas person-to-person infection is uncommon. Secondary cases form a very small proportion of an epidemic; so serial transmission in an unhygienic environment is not a feature.

Carriers The carrier state is the most important epidemiological feature, with persistence of the organism in some individuals for periods in excess of 50 years. Three per cent of typhoid cases are found to still be excreting organisms after 1 year. People become more prone to act as carriers if they have a chronic irritational process, such as cholecystitis, and especially the presence of gallstones (in which *S. enterica* are able to survive). *Opisthorchis sinensis* has also been associated with the development of faecal carriers. Urinary carriers often suffer from an abnormality of the urinary tract such as calculus and *Schistosoma haematobium* is a predisposing cause.

Incubation period is 3–30 days, with a mean of 8–14 days. The length of the incubation period is inversely proportional to the infecting dose.

Period of communicability From 1 week after the start of illness for a period of 3 months, except in the chronic carrier where it continues for years.

Occurrence and distribution In most tropical areas, the disease is endemic with seasonal outbreaks. Water is probably the main vehicle of transmission, but may be more related to the gathering of people at scarce water sources (as occurs in the dry season), rather than epidemics occurring with the early rains. Endemic typhoid is maintained by sub-clinical infections, especially in undiagnosed children, who obtain a degree of immunity. It has been suggested that these sub-clinical infections result from persons swallowing lower bacterial doses than the critical threshold. In endemic areas, the peak of infection is in children between 5 and 12 years of age.

Typhoid is a worldwide disease and serious outbreaks, generally epidemic in nature, have occurred in developed countries from contamination of the water supply or food produce. Repair work on water supplies or an accidental interruption of chlorination has led to epidemics. Typhoid organisms have persisted in canned meat cooled in infected water thousands of miles away from the outbreak. Many well-known outbreaks have been due to ice cream. The movement of carriers can be followed from the outbreaks they produce as they travel around.

Control and prevention Control relies on the protection of water supplies and the sanitary disposal of faeces. Placing latrines too close to wells, fractures in water mains and accidental contamination by sewage are ways in which outbreaks occur. Drinking water taken from polluted streams can be boiled, chlorinated or left to stand (the three-pot system in Fig. 3.7). Reservoirs and settling tanks can reduce the level of organisms below the infecting dose.

Where the outbreak can be traced to a food source, a search for carriers can be made. Stool specimens should be obtained from persons involved in the preparation of the food. If a carrier is discovered, they should be prohibited from preparing food. This cannot always be applied to domestic catering, so careful instruction in personal hygiene should be tried. The organism can persist under the nails, so these should be kept short. Food must be protected from flies and stored only for limited periods. All shellfish must be properly cooked.

An infecting dose of at least 10^3 organisms is required (except in persons suffering from achlorhydria), but may need to be as high as 10^9. The main effect of vaccination appears to be to offer protection against lower dose infecting inocula (less than 10^5 organisms).

Typhoid vaccine has a variable effect, offering protection to persons who receive a low infecting dose, but none to those who ingest a high dose of organisms. It may, therefore, be useful for individual protection, but is limited on a mass immunization basis, except to selected groups such as school children. The live oral vaccine (Ty 21a) gives protection for at least 3 years and may also give cross-immunity against *S. enterica* Paratyphi B. It is administered in three capsules taken orally on days 1, 3 and 5. A vaccine containing the polysaccharide Vi antigen is administered parenterally by a single injection. Both of these methods produce less reaction than the whole-bacteria vaccine. A booster dose is required every 3 years in travellers or persons from non-endemic areas living in countries where typhoid is common. The oral vaccine is probably more effective in young children and in mass programmes, given as a liquid formulation rather than in capsules, but proguanil, mefloquine and antibiotics should be stopped 3 days before administration.

Treatment is with ampicillin or co-tri-moxazole, but multiple resistant organisms have meant that more expensive antibiotics, such as the quinalones (e.g. ciprofloxocin and ofloxacin) and third-generation cephalosporins, are now required. Prolonged treatment of the carrier with ampicillin, 1 g three times a day for 11 weeks has been successful, or if available, one of the quinalones can be used. Relapse occurs in about 5% of treated acute cases.

Surveillance Once a carrier has been identified they should be warned of the danger they pose to others and told to report their condition to any medical people they come in contact with. Carriers are sometimes registered by health authorities.

8.7.1 Paratyphoid

Organism *Salmonella enterica* Paratyphi A, B and C. Paratyphi B is the commonest.

Clinical features Paratyphoid is similar to typhoid, but with less systemic effects and diarrhoea a more important feature. A rash is less commonly seen, but when it does occur, it is more extensive involving the limbs and face as well as the body. Ulceration of the gut can occur, but less commonly than in typhoid.

Transmission Infection originates from a carrier or a person with the illness, more commonly food-borne than by other means (see under food poisoning, Section 9.1).

Diagnosis See typhoid.

Incubation period 1–10 days.

Period of communicability 1–2 weeks.

Occurrence and distribution Paratyphoid has a similar distribution to typhoid with an endemic pattern in developing countries and epidemic in developed, but is less commonly detected.

Control and prevention See typhoid.

Treatment See typhoid.

Surveillance See typhoid.

8.8 Hepatitis A (HAV)

Organism Infectious hepatitis is a viral infection caused by a member of the *Picornaviridae*, which includes both enteroviruses and rhinoviruses.

Clinical features The main pathology is inflammation, infiltration and necrosis of the liver, resulting in biliary stasis and jaundice. The infection generally starts insidiously, the person feels lethargic, anorexic and depressed. Fever, vomiting, diarrhoea and abdominal discomfort ensue before the appearance of jaundice reveals the diagnosis. Once jaundice appears, the person generally starts to feel better. Hepatitis A is a mild disease leading to spontaneous cure in the large majority, with only a few cases developing acute fulminant hepatitis and even rarely severe chronic liver damage. There is an increase in symptomatic and severe cases with increasing age.

Diagnosis is made on clinical grounds and by the demonstration of IgM antibodies to HAV (IgM anti-HAV) in serum.

Transmission The early case is highly infectious contaminating food and water. Infection can also be transmitted directly from poor personal hygiene such as by hand-shaking. Intra-familial transmission is the commonest pattern generally due to contamination of food and utensils by a food handler, but large epidemics can occur where a person in the early stages of the illness prepares community food. Because of its insidious nature, the disease is not generally recognized until jaundice appears, by which time infection may have been widely transmitted.

Hepatitis is mainly a disease of poor sanitation, with water and food as the principal vehicles of transmission, but can also occur when sanitation is good. Salads, cold meats and raw sea food are common vehicles of transmission.

The carrier state is not important, but a large number of asymptomatic cases are produced. Epidemics occur when sewage contaminates water supplies producing infection in people who have previously acquired some immunity, suggesting that the disease may be dose-dependent. Where there is a large infecting inoculum, infection can occur despite previous experience of the disease. Chimpanzees and other animals have been found infected, but probably have no epidemiological significance.

Incubation period is 15–50 days, generally about 28 days.

Period of communicability is the later half of the incubation period until about 1 week after jaundice appears, so that most cases have already transmitted the virus to family and contacts before they report for medical attention.

Occurrence and distribution Hepatitis is endemic in most tropical countries, with children coming into contact early in life and developing a degree of immunity. Non-immune persons, such as from an area of good sanitation coming into this environment, are likely to develop the disease. Epidemics occur in developed countries, especially in institutions, such as schools and prisons, due to poor food hygiene.

Control and prevention During an outbreak of hepatitis A, extra effort should be made to encourage scrupulous personal hygiene with hand-washing. Anybody who starts to feel unwell should be temporarily relieved

of preparing food. In an epidemic situation, search should be made for the origin of the outbreak and preventive measures taken. In the long term, water supplies and sanitation should be upgraded.

HAV vaccine protects the individual at risk and should be mandatory for those going from an area of good sanitation to one of poor sanitation, such as tourists and expatriates. Two doses are required to be given 6–18 months apart, although one dose still gives high levels of immunity. Immunity from a two-dose regime may be lifelong, but a booster at 10 years is currently recommended. As most of the population in an endemic area would have met the infection as children and either had no symptoms or just a mild infection, there is no case for mass vaccination, except for high-risk groups.

Treatment There is no specific treatment and supportive measures should be undertaken. Fatty foods should be avoided and a good fluid intake maintained.

Surveillance Once hepatitis has been detected, health authorities should notify central authorities and surrounding areas.

8.9 Hepatitis E (HEV)

Organism An enteric (E) virus provisionally classified as a calicivirus.

Clinical features Hepatitis E is very similar to hepatitis A except that it nearly always occurs in large epidemics. The main difference is that hepatitis E results in a high mortality in pregnant women (up to 20%).

Transmission Similar to hepatitis A, although the main means of transmission is via water. A reservoir has been found in wild and domestic pigs, suggesting a zoonotic pattern of transmission.

Diagnosis is by the detection of IgM and IgG anti-hepatitis E virus (anti-HEV) in serum.

Incubation period 3–9 weeks.

Period of communicability From 14 days after the appearance of jaundice for a further 2 weeks.

Occurrence and distribution Hepatitis E has been responsible for large epidemics in South and Southeast Asia, especially Myanmar and Vietnam, where it appears to be endemic. Epidemics have also occurred in North Africa, Ethiopia, China and Mexico.

Control and prevention The same as hepatitis A, but extra precautions should be taken to protect pregnant women. There is no specific vaccine.

8.10 Poliomyelitis (Polio)

Organism Poliovirus (*Enterovirus*) types 1, 2 and 3.

Clinical features Infection commences with fever, general malaise and headache, the majority of cases resolving after these mild symptoms, but approximately 1% proceed to paralytic disease. The virus has a predilection for nerve cells, especially those with a motor function (the anterior horn cells of the spinal cord and the motor nuclei of the cranial nerves). These cells are destroyed and a flaccid paralysis results.

As a generalization, paralysis is more common in the lower part of the body, becoming less common the higher up it affects. Unilateral lameness is more common than bilateral lameness. The severe form of bulbar poliomyelitis is generally fatal in poor countries where respirators and intensive nursing care are not available. Site of paralysis is associated with injections or operations and such procedures should be avoided if there is any suggestion of poliomyelitis.

Diagnosis of the disabled case is made on clinical grounds, differentiating from the spastic paralysis of birth injury with which it is commonly confused. In polio, there will be a history of normal birth with commencement of walking, followed by a feverish illness and the development of flaccid paralysis. The paralysis is limited to well-demarcated muscle groups and there is no sensory loss. A similar history may be given for meningitis, but the damage will be central with accompanying mental deficiency.

Transmission is generally via the faecal–oral route, although the virus initially multiplies in the oro-pharynx; hence airborne transmission can also occur. The virus then invades the gastro-intestinal tract, where it is excreted for several weeks.

A disease of low hygiene, young children (4–5 months) meet the virus with only a small proportion showing overt disease. Of these, 80–90% have an inapparent subclinical disease, 5–10% suffer from fever, headache and minor clinical signs, with only 1% going on to paralysis. Paralysis is more common with older age. Therefore, a non-immune person going into an endemic environment is at far greater danger of developing paralytic poliomyelitis. Raising standards of hygiene will also have the same effect because it spares people from meeting the virus as young children and allows a pool of susceptibles to develop. In the course of time, the number of non-immunes will be sufficient for an epidemic to take place. There will also be a higher proportion of paralysed cases (peak age 5–9 years) and many deaths. Sadly, the raising of living standards will change polio from an endemic disease with a few paralysed cases to an epidemic disease of increased severity. In epidemic poliomyelitis where sanitation is good, pharyngeal spread becomes a more important method of transmission.

Poliovirus strains vary in their neurovirulence with the more virulent strains having a greater tendency to spread. This could be due to a lower infective dose of the virulent virus being required to produce disease.

Incubation period is from 5 to 30 days with a mean of 10 days.

Period of communicability From 2 days after exposure up until 6 weeks.

Occurrence and distribution Poliomyelitis formerly occurred throughout the world, endemic in the poorer regions and epidemic in those with good sanitation, but this has changed considerably with the WHO programme of eradicating polio from the world. The Americas, Europe and Western Pacific are now free of infection, while there are very few cases remaining in the rest of the world. The end of 2005 has been set as the target date for global eradication of polio.

Control and prevention The main method of prevention and control is with polio vaccine. Two types of vaccine are available, the killed (Salk) and the attenuated living (Sabin). The Salk vaccine is given by intramuscular injection, inducing a high level of immunity not antagonized by inhibitory factors in the gut, but is expensive to produce because it contains many organisms. The Sabin vaccine is administered orally making it easier and cheaper as well as producing intestinal immunity, which can block infection with wild strains of poliovirus. Multiplication of the virus in the intestine makes it very useful in preventing epidemics and allows it to spread to non-vaccinated persons in conditions of poor hygiene, thereby protecting them as well. Unfortunately, the inhibiting action of antibodies in breast milk and colonization of the gut by other entero viruses can reduce its effectiveness. Increasing the dosage and telling mothers not to breast-feed for at least an hour after administration can help.

Because there are three strains of the poliovirus, the vaccine should be given on three separate occasions, separated by periods of at least 1 month to ensure that immunity develops to each of the strains. Polio vaccine is conveniently administered at the same time as DTP. A preliminary dose can be given soon after birth in areas where wild poliovirus is circulating.

There is a slight risk of a live attenuated virus becoming more virulent, so it is preferable to vaccinate the majority of the population all at one time. Also, in a situation of raising sanitary standards, epidemic poliomyelitis will only be prevented if there are sufficient people immunized to produce 'herd immunity'. For these reasons, mass campaigns can be effective. These should always be followed up by static clinics vaccinating newborns and missed persons. The WHO, in its bid to eradicate polio from the world, recommends National Immunization Days (NID) on which all children under the age of 5 years are vaccinated, irrespective of previous immunization status. Two doses are given at a month's interval followed by mop-up operations in areas of low coverage or where continuing transmission has been identified.

School children and adults, who have received a full course of childhood vaccinations, should have booster doses every 10 years. Maintenance of vaccination coverage should continue even in countries now free of infection and is essential for travel to parts of the world where polio has not yet been eradicated.

The long-term aim of prevention should be to raise standards of hygiene with the provision of water supplies and sanitation, but as mentioned above, this must proceed at the same time as an adequate vaccination programme.

Treatment There is no specific treatment for the acute stage, but rest and the avoidance of physical activity are beneficial. Specific supportive measures can be given to those with disabilities.

Surveillance developed for poliomyelitis eradication looks for cases of acute flaccid paralysis (AFP) in children under 15 years of age. These are investigated by stool examination, inquiry and search for other cases in the area. Remedial measures are carried out around the case, vaccinating all contacts.

8.11 *Enterobius* (Pin Worm)

Organism A nematode worm *Enterobius vermicularis.*

Clinical features The main symptom is intense pruritis ani. Heavy infections can rarely cause appendicitis or salpingitis in the female.

Transmission The gravid female migrates out of the anus at night to lay her eggs on the perianal skin before dying. This activity of the female causes the patient to scratch so that eggs are transferred to the fingers where they are swallowed or passed on to someone else. Eggs are thrown into the air such as during bed making or sweeping and so are often inhaled. Masses of eggs are liberated on each occasion so that infection of family groups, dormitories of school children, etc. occur at the same time.

Diagnosis Eggs can be collected from the perianal skin by using an adhesive tape slide. This is examined directly by microscope, the characteristic oval egg with flattened side measuring 50–60 μm by 20–30 μm (Fig. 9.1) being seen.

Incubation period 2–6 weeks.

Period of communicability As long as adult female worms discharge eggs until 2 weeks after treatment.

Occurrence and distribution This very common infection is more prevalent in the temperate than tropical regions of the world, favouring conditions where poor hygiene prevails.

Control and prevention Good personal hygiene, particularly cutting of finger nails and washing hands, is the means of control. Bedding and underclothes need to be washed frequently at the same time as treatment is given.

Treatment is with piperazine 65 mg/kg for 7 days, pyrantel pamoate in a single dose of 10 mg/kg (maximum 1 g), repeated after 2 weeks, or albendazole or mebendazole 100 mg single dose repeated after 2 weeks. It is preferable to treat everyone in the group at the same time to break the transmission cycle.

Surveillance Regular checks in an institutional situation, especially on individuals with repeat infections will prevent spread throughout the establishment.

9

Food-borne Diseases

The faecal–oral mechanism for transfer of infection often includes food as a mechanism of infection, but in addition, there are other diseases that are only transmitted by food. These can infect foods in general, such as with food poisoning, or be very specific in a particular food, such as certain helminth infections. As the method of infection is very specific so are its methods of control, which include food hygiene, the proper cooking of foods and sanitary methods to prevent the food from being contaminated.

9.1 Food Poisoning

9.1.1 Food poisoning due to bacteria

Organism Food poisoning can either be due to bacteria, viruses, organic or inorganic poisons (Table 9.1). The most common poisoning is that produced by bacteria. The main types of bacterial food poisoning are due to *Salmonella*, *Staphylococcus* or *Clostridia*.

Clinical features Due to the similarity of presentation, it is more convenient to consider them as a group, rather than individually. Onset is sudden with fever, generally vomiting and/or diarrhoea in a family or group of persons who have shared the same meal. Sometimes, a sub-normal temperature or lowered blood pressure is the presenting symptom. The incubation period is very short and sufficiently precise for the type of food poisoning to be suspected by the length of time since the food item was eaten.

Incubation period With staphylococcal food poisoning, it is between 1 and 6 h; *Salmonella* over 6 h, usually 12–36 h, and for *Clostridia*, 12–24 h or several days. Less commonly, food poisoning can be due to *Bacillus cereus* (1–12 h) and *Vibrio parahaemolyticus* (12–48 h).

Transmission is through the consumption of food contaminated with the bacteria or its toxins. Infection can sometimes result from a contaminated water supply and via milk that has not been pasteurized. *Salmonella* generally infects the food in the living state, such as cattle, poultry or eggs, but unhygienic practice in the slaughtering of animals or preparation of foodstuffs can also be responsible. The bacteria are killed by proper cooking and no toxins are produced; so examination of the meal should reveal an improperly cooked source.

Staphylococcal food poisoning results from toxin produced by the bacteria so the

© R. Webber 2005. *Communicable Disease Epidemiology and Control*, 2nd edition (Roger Webber)

Table 9.1. Food poisoning.

Agent	Period of onset (h)	Symptoms	Types of food
Bacterial food poisoning			
Staphylococcal	1–6	Sudden, vomiting more than diarrhoea	Stored food
B. cereus	1–12		
Salmonella	12–36	Vomiting, diarrhoea and fever	Improperly cooked meat, eggs and milk produce
C. perfringens	9–24	Abdominal cramps, diarrhoea, shock	Cooked meat, especially pig
C. botulinum	9–24	Ptosis, dry mouth, paralysis	Preserved foods
V. parahaemolyticus	12–48	Abdominal pain, diarrhoea and fever	Undercooked or raw fish
Fish poisoning			
Ciguatera	1–30	Parathesiae, malaise, sweating, diarrhoea and vomiting	Barracudas, snappers, sea bass, groupers
Scombroid	1–12	Burning sensation, nausea, vomiting	Tuna, mackerel, salmon or cheeses
Tetraodontoxins	0.5–3	Hypersalivation, vomiting, parasthesiae, vertigo, pains	Puffer fish
Shellfish, paralytic	0.5–3	Parasthesiae and paralysis	Clams and mussels
Shellfish, diarrhetic	0.5–3	Diarrhoea and vomiting	Clams, scallops, etc.
Plant foods			
Akee (*Blighia sapida*)	2–3	Vomiting, convulsions, death	Unripe fruit
Cassava (Cyanide)	Hours	Vomiting, diarrhoea, abdominal pain, headache, coma	Improperly processed root
Contaminants			
Triorthocresyl-phosphate	Days	Neuropathy	Cooking oil

food may be adequately cooked and no bacteria isolated from the suspected food source. It is commonly transmitted by food handlers with an infected lesion or unhygienic habits, such as transferring bacteria from the nose. *V. parahaemolyticus* is particularly associated with seafood or food that has been washed with contaminated seawater.

Clostridia food poisoning can be caused by several types of organisms. *C. botulinum* infection results in a severe disease, botulism, which is characteristic of home-preserved foods (see further Section 18.5). *C. perfringens* generally produces a mild disease of short duration, but in New Guinea and the Western Pacific Islands, it is responsible for enteritis necroticans or pigbel, in which there is an acute necrosis of the small and large intestines with a high fatality rate. This is associated with feasting, generally of pig meat, but also from other animals such as cattle. Children, particularly boys, are mainly affected. The disease is probably accentuated by a protease inhibitor contained in sweet potato, preventing breakdown of the toxin.

Clostridia have resistant spores, which can remain in the soil for long periods, and their contamination of partly cooked and re-heated food allows multiplication and production of the toxin.

There is often a seasonality of food poisoning, *Salmonella* in the summer months and *C. jejuni* in spring and autumn. *C. perfringens* occurs throughout the year.

Diagnosis and investigation of the outbreak The epidemiologist is concerned with diagnosing the cause of the outbreak and, therefore, a search is made to discover a common food that has been eaten by all the persons who have succumbed to the illness. The foodstuff is likely to be one particular ingredient of the meal, rather than the whole meal and samples should be taken for culture. If nothing is grown, this does not rule out a *Staphylococcal* or *Clostridia* food poisoning cause and finer questioning on foodstuffs consumed might be the only way to discover the offending item. (See Section 2.2.5 on how to analyse the relative importance of different foods eaten.)

Period of communicability In *Salmonella* infection, organisms can be excreted for up to 1 year although it is generally just for a period of weeks.

Occurrence and distribution Food poisoning is found worldwide with large outbreaks associated with gatherings of people, such as celebrations and weddings. Many small outbreaks and those occurring in the home go unreported unless individuals are ill enough to be hospitalized. Sometimes a batch of food is infected and distributed to several outlets, so as soon as the food-poisoned item is discovered, all of it must be traced and destroyed.

Control and prevention All suspect food must be destroyed and if it is part of a common foodstuff, then all must be traced and disposed of. The source of contamination, such as an abattoir, must be looked for and control measures implemented. Prevention is by proper cooking of food and personal hygiene. Where repeated attacks occur, a search for a carrier should be made amongst food handlers. Anyone with a septic or discharging sore should be banned from handling and preparing food.

Food must be stored, prepared and cooked properly (Section 3.3.2). Establishments that prepare food, such as restaurants and hotels, should be regularly inspected and certified.

Treatment The treatment of cases of food poisoning is supportive with fluids and electrolytes (either orally or intravenous).

Surveillance Food handlers should be checked by supervisors and food establishments visited on a regular basis by health inspectors.

9.1.2 Fish poisoning

Organism Fish poisoning is a specific form of food poisoning caused by toxins present in the fish or shellfish when they are caught or which develop due to partial decomposition taking place if they are not eaten straight away or refrigerated. Ciguatera toxin is produced by the dinoflagellate *Gambierdiscus toxicus*, which is present in algal blooms, often called red tides, while shellfish poisoning can de due to the dinoflagellates *Gonyaulux*, *Gymnodinium*, *Dinophysis* or *Alexandrium*.

Clinical features Symptoms are normally mild with paraesthesia (tingling and burning sensations or pain and weakness), malaise, sweating, diarrhoea and vomiting, but in the young or those who have consumed a large quantity of poison, the condition is more serious. Respiratory and motor paralysis can occur, often resulting in fatalities. Neurological symptoms can persist for some time after the original illness.

Transmission is through eating fish that has not been refrigerated or already contains the toxin. At certain times of the year and when hurricanes, seismic shocks or similar disturbances of the coral reef occur, an algal growth containing the dinoflagellate develops. Fish feed on the algal bloom, or it is inadvertently filtered by shellfish, and their flesh becomes poisoned. Fish that are normally quite edible, such as barracuda, snappers, sea bass and groupers, become poisonous at these periods. The commonest poison is ciguatoxin, which is not destroyed by cooking.

Incubation period 0.5–3 h after eating fish or shellfish.

Period of communicability Not transmitted from person-to-person.

Occurrence and distribution Fish poisoning is commonly found amongst island communities or coastal people in which fish is a major item of diet. It is an important problem in Pacific Islands, the Caribbean, Southeast Asia and Australia.

Control and prevention All freshly caught fish should be gutted and refrigerated as soon as caught, unless cooked and eaten straight away. Red tides (algal blooms) occur as a result of some disturbance of coral reefs, such as hurricanes, earthquakes and El Niño climatic disturbances. Algal blooms and hence fish poisoning are related to the surface temperature. As a result, where this is abnormally increased during an El Niño event, there is an increase in fish poisoning and the converse when the temperature is less than expected.

Treatment There is no specific treatment; supportive therapy being given.

Surveillance When red tides are reported, eating reef fish should be avoided.

9.1.3 Food poisoning due to organic or inorganic toxins

More generalized outbreaks involving large numbers of people not necessarily associated with each other and presenting with bizarre symptoms, such as paralysis, may be caused by an organic or inorganic poison contaminating the food. Examples are cyanide poisoning from poorly processed bitter cassava, eating unripe akees (a fruit popular in the Caribbean) or contaminants in cooking oil.

Although very localized, such outbreaks can be serious with considerable morbidity and sometimes mortality, necessitating the identification of the source as a matter of urgency and banning them from human consumption.

9.2 *Campylobacter* Enteritis

Organism *Campylobacter jejuni.*

Clinical features An acute diarrhoeal disease with abdominal pain, malaise, fever and vomiting. It is often self-limiting within 4–7 days, but in severe cases, pus and blood are found in the stools, with a presentation similar to bacillary dysentery. With its association with a food source, it is often thought to be a case of food poisoning until the organism is identified. *Campylobacter* enteritis is an important cause of traveller's diarrhoea.

Diagnosis The organism can be isolated from the stools using selective media. A preliminary diagnosis can be made by examining a specimen of stool with phase-contrast (dark-ground) microscopy, where an organism similar to a cholera vibrio will be seen. The presence of faecal material and absence of cholera-like symptoms will differentiate it from cholera.

Transmission Domestic animals including poultry, pigs, cattle, sheep, cats and dogs are reservoirs of the organism and their consumption or human's close association with them is responsible for much of the transmission. Most infections are due to faecal contamination by animals or birds, especially of unpasteurized milk and unchlorinated water. Water can be contaminated by bird droppings in which the organism is able to survive for several months at a temperature below 15°C. Many infections are transmitted by pets, especially puppies and person-to-person transmission can occur in a similar way.

Incubation period 1–10 days. The larger the dose of organisms ingested, the shorter the incubation period.

Period of communicability 2–7 weeks, but person-to-person transmission is uncommon.

Occurrence and distribution Children under 2 years of age are most commonly infected in developing countries, immunity developing to further infection in those over this age. There is a worldwide distribution with many of the cases in developing countries not being identified. There has been a progressive increase in *Campylobacter* for no explainable reason. It is one of the commonest causes of gastroenteritis (Section 8.1).

Control and prevention Proper cooking of foodstuffs and control of pets are the main preventive methods. Wherever possible, water should be chlorinated and milk pasteurized.

Treatment Oral rehydration.

Surveillance and investigation An outbreak of *Campylobacter* should be investigated in the same way as a food-poisoning outbreak and remedial measures taken around the source.

9.3 The Intestinal Fluke (*Fasciolopsis*)

Organism The large human fluke *Fasciolopsis buski*.

Clinical features The adult worm lives in the small intestines and produces damage by inflammatory reaction at the site of attach-

ment. This sometimes leads to abscess and haemorrhage, but as well as these local effects, the parasite produces toxins. These can lead to oedema, weakness and prostration, ending fatally in the debilitated child.

Diagnosis is made by finding the egg in faeces, a giant among parasites (Fig. 9.1). The egg is indistinguishable from *Fasciola hepatica* (see Section 9.4).

Transmission The eggs are passed in faeces either directly into water or are washed there following rains, where they hatch and liberate a miracidium, which must find a snail of the genus *Segmentina*. Developing first into a sporocyst, then a redia, numerous cercaria are produced. On leaving the snail, the cercaria encyst on water plants that are subsequently eaten raw by humans (Fig. 9.2). These plants include the water calthrop (*Trapa* sp.), the water chestnut (*Eliocharis tuberosa*) and the water bamboo (*Zizania aquatica*). Beds of these water plants are often grown in ponds fertilized by human sewage, providing considerable opportunity for transmission. Even if the foods are subsequently cooked, they are often first peeled with the teeth so that cercariae are still swallowed.

A reservoir of infection is maintained in pigs, sheep, cattle and other domestic herbivores. Infection is particularly high in pig-rearing areas. Humans also act as reservoirs.

Incubation period 2–3 months.

Period of communicability is 12 months, but animals act as a permanent reservoir.

Occurrence and distribution East Asia, especially China, Taiwan, Thailand, Borneo and Malaysia, in some 15 million people.

Control and prevention is by the proper preparation and cooking of water plants. Much can be done to reduce transmission by regulating the use of human faeces as a fertilizer. Domestic animals should be kept away from water plant cultivation ponds.

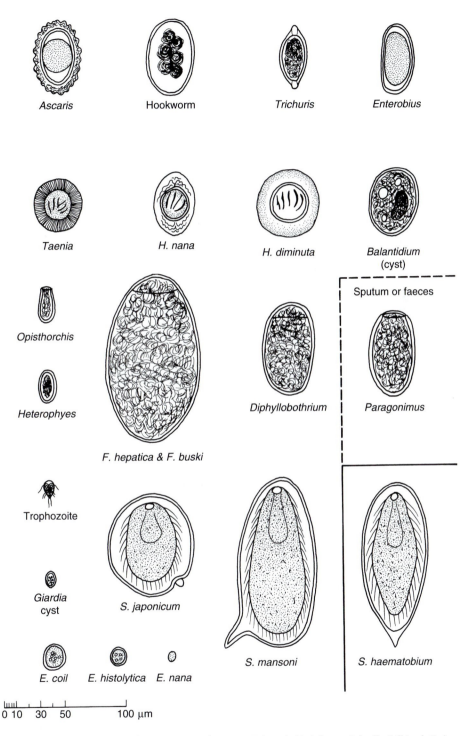

Fig. 9.1. Parasite eggs found in faeces, urine and sputum. *E. (nana), Endolimax; E. (coli), E. (histolytica), Entamoeba; F. (hepatica), Fasciola; F. (buski), Fasciolopsis; H. (diminuta), H. (nana), Hymenolepis; S. (haematobium), S. (japonicum), S. (mansoni), Schistosoma.*

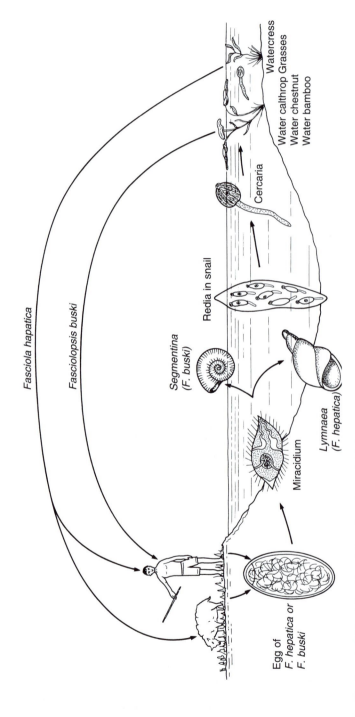

Fig. 9.2.   The intestinal (*Fasciolopsis*) and sheep liver (*Fasciola*) flukes.

Treatment is with praziquantel 25 mg/kg three times a day for 1–2 days.

Surveillance When a case is diagnosed, other members of the family should be investigated and a common food source looked for.

9.4 The Sheep Liver Fluke (*Fasciola hepatica*)

Organism The sheep liver fluke *Fasciola hepatica*. Less commonly *F. gigantica*.

Clinical features The parasite has a predilection for the liver, piercing the gut wall and migrating through the liver substance to lie in the biliary passages. This migration and residence in the liver causes extensive damage, leading to fibrosis and cirrhosis.

Diagnosis is made by finding the very large egg in the stool, which is almost identical to that of *Fasciolopsis* (Fig. 9.1).

Transmission The life cycle is similar to *Fasciolopsis* in that eggs passed in the faeces liberate a miracidium on contact with water. The miracidium searches for and invades snails of the genus *Lymnaea*. After passing through sporocyst and redia stages, the cercaria encyst on grass or water plants (e.g. water cress). The normal life cycle is in sheep, humans becoming incidentally infected when contaminated water plants are eaten (Fig. 9.2). Cattle and goats also act as reservoirs.

Incubation period Probably 2–3 months.

Period of communicability Not transmitted from person-to-person.

Occurrence and distribution Worldwide distribution in sheep-rearing areas, especially the Andean highlands of Bolivia, Ecuador and Peru, the Nile delta region of Egypt and northern Iran. *F. gigantica* is found in Africa and the Western Pacific; 2.5 million are probably infected in the world, with up to 60% of the population in highly endemic areas.

Control and prevention In known endemic areas, careful control is required in the growing and consumption of water plants such as cress. Animal faeces should not be used to fertilize water plants. The close association of humans and sheep or other domestic animals greatly increases the opportunity for infection.

Treatment Triclabendazole at 10 mg/kg single dose, which can be repeated after 12 h.

Surveillance Sheep should be examined at regular intervals and treated.

9.5 The Fish-transmitted Liver Flukes

Organism The trematode fluke *Opisthorchis sinensis* (previously called *Clonorchis*).

Clinical features The adult fluke lives in the branches of the bile duct resulting in trauma and inflammation. Dilation of the biliary system causes a distortion of the liver architecture, which can lead to biliary stasis, hepatic engorgement, fatty infiltration and finally cirrhosis. *O. sinensis* is a risk factor for cholangiocarcinoma. Migration of the flukes up the pancreatic duct can damage the pancreas leading to recurrent pancreatitis.

Diagnosis The small operculated egg is found on faecal examination (Fig. 9.1).

Transmission Humans are infected by eating raw fish, which includes pickled, smoked or undercooked fish. Eggs passed in the faeces develop into miracidia, which are swallowed by snails of the genus *Bulimus*, *Bithynia* or *Parafossarulus*. These pass through the sporocyst and redia stages in the snail and produce free-swimming cercaria. Seeking out a suitable fish, cercaria penetrate between the scales and encyst in the flesh. The parasite also attacks dogs, cats, rats and pigs, which form reservoirs of infection (Fig. 9.3).

Incubation period Approximately 4 weeks.

Period of communicability Eggs may be passed for as long as 30 years, but reservoir animals are also an important source of human infection.

Occurrence and distribution Distribution is very similar to *Fasciolopsis*, being found in China, Japan, Korea, Taiwan, Thailand,

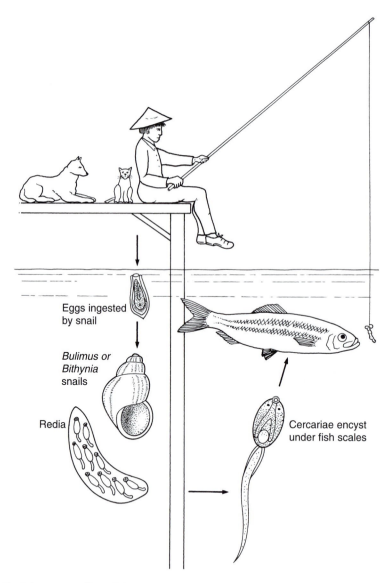

Eggs ingested
by snail

*Bulimus or
Bithynia*
snails

Redia

Cercariae encyst
under fish scales

Fig. 9.3. The fish-transmitted liver flukes, *Opisthorchis sinensis, O. felineus, O. viverrini, H. heterophyes* and *M. yokogawai.*

Laos, Cambodia and Vietnam (lower Mekong valley). Some 30 million people suffer from the disease.

Control and prevention Control is by the proper cooking of fish. Members of the carp family (*Cyprinidae*), the so-called 'milk fish', are eaten raw as a delicacy. They are grown in fish farms as part of a system of aquaculture, fertilized by human faeces. Regulation of this practice is required to reduce this unpleasant infection. Other foods, such as fish paste often added to food after it has been cooked to improve the taste, are made from raw fish and are a potent source of infection.

Treatment Treatment is with praziquantel 25 mg/kg three times a day for 1–2 days.

Surveillance When a case is identified, search should be made for the culprit food source.

There are a number of less common trematodes that have the same life cycle as *O. sinensis* (Fig. 9.3). *O. viverrini* is found in Thailand and Laos where raw fish paste is a favourite food additive. *O. felineus* occurs in Central and Eastern Europe, similarly causing disease of the liver. As suggested by its name, it is mainly a disease of cats, but humans can become infected. *Heterophyes heterophyes* and *Metagonimus yokogawai*, found in Asia and the Far East, do not attack the liver, but remain in the intestines. The eggs of all of these flukes are very similar (Fig. 9.1).

9.6 The Lung Fluke

Organism Unique amongst all the helminths, the trematode *Paragonimus westermani* selectively inhabits the lung.

Clinical features Foreign body reaction to the parasite in the lung results in fibrosis, compensatory dilation and abscess formation. Haemoptysis is often an important feature, mimicking tuberculosis. Symptoms include cough and chest pain. If the parasite migrates to a site other than the lung, it can cause CNS, liver, intestinal, genitourinary or subcutaneous disease.

Diagnosis is by finding eggs in the sputum, or if swallowed, in the faeces (Fig. 9.1). Any case of haemoptysis without other signs of tuberculosis should have a sputum examination, on which an acid-fast bacilli (AFB) stain has not been used, as this destroys the eggs.

Transmission The egg on reaching water softens and a miracidium frees itself from the egg capsule and searches for a snail of the genus *Semisulcospira*. Passing through the sporocyst and redia stages, the cercaria encysts in the gills and muscles of freshwater crabs and crayfish. Humans are infected by eating uncooked, salted or pickled freshwater crab (*Eriocheir* and *Potamon*) or crayfish (*Cambaroides*), while an animal reservoir (mainly cats and dogs) helps to maintain the disease. The liberated metacercaria pass through the intestinal wall and penetrate the diaphragm to enter the lung. Adults develop in the lungs to produce eggs, which are liberated into the sputum. Occasionally they find their way to unusual sites, the brain being particularly serious (Fig. 9.4).

Incubation period 6–10 weeks.

Period of communicability Up to 20 years.

Occurrence and distribution *P. westermani* disease is found mainly in China, other parts of Asia, Africa and the Americas. Closely related species are *P. africanus* and *P. uterobilateralis* in West Africa, *P. pulmonalis* in Japan, Korea and Taiwan, *P. philippinensis* in the Philippines, *P. heterotremus* in Thailand and Laos, *P. kellicotti*, *P. caliensis* and *P. mexicanus* in Central and South America. In all, it has been calculated that some 30 million people suffer from the lung fluke.

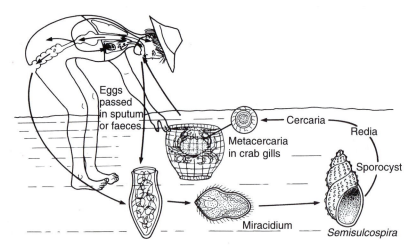

Fig. 9.4. The lung fluke – *Paragonimus westermani.*

Control and prevention Control is most effectively achieved by ensuring that all crab and crayfish meat is properly cooked. Much can be achieved by teaching people about the life cycle of this and other trematode infections, stressing that all food must be cooked and faeces disposed of properly. Spitting should be outlawed.

Treatment is by praziquantel 25 mg/kg three times a day for 2 consecutive days. Alternatively, triclabendazole 10 mg/kg, repeated in 12 h, can be used.

Surveillance It is a focal disease so that identifying a case will often lead to a foci of infection and preventive action can then be instituted.

9.7 The Fish Tapeworm

Organism The large tapeworm *Diphyllobothrium latum.*

Clinical features The presence of such a large worm (10 m or more) in the intestines can consume a considerable quantity of nutrients, but the main pathology is due to its selective absorption of vitamin B_{12}, resulting in a megaloblastic anaemia in the host.

Diagnosis is made by finding the egg in the faeces (Fig. 9.1). Sometimes, worm segments (proglotids) are also passed.

Transmission The adult worm is found in the intestines of humans, dogs, cats, foxes and bears, and a number of other mammalian hosts. Eggs are passed in the faeces, which on contact with water liberate a coracidium, which is ingested by a copepod (*Cyclops* and *Diaptomus*). The coracidium develops in the copepod to a larval form, a procercoid, which when eaten by a freshwater fish finds its way into the muscles and develops into a plerocercoid. When the raw or improperly cooked fish is eaten, the liberated plerocercoid attaches itself to the intestinal wall and develops into an adult tapeworm (Fig. 9.5).

Incubation period 3–6 weeks.

Period of communicability Humans can continue to liberate eggs into the environment for many years, but most of the infective source is from the animal reservoir.

Occurrence and distribution The parasite is found in the cooler parts of the world, around lakes of Europe, America, China and Japan. It is also found in indigenous tribes living in the Arctic and sub-Arctic

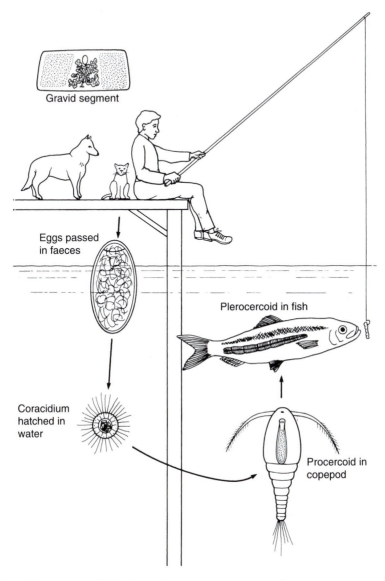

Fig. 9.5. The fish tape worm – *Diphyllobothrium latum*.

regions. It is a disease of some 13 million people.

Control and prevention Control is by ensuring that fish are properly cooked. Deep-freezing fish will also kill the parasite. Sanitation will decrease the human cycle and animal faeces should be prevented from entering water sources.

Treatment Niclosamide as a single dose of 2 g or praziquantel as a single dose of 5–10 mg/kg.

9.8 The Beef and Pork Tapeworms

Organism *Taenia saginata*, the beef tapeworm and *T. solium* the pork tapeworm.

Clinical features The adult worm of both species can live in the intestines producing little pathology, being diagnosed often by accident. It does, however, share the food supply of its host so that when intake is inadequate, debility can occur. The serious problems are due to the *Cysticercus cellulosae* (from *T. solium*). The cysts die and calcify, those in the brain being a common cause of epilepsy or mental disorder.

Diagnosis is made by finding the proglottids (worm segments) in the faeces, the patients often making their own diagnosis. It is very important to distinguish between *T. saginata* and *T. solium* in view of the danger of inducing cysticercosis. *T. saginata* has 18–30 compound branches of the uterus on each side whereas *T. solium* has only 8–12 (Fig. 9.6).

Transmission The adult worm lives in the small intestine of man and as it matures, gravid segments break off and are passed in the faeces. Cattle or pigs inadvertently eat the proglottids (mature segments) or the discharged eggs contaminate the pasture. Alternatively, the animal can become infected by drinking water polluted by sewage. It has

also been found that birds feeding on sewage can carry eggs for long distances and then deposit them on pasture land. Flies might have a place in transmission. The eggs develop into cysticerci in the muscles, favouring the jaw, heart, diaphragm, shoulder and oesophagus. Humans acquire the disease by eating improperly cooked beef or pork containing the cysticercus.

Both the beef tapeworm (*T. saginata*) and the pork tapeworm (*T. solium*) have the same life cycle except that the intermediate stage, the cysticercus of *T. solium*, can also occur in humans. This happens by swallowing eggs directly, either by autoinfection, from eggs in food or water or through sewage contamination. Also any gastric disturbance that might cause the regurgitation of proglottids into the stomach (including improper treatment) can lead to the liberation of vast quantities of eggs, with the result that cysticerci are produced anywhere in the body including the brain, orbit and muscle.

Incubation period 8–14 weeks.

Period of communicability Adult worms can live for as long as 30 years, their eggs

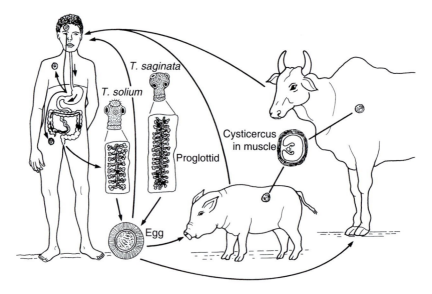

Fig. 9.6. The tape worms – *Taenia solium* and *T. saginata*.

contaminating the environment and in *T. solium* a direct threat to any other person.

Occurrence and distribution These are the commonest and most cosmopolitan of all the tapeworms, with a worldwide distribution in beef- and pork-eating areas, especially in the tropical belt and Eastern Europe. Over 60 million people are thought to be infected.

These two worms are found in areas of beef and pork eating where there is a ready transmission cycle in operation. Finding the worm in humans means that it is probably reasonably common in that area, whereas other places where beef and pork eating are just as much part of the usual diet, they are not found. *T. saginata* is increasing in Europe probably because of human sewage contamination of animal drinking water. *T. solium* is common in Mexico, Chile, Africa, India, Indonesia and Russia.

Control and prevention The main means of control is the proper cooking of meat. The underdone steak or joint of meat where internal temperatures are not high enough to kill the cysticercus are common ways in which transmission can still take place despite cooking. Proper control of slaughter-ing in official abattoirs, with meat inspection, can prevent the dissemination of infected meat. Condemned carcasses must be burnt.

Treatment for both worms is with niclosamide 2 g as a single dose. Alternatively, praziquantel as a single dose of 5–10 mg/kg can be given. Praziquantel at a dose of 50 mg/kg for 15 days can be used for cerebral cysticercosis in conjunction with corticosteroids, as an in-patient.

Surveillance Where a localized cycle of infection is occurring, investigation may reveal a sewage leak or other source of contamination that could easily be rectified.

9.9 Trichinosis

Organism *Trichinella spiralis* (Fig. 9.7), *T. nelsoni, T. nativa, T. britovi* and *T. pseudospiralis,* nematode worms.

Clinical features The severity of the disease depends upon the dose of larvae that have encysted in the tissues. During the second week of infection, there is headache, insomnia, pain, dyspnoea and pyrexia with

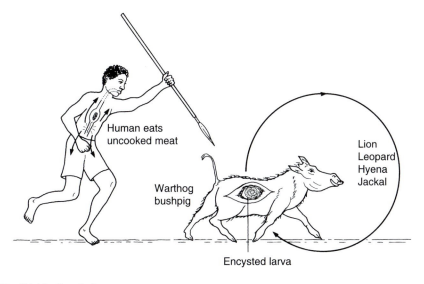

Human eats uncooked meat

Warthog bushpig

Lion Leopard Hyena Jackal

Encysted larva

Fig. 9.7.   *Trichinella spiralis.*

oedema of the orbit and eosinophilia. If the symptoms are sufficiently severe, death can result; otherwise, once the attack is over, the cysts cause no further trouble, gradually die and calcify.

Diagnosis is made by muscle biopsy of the deltoid or thigh muscles where the encysted larvae are found.

Transmission The life cycle is a simple one, encysted larvae in the muscles are eaten by another animal and the liberated larva develops into an adult to produce numerous new larvae, which are then carried to all parts of the body in the circulation. Only the larvae that reach striated muscle survive, the diaphragm, tongue, throat, eye and thorax being the favoured sites.

In the different climatic zones of the world where different groups of animals live off each other, several transmission cycles have evolved. In Africa, the warthog and the bushpig form the vital link in the cycle. Being the favoured prey of lions and leopards, these carnivores, with the hyenas and jackals that finish off the remains, become infected. The general scavenging nature of the warthog and pig inadvertently eating the remains of dead animals allows the cycle to be completed. Humans come in as intruders, a dead end to the cycle when they feast on a recently killed bushpig.

In Europe and Asia, the rat is the reservoir of infection, but by its scavenging nature, the pig acquires infection and when cooked on a spit or otherwise eaten in an improperly cooked way, humans become infected. Sausages made from food scraps or hamburgers contaminated with bits of pork can be potent sources. In the Arctic, the seal and polar bear are involved in the transmission cycle; the latter acquires very high levels of infection. The death of some Arctic explorers has been attributed to killing and eating polar bears infected with trichinosis.

Incubation period 8–15 days.

Period of communicability Not transmitted from person-to-person, but once infected animals are infectious, probably for the rest of their life due to repeated doses of infecting nematodes.

Occurrence and distribution Approximately 40 million people of the world's population are affected although trichinosis commonly occurs as a localized outbreak with a group of people all contracting the disease at the same time. A classic example is for a wild pig to be killed and cooked over a fire by turning it on a spit. By this means, only the outside meat is well cooked and inside, the temperature has not been sufficient to kill the larvae. Outbreaks in the industrialized countries and in the urban areas of developing countries are commonly caused by eating sausages, especially of the salami type.

Control and prevention All meat for human consumption should be inspected. The calcified cysts can be detected with the naked eye and by cutting into the muscle. Where an outbreak occurs, such as with eating sausages, the source should be investigated and food hygiene practices enforced.

All meat must be properly cooked until there is no redness in any part of the joint. Cooking slowly for a long time is preferable to cooking quickly or on an open fire where the outside gets overcooked while the inside remains almost raw. Deep freezing of meat for 20 days or irradiation can kill the cysts.

Treatment is symptomatic with steroids. Mebendazole or albendazole should also be given for 4 days.

Surveillance Where an outbreak occurs, the participants at the feast will all start having symptoms at much the same time. By counting back 2 weeks from these cases, the source of infection can be localized.

9.10 Other Infections Transmitted by Food

A number of other infections are also transmitted by food although their principal method of transmission is by other means. Any of the faecal–oral diseases covered in Chapter 8 can be transmitted this way – bacillary dysentery, typhoid, hepatitis A, *Giardia* and El Tor type cholera being spread by eating salad vegetables, raw fish or other food. The parasitic worms transmitted by soil contact, *Trichuris*, *Ascaris*, *Strongyloides* and the hookworms (Chapter 10) can also be transmitted by food, especially that grown in soil such as root crops and vegetables. Hydatid disease (Section 17.2) and *Toxoplasma* (Section 17.5) can be acquired through food. Brucellosis (Section 17.6) is often transmitted in goat's milk or cheese made from it, while anthrax (Section 17.7) can rarely be caught by eating the meat of a cow that has died from the disease.

10

Diseases of Soil Contact

_____

The soil can be a source of infection for several diseases particularly those caused by nematodes and the bacterial infection, tetanus. Transmission can either be direct from contamination with the soil as with tetanus bacilli, by swallowing nematode eggs, or the larvae can penetrate the skin when it comes into contact with the soil. Developmental stages often take place in the soil, which becomes a necessary environment for the life cycle. The promotion of personal hygiene and preventing contamination of soil through sanitation are the main methods of control for the nematode infections and vaccination for tetanus.

Since there is a common mode of transmission for the three main nematode infections (*Trichuris, Ascaris* and the hookworms), they nearly always go together. As a result, if the person is infected with one nematode, he or she is likely to have all three infections. It is this combined effect that causes considerable morbidity in children in developing countries and if one looks again at Table 1.1, it will be noticed that having all three infections bring their importance in terms of DALYs to the 12th position.

10.1 *Trichuris* (Whip Worm)

Organism The nematode *Trichuris trichiura*, which has a characteristic egg (elongated and with a knob at each end) when seen in faecal specimens (see Fig. 9.1).

Clinical features A large number of people carry this infection quite asymptomatically, but it has been realized that the debilitating effect of this infection, especially in children in developing countries, can be quite considerable. This is especially the case when trichuriasis is associated with other common infections, the combined effect leading to much ill health. When there are over 16,000 eggs/g of faeces, a chronic bloody diarrhoea, anaemia, rectal prolapse and occasionally, appendicitis can result. These infections tend to occur when the child eats earth (pica), which can be a result of iron deficiency. Heavy infections are probably potentiated by nutritional deficiencies, especially of zinc.

Diagnosis The characteristic egg is easily seen in a fresh faecal specimen (Fig. 9.1).

Transmission The egg develops in the soil and when swallowed directly or as a contaminant of food, it changes into an adult in the caecum. Eggs are most commonly carried on the fingers or swallowed when the fingers are licked. The soil is readily contaminated from indiscriminate defecation, especially where the faeces are not buried or a latrine used. Villages often have traditional places for defecation, thereby increasing the potential for infection than when such customary places are not the rule.

Incubation period It takes 2–3 months for eggs to be found in the faeces after eggs are first swallowed, with symptoms occurring about 1 month after ingestion.

Period of communicability Persons can remain infected for several years if not treated, continually contaminating the environment if they have poor defecating practices.

Occurrence and distribution It is a very common parasite (perhaps 540 million people are infected) and causes far more disability than previously thought to be the case (see Table 1.1). Most of the infection with debilitating consequences occurs in developing countries, but the parasite is found worldwide.

Control and prevention Washing hands before having food and the careful preparation of food are the main methods of control. Vegetables and root crops, in particular, must be washed carefully to remove all earth. Parents should discourage their children from eating earth and have anaemia treated with iron supplementation. Proper sanitation should be installed to prevent soil contamination.

Treatment is with mebendazole or albendazole. (See under hookworm for dosage.)

Surveillance Routine stool investigation of children admitted to hospital will show a number of nematode infections.

10.2 *Ascaris*

Organism The nematode worm *Ascaris lumbricoides*.

Clinical features The fertile egg, when swallowed, hatches in the stomach and the larva penetrates the intestinal mucosa to enter the blood stream, passing through the venous and pulmonary circulations to the lungs where it breaks through the alveolar wall to emerge in the bronchioles. Migrating up to a main bronchus, it ascends the trachea and is swallowed back into the gastro-intestinal tract. By the time it reaches the intestines, it has developed into an adult, the fertilized female laying eggs into the excrement (Fig. 10.1). This common intestinal parasite can occur in considerable numbers without causing any symptoms and is often found when a routine stool examination is performed. When the larvae pass through the lungs, pneumonitis and possible haemoptysis can occur, otherwise the sheer number of worms can cause intestinal obstruction or blocking of vital structures, such as the common bile duct. Where nutrition is marginal, the loss of nutrient can be sufficient to tip a child into malnutrition. It has been calculated that 25 worms can produce a loss of 4 g protein daily from a diet containing 40–50 g protein. Deficiency of vitamins A and C can also occur. Academic performance in school decreases with heavy *Ascaris* infections.

Diagnosis Direct smear examination of the stool is sufficient for diagnosis (Fig. 9.1). The egg has a strong outer coat, which is stained brown from bile pigments, thus differentiating it from hookworm eggs, which are of a similar size.

Transmission The eggs are not infective until they have undergone development in the soil for 1–2 weeks. They require warmth and moisture to develop and will remain viable in the soil for a considerable period of time awaiting the right conditions. The infective larva goes through stages of

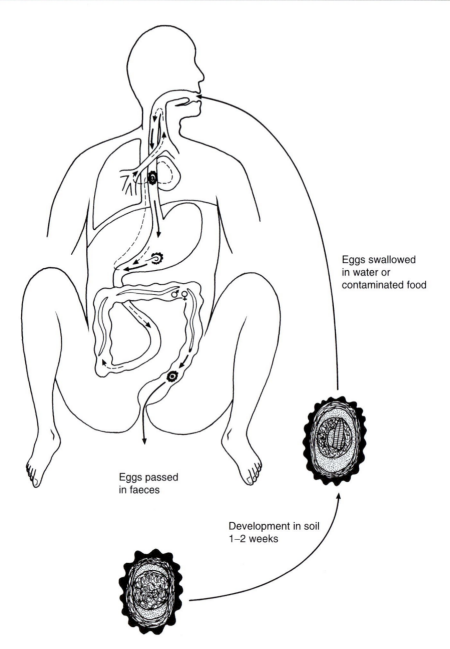

Fig. 10.1. *Ascaris lumbricoides* life cycle.

development within the egg casing and if swallowed, infection occurs. Eggs are normally swallowed in polluted water, on vegetables that have been washed with polluted water or by swallowing earth directly. Eggs are passed during indiscriminate defecation.

Incubation period 10–20 days

Period of communicability From 2 months after infection up until about 1 year.

Occurrence and distribution *Ascaris* is a very common nematode infection found in all parts of the world and in all strata of the society (1000 million people are estimated to be infected). Children aged 3–7 years have the highest prevalence.

Control and prevention is with personal hygiene, food hygiene and proper sanitary facilities. The egg is extremely resistant, being unaffected by cold, drying and disinfectants. A temperature of 43°C or higher is required to kill them; therefore, any composting process using human excreta must maintain this temperature for at least 1 month (Fig. 1.2).

Treatment is with pyrantel pamoate or mebendazole. (See under hookworms for dosage.)

Surveillance As with *Trichuris* infection, it is worth doing routine stool examination on children admitted to hospital as any lessening of the worm burden will improve health.

10.3 Hookworms

Organism *Ancylostoma duodenale* and *Necator americanus* cause the two common hookworm infections of humans.

Clinical features The infective (filariform) larvae directly penetrate the skin and migrate to a blood vessel or lymphatic vessel from where they are carried in the circulation to the lungs. In the lungs, they break out of the alveoli, find their way up the trachea and enter the gastro-intestinal tract. The adult stage is finally reached in the duodenum or jejunum, where the male and female worms mate and produce eggs (Fig. 10.2).

Despite its extensive journey through the human body, like *Ascaris*, the hookworms are very well adapted to their host and only produce symptoms when heavy infections occur. The passage through the skin can result in a transient urticaria (ground itch), while that through the lungs pneumonitis and haemoptysis. Occasionally, the haemoptysis can be sufficient to

suggest a diagnosis of tuberculosis. The main effect results from the adult worms attaching to the intestinal wall where they invaginate a piece of mucosa, extracting blood and nutrients. Anaemia results from frank blood loss and depletion of iron reserves. The degree of anaemia produced depends upon the worm load and one estimate calculates that 60–120 worms (measured by 30 worms excreting 1000 eggs/g faeces) will result in slight anaemia, whereas over 300 worms (10,000 eggs/g faeces) will cause severe anaemia. The newly established worm may produce several bleeding points and if the sexes are unbalanced, the search for a mate can result in increased activity. These effects will naturally be most profound in the growing child and the pregnant woman. It is the combination of malaria, malnutrition and other intercurrent infections, in combination with hookworms, that accentuate the seriousness of this infection.

Diagnosis Eggs are found in faecal examination. They are oval and have colourless thin walls differentiating them from *Ascaris,* which has a thick brown exterior (Fig. 9.1). The eggs of the two species are identical and only the adults can be differentiated, mainly from their characteristic mouthparts (Fig. 10.2).

Transmission The eggs are passed in the faeces and hatch within 24–48 h to liberate an intermediate (rhabditiform) larva. After some days, it moults to produce the infective filariform larva. In suitable conditions of moist, warm but shaded soil (30°C for *N. americanus* and 25°C for *A. duodenale*), this stage of the larva can live for several months awaiting the opportunity to penetrate through the skin of a new host. (The ingested third stage larvae of *Ancylostoma* can also produce infection.) The larva commonly penetrates the foot of the unshod person and intense infection can occur where areas of beach or bush are demarcated for defecation purposes. Non-human hookworms can also penetrate the skin and produce cutaneous larva migrans (see Section 17.4).

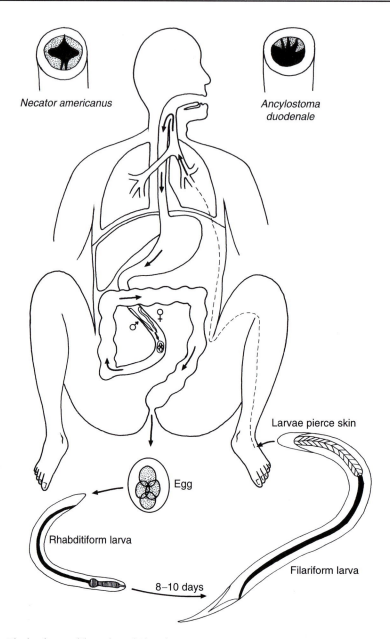

Necator americanus

Ancylostoma
duodenale

Larvae pierce skin

Egg

Rhabditiform larva

Filariform larva

8–10 days

Fig. 10.2. The hookworm life cycle and identification.

Incubation period 8–10 weeks.

Period of communicability From about 2 months after infection to up to 5 years; generally 1 year.

Occurrence and distribution N. *americanus*, despite its name, is the more widely distributed, being found extensively throughout the tropical belt and well north of the Tropic of Cancer in America and the Far East. *A. duodenale* is found in the Far East, the Mediterranean and the Andean part of South America (Fig. 10.3). It has been suggested that N. *americanus* was carried from Africa to the Americas as a

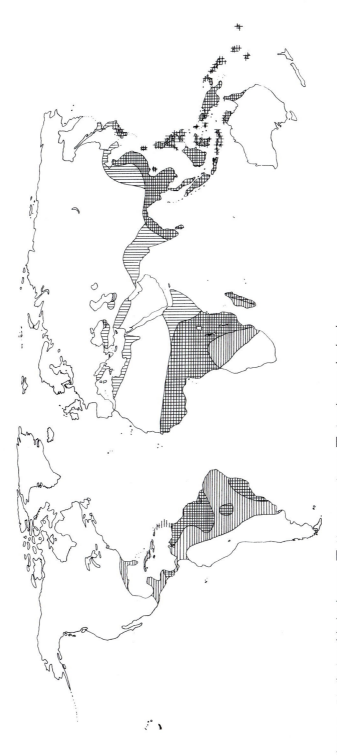

Fig. 10.3. Distribution of the hookworms. ▦, *Necator americanus*, ▨, *Ancylostoma duodenale*.

result of the slave trade. Altogether, some 720 million of the world population have hookworms.

Control and prevention is by use of pit latrines or other methods of sanitation. The wearing of footwear effectively prevents penetration by the larvae. The open sandal type of footwear often worn (thongs, flip-flops) is not effective and infection can readily occur. Mass treatment can be given to reduce the parasite load, but without health education and the proper use of latrines, it will only produce a temporary improvement.

Treatment A number of drugs are effective in treatment. Albendazole 400 mg single dose, mebendazole 500 mg single dose or 100 mg twice a day for 3 days, levamisole 2.5 mg/kg daily for 3 days, oxantel 10 mg/kg daily for 3 days or pyrantel pamoate 10 mg/kg daily for 3 days. The treatment should be repeated 12 weeks after the previous treatment. There is concern that resistance could develop as in veterinary practice; therefore, combinations, such as mebendazole+levamisole or pyrantel+oxantel, have been advocated. In the debilitated child, supporting therapy will need to accompany deworming. Iron supplementation, or in the severe case blood transfusion, will be required to treat anaemia.

Surveillance When mass treatment is planned, an initial survey will delineate the size of the problem. Follow-up spot checks of individual stool specimens can be made to assess progress.

10.4 *Strongyloides*

Organism The nematode *Strongyloides stercoralis*, which is morphologically similar to the hookworms. Far less common is *S. fülleborni*.

Clinical features There are several alternative cycles of development and it is the type of cycle which determines the nature and degree of pathological change and hence the clinical features.

An infective filariform larva develops in warm moist soil, penetrates the skin, and follows the same internal route as the hookworms to the final resting site in the small intestine. However, no eggs are passed to the outside, only rhabditiform larvae are found in the faeces. If environmental conditions are favourable, a free-living cycle takes place, with the rhabditiform larvae developing into adults in the soil. This cycle can be repeated and the number of potential parasites increases with each completed cycle. If conditions change, filariform larvae are produced or if unsuitable for the free-living cycle, then the rhabditiform larvae passed in the faeces change directly into filariform larvae. Direct autoinfection can also occur, with the rhabditiform larvae penetrating the intestinal mucosa to enter the blood stream without ever leaving the body. Swallowed larvae can as well complete their development by entering the body through the intestinal mucosa (Fig. 10.4). Achlorhydria, as occurring in malnutrition, makes infection easier by the oral route.

It is the abnormal cycle of autoinfection that can lead to wandering larvae producing linear urticaria (larva currens) or 'eosinophilic lung'. Larva currens can persist for periods in excess of 40 years. Immunocompromised persons, such as those with HIV infection or malignant disease, can get widespread dissemination of worms with serious consequences.

Diagnosis is made by finding the rhabditiform larvae in the faeces or in the aspirate of the duodenal string test. Serological tests can be of value, but where positive, repeat stool examinations should be made.

Transmission is from direct penetration of the skin by infective stage (filariform) larvae or being swallowed from contaminated food, water or fingers. Soil is contaminated by faeces deposited directly on the ground or inadequately buried.

Incubation period 2–4 weeks.

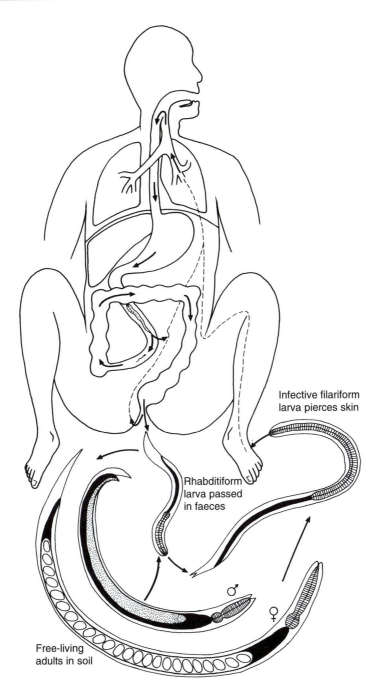

Infective filariform
larva pierces skin

Rhabditiform
larva passed
in faeces

♂

♀

Free-living
adults in soil

Fig. 10.4. *Strongyloides stercoralis* life cycles.

Period of communicability Due to autoinfection and long-living adult worms, once infected, a person can continue to produce larvae for 30–40 years.

Occurrence and distribution Mostly found in the warm wet tropics, the parasite also occurs in temperate areas. *S. fülleborni* has only been reported from Africa and Papua

New Guinea. Adults, rather than children, manifest the clinical symptoms, either acquiring the parasite when they were children or in adult life.

Control and prevention All the methods applicable to the other soil-based nematode infections are applicable, such as personal hygiene, careful washing and preparation of vegetables and the wearing of adequate footwear. Soil contamination can be prevented by good sanitation.

Treatment is the same as for hookworm infection or any of these treatments can be combined with ivermectin or diethylcarbamazine (DEC, see under filariasis, Section 15.7).

10.5 Tetanus

Organism The bacillus *Clostridium tetani*, which is a Gram-positive rod with spherical, terminal spores, giving it a characteristic drum-stick appearance.

Clinical features Infection results from the organism entering an abraded surface, such as a cut or scratch. It favours anaerobic conditions, liberating toxin, which produces severe muscle spasms. It is a serious condition in the neonate due to infection of the umbilical cord stump.

The adult presents with muscle spasm and rigidity. There may be trismus, in which the muscles of the jaw and later the back become rigid leading to lock jaw and opisthotonos. Muscle spasms can produce the characteristic half smile, half snarl of 'risus sardonicus' or generalized opisthotonos. These spasms are initiated by external stimuli, such as touch or attempts at intubation, and every care must be taken to protect the patient from such stimuli. Neonatal tetanus generally presents as a difficulty in sucking; then the rigidity of muscles and generalized convulsions develop. It usually commences within 5–10 days of birth.

Diagnosis is on the clinical presentation.

Transmission The organism is introduced into a wound from soil, dust or animal faeces. Cutting the umbilical cord with an unsterile instrument, such as a bamboo knife, or traditional practice of treating the umbilical stump are potent methods of causing neonatal tetanus. These can involve covering the stump with an unsterile dressing or customary practice of using a cow dung or earth poultice.

The bacillus is found naturally in the soil where it survives in anaerobic conditions. Many types of soils have been found to harbour *C. tetani*, but it is more common in cultivated soils, especially those manured with animal faeces. The organism is found in horse and cattle dung and less commonly in pig, sheep and dog faeces. It is occasionally found in human excreta, particularly in people associated with animals.

The vegetative form of the organism is sensitive to antibiotics, disinfectants and heat, but as a spore, it is resistant to all but the super-heated steam of an autoclave. Indeed, the spores of *C. tetani* are used to test the effectiveness of the sterilizing process because if it cannot survive, then no other organism can (apart from anthrax).

Spores can survive for considerable periods of time, but when they enter a wound or umbilical stump in which there is a low oxygen reduction potential, they release the vegetative form, which grows anaerobically and infection takes place. It is the moist, contaminated umbilical stump or the traumatized wound that provides suitable conditions.

The replication of the organism is not important, but toxin is produced that can have a profound effect out of all proportion to the initial infection. The exotoxin has a high affinity for nervous tissue and as little as 0.1 mg is sufficient to kill a person. Toxin is absorbed along the nerves, reaching the spinal cord where the generalized features of the disease are produced.

Incubation period is from 4–21 days, but most cases occur within 14 days. There is a relationship between incubation period and severity, with an incubation period of less than 9 days having a mortality of 60% and more than 9 days 25% mortality. This is due to the dose of the toxin.

Period of communicability Not transmitted from person-to-person directly or indirectly.

Occurrence and distribution Tetanus occurs worldwide, with higher rates in Africa, Asia (especially Southeast) and the Western Pacific. Neonatal tetanus is a serious problem in Africa, especially where birth practices are rudimentary. There is an association with agricultural areas where animal excreta is commonly used for fertilizing the soil, as a fuel or as a plaster on the walls of houses. Domestic animals either share the same house as their owners or live in such close proximity that their faeces contaminate the surrounding soil.

Control and prevention The aim should always be to prevent tetanus with vaccination and good hygiene practices, especially with the newborn.

The most effective way of preventing neonatal tetanus is the vaccination of all women of childbearing age. The policy is to give all women a lifetime total of five doses of tetanus toxoid. This is preferable to waiting until the woman becomes pregnant because many women do not attend antenatal clinic, especially those who are likely to use traditional applications to the umbilical cord stump. The effectiveness of various strategies is shown in Fig. 10.5. Women should, therefore, be given their first dose of tetanus toxoid at first contact or as early as possible during pregnancy. The second is given 4 weeks later and the third 6–12 months after the previous dose or during the next pregnancy. Doses four and five are given at yearly intervals. Where a woman has a certificate to say that she has received vaccination as a child, then she only needs to have two doses during the first pregnancy and one more before or during the second pregnancy.

Infants are given tetanus toxoid as part of their childhood vaccination programme as DTP at 6, 10 and 14 weeks of age. An additional booster dose of DTP can be given at 18 months to 4 years of age. School

children or adults who have not been vaccinated before should be given two doses of adsorbed tetanus toxoid (0.5 ml), separated by 4 weeks and a third dose of 1 ml 6 months later. Booster doses every 10 years will maintain a high level of immunity.

In the event of a person being injured and presenting with a contaminated wound that could produce tetanus, the following action should be taken – clean out the wound, give penicillin, then the following:

- If the person has been fully vaccinated in the past, a booster dose of toxoid is required only if this is more than 10 years ago.
- If there is no record of tetanus vaccination or protection is in doubt, then give the first dose of tetanus toxoid plus 250 units of human tetanus immune globulin or 1500 units of equine tetanus antitoxin, following a test dose. Instruct the person to return at 4 weeks and then 6 months to complete the course of vaccination.

Good birth practices are important in preventing neonatal tetanus and several countries have developed systems for contacting traditional birth attendants (TBAs) and giving them courses of instruction. Prepacked sterilized blades for cutting the cord can be given and iodine, spirit or similar antiseptic provided to apply to the cord stump. Where there is no system of TBAs but delivery takes place at home with the assistance of mother or other female relative, then an instruction sheet in the local language can be given to the pregnant woman when she attends the antenatal clinic or at any other contact with the health services. Figure 10.6 illustrates several strategies for reducing neonatal tetanus as tried out in rural Haiti.

Treatment Tetanus is a self-limiting disease and if the patient can be kept alive for 3 weeks, then complete recovery should take place, but keeping the patient alive for this period of time is the problem. It is the toxin that is causing the symptoms and once this is fixed in the nerves, only support can be given to the patient to

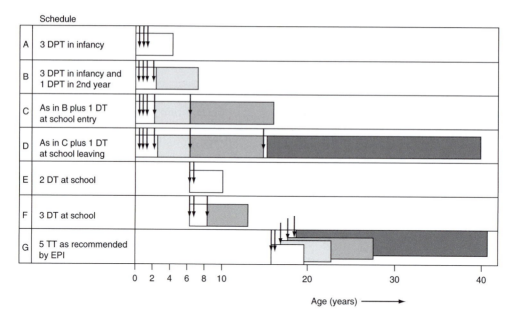

Fig. 10.5. Expected duration of tetanus immunity after different vaccination schedules. DPT, diphtheria, pertussis and tetanus; DT, diphtheria and tetanus; TT, tetanus toxoid; EPI, Expanded Programme of Immunization. (Reproduced by permission of the World Health Organization, Geneva.)

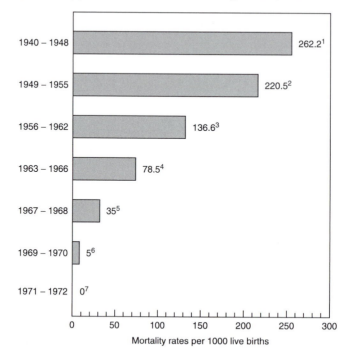

Fig. 10.6. Neonatal mortality per 1000 live births in rural Haiti, 1940–1972, from a retrospective study of 2574 mothers. 1, before national programme for training TBAs; 2, national programme for training TBAs; 3, hospital treatment for tetanus, training of TBAs by hospital nurse; 4, immunization of pregnant women in hospital clinics; 5, immunization of women in market places by hospital team; 6, immunization after door-to-door invitation by community workers. (Reproduced by permission of the World Health Organization, Geneva.)

maintain respiration, urinary output and nutrient intake. The patient is sedated to reduce spasms and in all ways, expertly nursed. The contaminated wound must be cleaned and excised, antitoxin or immuno-globulin administered and penicillin given to kill any remaining organisms. Sadly, the mortality from tetanus is high – 40% in adults and 90% in neonates, so the objective should always be to try and prevent it.

Surveillance WHO has set out to eliminate maternal and neonatal tetanus (it can never be eradicated because *C. tetani* will always remain in the environment) as a health problem by 2005, by intensified vaccination, the promotion of clean delivery practices and a programme of school vaccination. High-risk areas need to be identified from a knowledge of the birth practices, lack of health facilities or preponderance of cases. All children at school entry should be required to bring their vaccination certificates with them and if these are not adequate, receive a course of tetanus toxoid.

11

Diteases of Water Contact

Water is an important medium for the transmission of disease processes. Normally it is
through drinking water, which has become
polluted by faecal material, that infection is
transmitted, or through water used to wash
food and the food subsequently consumed.
It also serves as a medium for fish or other
organisms to live, which may carry a parasitic stage that is transmitted when they are
eaten (as covered in Chapters 8 and 9). In
this chapter, we look at one important disease and one almost eradicated that are
transmitted by contact with water, in
which the intermediate stages are free
living. Minimizing water contact is, therefore, the best method of control if it can be
applied.

11.1 Schistosomiasis

Organism The main parasites are *Schistosoma haematobium, S. mansoni* and *S.
japonicum.* Other species, such as
S. intercalatum and *S. mekongi* do occur,
but they are only important in well-
defined areas and their epidemiology and
control are similar to one of the three main
types.

Clinical features Infection normally starts
in childhood, with often very little signs of

the disease until adulthood. Passing blood
in the urine is one of the first signs of *S.
haematobium* disease, but because it is so
common in the local area, it is generally
ignored, with boys assuming it quite normal
that they should have period bleeding like
girls do. Infection and egg output increases
up to about 15 years of age and then declines. Individuals vary in their response,
with some persons acquiring heavy infections and developing severe pathological
changes, while others have only minor
symptoms. The more serious manifestations
are liver fibrosis, portal hypertension and
obstructive urinary problems, with the pathology depending upon the species of parasite and the number of eggs deposited in the
tissues. Infections with *S. mansoni* and *S.
japonicum* lead to intestinal and liver
damage, while that with *S. haematobium*
results in bladder complications, including
bladder cancer.

Diagnosis is made by finding the characteristic eggs (Fig. 9.1) of *S. haematobium* in
the urine and those of *S. mansoni* and *S.
japonicum* in the faeces or from a rectal
snip. Urine samples are best collected between 1100 and 1500 h when egg output is at
a maximum. Leaving the urine to stand, cen-
trifuging it, or passing it through a filter increases the chance of finding eggs. While the

© R. Webber 2005. *Communicable Disease Epidemiology and Control,* 2nd edition (Roger Webber)

qualitative diagnosis is required in the individual case, quantitative estimates are more valuable in epidemiological investigations. In *S. haematobium*, the simplest method is to pass 10 ml of urine through a filter in a Millipore holder. The paper or membrane is taken out, dried and stained with ninhydrin and the eggs counted directly. Immunological methods, indirect fluorescent antibody test (IFAT) and enzyme-linked immunosorbent assay (ELISA) test have also been developed for schistosomiasis, but they only indicate recent or past infection, so eggs must be looked for to confirm the diagnosis. They are useful in epidemiological surveys for rapidly defining the extent of the infected area.

Pathology is related to the number of worms, which can be measured by the number of eggs produced. In *S. haematobium*, the production of 50 eggs/ml of urine or above is regarded as the level of severe pathology and much of present day control strategy is aimed at reducing the egg count below this level.

Transmission Infection results from cercariae directly piercing the skin of a person when they go into the water. On penetrating the subcutaneous layer of the host, the cercaria becomes a schistosomule, migrates to the lungs and finally develops into an adult in the portal vessels of the liver. Both male and female worms are required so that pairing can take place prior to migration to the final destination in the mesenteric or vesical plexus. Adult worms can live for 20–30 years, but are active egg producers for 3–8 years, although some have produced viable eggs for over 30 years. The egg output per day in *S. haematobium* is some 20–250, in *S. mansoni* 100–300 and in *S. japonicum* 1500–3500. It is this massive output of eggs in *S. japonicum* that leads to the more rapidly developing and severe pathology.

Less than 50% of eggs manage to pass through the bladder or intestinal wall to develop further, the remainder being trapped in the tissue. On reaching water, a temperature of 10–30°C and the presence of light induce hatching, resulting in miracidia swimming out. They actively search out a snail using geotactic and phototactic behaviour, homing-in on a chemical substance 'miraxone' inadvertently liberated by the snail. The miracidium must penetrate a snail within 8–12 h, but their chance of success decreases with age. Some 40% of snails are infected at a distance of 5 m in still water, but where the water is flowing, similar infection rates can occur at a far greater distance. Normally, infection occurs in water flowing at 10 cm/s or less. Even after the rigours of the journey when miracidia have entered the correct species of snail, many are inactivated and only a small proportion develop into sporocysts. This is determined by the part of the snail entered and immunity to reinfection developed by the snail (Fig. 11.1).

Cercariae are stimulated by light to emerge from the snail when the ambient temperature is between 10°C and 30°C. Cercarial emergence increases as daylight penetrates the watery environment producing a peak for *S. mansoni* at 1200 noon and for *S. haematobium*, mid-to-late afternoon. With *S. japonicum*, the stimulus produced by light is delayed and maximal cercarial liberation occurs at 2300 h. The number of cercariae issuing from a snail can be immense, in the order of 1000–3000/day, but this depends upon the species and relative size of the snail. Where more than one miracidium has penetrated a snail, there is depression of cercarial production; this may also occur if the snail is host to other trematode infections. Cercarial output is greatest in *S. mansoni*, less in *S. haematobium* and least of all in *S. japonicum*. Cercariae survive for 24 h, but their greatest chance of penetrating the host is when they are young. When cercariae enter within 2 h of release, only 30% die, but this rises to 50% at 8 h and 85% at 24 h.

The snail intermediate hosts are species specific, *Bulinus* spp. in *S. haematobium*, *Biomphalaria* spp. in *S. mansoni* and *Oncomelania* spp. in *S. japonicum*. They are illustrated in Fig. 11.1. They can adapt to a wide range of habitats from natural waterways to temporary ponds and cultivated rice fields. Whenever there is sufficient organic matter on which to feed, snails will be found. Within a body of water, distribution

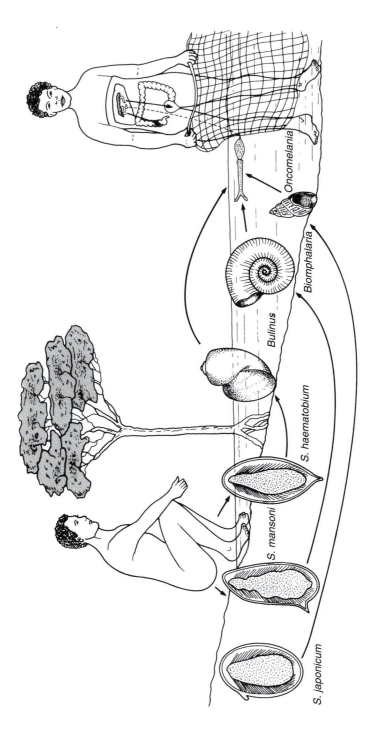

Fig. 11.1. Schistosomiasis species and life cycles.

may be quite irregular with dense colonies in some places and complete absence in others. Various factors, which may influence snail colonization, are:

- *Electrolyte concentration.* Snails demand a minimum calcium concentration, cannot tolerate high salt content or a low pH.
- *Light* is not required by the snail, and they can often survive in near total darkness.
- *Rainfall* may herald the end of the dry season and provide water in which snail populations can increase, but if the rainfall is too heavy, it may flush out the snails, resulting in a subsequent decrease. Snail populations, therefore, may follow a seasonal pattern.
- *Temperature* rise encourages expansion of the population up to a maximum of approximately 30°C.
- *Density* is a limiting factor and results in reduced growth.
- *Aestivation* or the ability of snails to survive out of the water for weeks or months allows populations of snails to continue from one season to another, possibly also transferring immature infections of *S. haematobium* and *S. mansoni*. The snail host of *S. japonicum* can survive conditions of desiccation best of all.

Snails are capable of self-fertilization, although cross-fertilization is more common. Their reproductive capacity is phenomenal and a single snail can produce a colony within 40 days and be infective in 60 days. When conditions are optimal, many species of snails will double their population in 2–3 weeks. In measuring the age of snail populations, size of snails is a useful indicator. A large number of small samples from many different areas are preferable to a few large samples in estimating the numbers and density in water courses. Infection rates in snails are generally low, with only some 1–2% of the colony being infective, but even so this level is sufficient to account for high prevalence rates in the human population.

Humans contaminate water either by urinating or defecating into or near water courses. Egg output is variable between individuals and their age, with a few individuals having heavy infections and egg outputs, while the majority have light infections. In areas of high endemicity, children between 5 and 14 years are responsible for over 50% of the contamination. As the infection rate declines, older age groups become more important.

People are infected by collecting water, washing (both clothes and the person), in their occupation (such as fishing) or during recreation. Children are most commonly infected when they play in water, while in adults, it is when they carry out their domestic duties or occupation. Infection is generally due to repeated water contact over a long period of time, but can occur from a single immersion if it coincides with a large number of cercariae in the water.

Animals, such as water buffalo, cattle, pigs, dogs, cats and horses, can also serve as reservoirs of *S. japonicum*, but they are less important than humans as sources of infection.

Incubation period 2–6 weeks.

Period of communicability 10–20 years.

Occurrence and distribution *S. haematobium* and *S. mansoni* were originally diseases of Africa, where they are widely distributed, but with the massive exodus of slaves that took place in the 17th and 18th centuries, this legacy was carried with them. The East African slave trade carried *S. mansoni* to the Arabian peninsula and *S. haematobium* to the Yemen and Iraq. The Western trade was solely in *S. mansoni*, which found a suitable snail host in South America and the Caribbean. *S. japonicum* probably originated in China, where it has been found in mummified bodies, but is also found in the Philippines, Taiwan and Sulawesi in Indonesia (Fig. 11.2). No cases have been found in Japan since 1978. A separate species *S. intercalatum*, pathogenically similar to *S. mansoni*, is found in Congo, Cameroon, Central African Republic, Chad, Gabon and São Tomé. *S. mekongi* is restricted to the Mekong River basin in Laos,

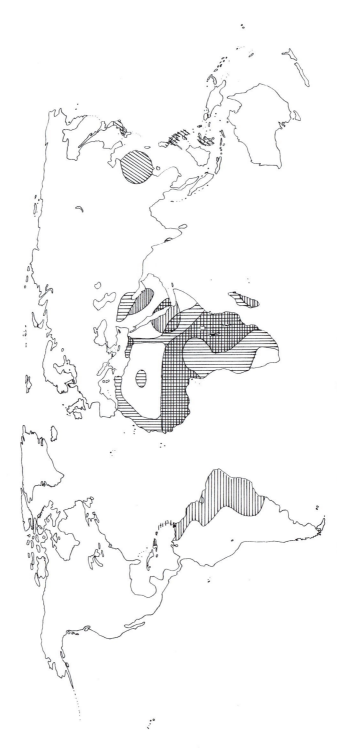

Fig. 11.2. Distribution of schistosomiasis. ▨ *S. mansoni*, ▤ *S. haematobium*, ▩ *S. japonicum*.

Thailand and Cambodia. Other localized species are *S. malayensis* in peninsular Malaysia and *S. mattheei* found in southern Africa.

Control and prevention There are two approaches to the control of schistosomiasis:

- reduce the transmission of the parasite;
- reduce the level of infection in individuals.

The first attempts to control the parasite, while the second aims at minimizing the pathological effects. The various methods of control are as follows.

REDUCTION OF CONTAMINATION OF THE ENVIRONMENT Humans pollute the environment by urinating or defecating into bodies of water. This can be minimized by encouraging the use of latrines. Unfortunately, it is very difficult to get everybody in a family or community to always use a latrine and the few non-users will be sufficient to maintain a level of pollution (see Section 2.4.2). There is also the longevity of the adult worms, meaning that prevalence rates will remain static in the community for a considerable period of time.

REDUCTION OF THE SNAIL INTERMEDIATE HOST   The snail is a vulnerable link in the life cycle of the parasite and can be attacked in an effort to break transmission. The various methods that can be used are:

- predators;
- biological control;
- water management and engineering;
- molluscicides.

Various kinds of fish (particularly *Tilapia* and *Gambusia*) are natural predators, but they will only reduce snails to a certain level unless they have an alternative source of food. Snails, especially of the *Marisa* and *Helisoma* genera, compete for food supplies and *Marisa* will even prey on eggs and juveniles of *Biomphalaria*. Another approach to biological control is the sterile male technique, but since many snails are hermaphrodite, it is only suitable with *Oncomelania*.

Where small and temporary ponds are foci of infection, they can be drained or filled (by controlled tipping of household refuse). Where canals and irrigation systems are responsible, concrete lining, increasing rate of flow and any method to reduce vegetation can discourage snail habitation. Unfortunately, these methods are rarely effective on their own and need to be combined with molluscicides (e.g. niclosamide, Bayluscide), which can be administered as a liquid, suitable for treating moving water, or as granules in lakes and ponds. Continuous application is required to make a sustained effect on the snail population. It has the disadvantage of killing fish and is expensive. Cheaper preparations, such as copper sulphate, are still in limited use and naturally occurring plant preparations, such as Endod (*Phytolacca dodecandra*), have shown promise. However, the remarkable recovery of snail populations once control methods are removed and the cost of molluscicides make snail reduction a less effective approach in schistosomiasis control.

REDUCTION OF WATER CONTACT   Preventing water contact can be highly effective in the individual. Various ways of encouraging this are:

- health education, especially to school children, but this is often ineffective unless an alternative (e.g. swimming pool), is provided;
- providing places to wash have been disappointingly ineffective for the cost involved;
- where areas of absent or minimal transmission occurs in occupational or recreational bodies of water, people can be encouraged to use these, rather than the heavily infected parts;
- wear rubber boots when wading through water, or if accidental exposure occurs, then rub vigorously with a towel and apply 70% alcohol;

- drinking water can be treated with iodine or chlorine or if left to stand for at least 48 h, cercarial die-off will be complete.

REDUCTION OF HUMAN INFECTION BY MASS CHE- MOTHERAPY   With the discovery of effective preparations, such as praziquantel, single-dose MDA is now a good method of control. A suitable target population is school children between 5 and 15 years of age where mass therapy is used. Alternatively, only the positive cases, or those with heavy infections, are treated following a simple diagnostic procedure. Individual treatment, based on worm load estimation, aims at disease control by reducing morbidity. It permits limited resources to be more widely spread and attempts the less ambitious target of disease rather than transmission reduction.

The anti-malarial drug artemethur is also valuable in the control of schistosomiasis and could be used in areas where there is no malaria, such as China, southern Brazil and Southwest Asia. It can be used in combination with praziquantel.

REDUCTION OF THE ANIMAL RESERVOIR   Animal reservoirs are responsible for maintaining *S. japonicum*. In order of importance they are dogs, cows, pigs, rats and water buffaloes. As most of these are domestic animals, proper animal management can reduce contamination of the environment. Vaccination of domestic animals could be done. Baboons and monkeys have been shown to be reservoirs of *S. mansoni* and could play a part in maintaining infection. There is little prospect of controlling these animals.

VACCINATION   There are difficulties in preparing a vaccine because the schistosome is able to absorb host antigen and mask its presence, but three vaccines are currently under trial for *S. mansoni*.

STRATEGIES FOR SCHISTOSOMIASIS CONTROL   Various approaches for the control of schisto-somiasis have been tried depending on the resources and nature of the disease as follows:

- Raising of economic standards by the provision of water supplies and sanitation, environmental engineering and water management has been shown to be effective on a long-term basis in countries such as Japan and China.
- In well-controlled irrigation schemes, mollusciciding on its own may be effective. Where discipline and motivation of the population are less certain, a double approach of mass chemotherapy and reduction of water contact is more effective.
- When resources are scarce and greatest benefit for limited finance is required, treatment of high worm load cases is the method of choice.

Surveillance Effectiveness of control strategies can be measured by:

- change in incidence rate;
- a shift in peak prevalence to an older age group;
- reduction in geometric mean egg output;
- greater awareness of socio-economic values (e.g. the use of water supplies and sanitation facilities).

11.2 Guinea Worm

Dracunculus medinensis, the largest of the nematode worms to attack humans, used to be a serious problem in India, Pakistan, southern Iran, most of West Africa, Southwest Asia and Sudan, infecting some 80 million people. It is spread by spilt-water washing larvae back into an unprotected well or by infected people using walk-in wells. WHO launched an eradication programme to make all wells safe with a surrounding wall and concrete apron so as to prevent all spilt-water from washing back into the well. Walk-in wells were converted into lift-wells or alternative water supplies provided. By these simple strategies, *Dracunculus* infection has been eradicated from most of the area. In 2003, there were 32,193 cases; 63% of these cases were in Sudan, where control was hampered by the continuing war, while most of the rest were in Ghana, Nigeria and Mali. This has been the most successful eradication programme to use such a simple strategy.

12

Skin Infections

The skin is a common site for several communicable diseases, presenting with rashes of various kinds. Infection is often transmitted from one person to another directly by skin contact or by other means, especially the airborne route. Control is by the avoidance of contact with infected individuals and where available the use of vaccines.

Some skin infections, tropical ulcers and those due to scabies and lice have been covered in Chapter 7 as they share common methods of control. Typhoid often has an accompanying skin rash, but is more appropriately covered with other faecal–oral diseases in Chapter 8. Meningococcal meningitis often presents with a petechial rash and is covered in Chapter 13. Many of the arbovirus diseases present with skin rashes, but as their method of transmission is by vectors, they are covered in Chapters 15 and 16.

12.1 Chickenpox/Shingles (Varicella)

Organism *Herpesvirus* varicella-zoster virus (VZV).

Clinical features A generally mild disease, chickenpox is a common infection of children. Illness commences with fever followed by a characteristic skin rash of macules, papules, vesicles, pustules and dried crusts. The lesions occur in groups, appearing over several days, so pox of different stages will be seen at the same time. In chickenpox, the rash is distributed centrally, appearing on the chest and abdomen and sparsely on the feet and hands.

The majority of people contract the disease in childhood when it is an inconvenience rather than a life-threatening condition, but if this has not occurred and if they subsequently develop the illness as adults, it can be very serious. This is a particular problem in island and isolated communities where varicella can be a fatal disease in the elderly. Pregnant women, who contract the disease in late pregnancy or shortly after delivery, are at risk of severe generalized chickenpox with a 30% mortality. Neonates who develop chickenpox within 10 days of birth are liable to a serious generalized infection. Chickenpox in early pregnancy may result in congenital malformations. Death results from generalized viraemia, pneumonia, haemorrhagic complications, encephalitis or cardiomyopathy.

The virus remains latent in the body, lodged in nerve bundles, and in later life, especially during a debilitating disease (such as HIV infection), the identical virus

(VZV) causes shingles. This presents as a vesicular rash with erythema in a well-defined area of skin supplied by the affected dorsal root ganglia. Pain and paraesthesia occur along the course of the affected nerve.

Diagnosis is on clinical criteria, especially the central distribution of the rash and the presence of lesions at different stages, differentiating it from smallpox. Any case of a pox rash that dies or has an unusual distribution should be a smallpox suspect (see Section 18.2).

Transmission The infection is transmitted by fluid from the vesicles. This can occur in the pharynx before the main rash, when transmission is by droplets; otherwise, the spread occurs by direct skin contact, airborne dispersion of vesicle fluid or through articles soiled by discharges.

Incubation period varies from 2 to 3 weeks.

Period of communicability is from 3 days before the onset of the rash to 6 days after its first appearance.

Occurrence and distribution Chickenpox occurs worldwide in an epidemic form often spreading serially (Section 2.2) from one place to another. It is a disease of children in the temperate regions, but is more commonly found in adults in the tropics.

Control and prevention One attack of chickenpox confers life-long immunity; so it is preferable for children to have the disease rather than be protected and run the risk of developing it as adults. Special groups, such as neonates, pregnant women and the sick, should be protected by preventing cases of chickenpox from coming into contact with them. In hospital, cases of chickenpox should be isolated from other patients.

A live, attenuated varicella virus vaccine has been developed, but is not widely available. It is useful for vaccinating high-risk groups, such as women of childbearing age, who have not had chickenpox as a child, and the immunocompromised. There is a risk in using vaccination by shifting the age of developing naturally acquired chickenpox to older age groups where the disease is more serious, making it unlikely to become part of the routine childhood vaccination programme.

Treatment Acyclovir and vidarabine can be used to treat adults, children with serious disease and older persons with shingles. Human varicella-zoster immunoglobulin (VZIG) is available in some centres and can be used within 10 days of exposure for contacts liable to develop severe disease, such as pregnant women, neonates and the immunosuppressed.

Surveillance Outbreaks should be reported so that susceptible individuals can be protected and given vaccination if available. Any suspect case of smallpox must be reported to WHO.

12.2 Measles

Organism Measles is a member of the Paramyxoviridae family of viruses.

Clinical features Measles normally commences with a prodromal fever, cough, conjunctivitis and small spots (Koplik's spots) most easily seen inside the mouth. The characteristic blotchy rash begins on the third to seventh day of the illness, generally on the face, but soon spreads to the whole body.

In developing countries, it is a serious disease and accounts for a considerable amount of mortality and morbidity in the childhood population. It particularly has a severe effect on the nutritional status of the child, resulting in the healthy child losing weight and the malnourished child becoming critically ill. The peak of infection is between 1 and 2 years of age, at the very time when breast milk alone is an inadequate source of food supply and weaning foods may not yet have been introduced. The association of nutritional change and measles can be, and often is, a lethal combination.

There are a number of reasons for the nutritional depletion produced by measles. Any disease process puts extra demands on the body, increasing catabolism. Fever and the desquamation of all epithelial surfaces demands protein replacement, which is handicapped by a sore mouth, often secondarily infected by *Candida*, thus preventing the child from sucking properly so that even breast milk is not taken. Then from the other end, diarrhoea, which is such a common feature of measles in developing countries, discharges the body reserves further. Perhaps the greatest weight loss is due to immunosuppression, much of which takes place after the child has recovered from the acute attack.

The disease process attacks all epithelial surfaces, producing most of its complications in the respiratory tract. Pneumonia is the commonest complication, while laryngo-tracheo-bronchitis is serious, with a high mortality. Acute respiratory infections (see Section 13.1) are one of the leading causes of childhood ill health and the sequelae of measles are responsible for a large component of this problem. If the acute pneumonia does not kill, the damage done makes the child more susceptible to further attacks of respiratory infection when the measles has long gone.

The effects on the eye can cause blindness. Corneal lesions result from epithelial damage, which can lead to ulceration, secondary infection and scarring. In severe cases, perforation or total disorganization of the eye can occur. These severe effects only result if there is concomitant vitamin A deficiency, so giving vitamin A to all measles cases is effective. Measles by its nutritional and direct effects has been regarded as the most important cause of blindness in a number of tropical countries.

Measles is an important cause of otitis media. It can also result in encephalitis, either in the acute form or a late slow-onset sclerosing panencephalitis, which is always fatal.

Diagnosis is on clinical criteria, but measles IgM can be found in the saliva with immunological tests.

Transmission Although the main feature of measles is the skin rash, it is transmitted by the airborne route from nasal and pharyngeal secretions. This can be by articles contaminated with secretions such as cloth or clothing used to wipe a running nose as well as by respiratory droplets produced in a coughing bout.

Measles is the most contagious of all infectious diseases and no age is spared. In the Fijian outbreak in the 1870s, adults as well as children succumbed, affecting families as a whole at the same time, causing deprivation and starvation that resulted in a high death rate. Now adults have experienced measles as children, with the age of infection getting younger. This is explained by greater contact of communities due to improvement of communication, while the intense social contact at a very young age (babies carried on their mother's back) gives maximum opportunity for early transmissions.

Incubation period 10–14 days.

Period of communicability From 1 day before the first signs of infection until 4 days after the rash starts (or 4 days before to 4 days after the rash begins).

Occurrence and distribution Measles has been a severe infection in Western countries for a considerable period of time, producing mortality in poor and slum populations similar to what is seen in developing countries. Introduced with European exploration, it caused devastating epidemics, particularly in island communities, some of which never recovered their former population numbers. However, in many developing countries in which it is a major problem, there is evidence that measles has been present for several hundred years, with the pattern having changed from sporadic epidemics with all ages involved to one of endemicity in which the under-5-year-olds are predominantly affected.

Control and prevention of measles is by vaccination. As measles is such an infectious disease, it can be reckoned that every child will develop it. Some 10% will either have such a mild infection or be partially protected by maternal antibodies as to appear not to have been infected. A further 10–20% will not have measles until the following year due to the epidemic effect; therefore, the expected number of cases of measles can be calculated from the birth rate minus 25%. If the birth rate in a developing country is 50,000, then 75% of this means that 37.5 cases of measles per 1000 can be expected each year, which represents 37,500 cases in an administrative unit of a million people. Calculations like these can be used to estimate the number of children to be vaccinated and hence the vaccine requirements.

Eighty per cent of susceptibles will need to be vaccinated to produce control of the disease, but a lower target may be acceptable in more isolated communities. This target will need to be achieved every year in rural areas, but as much as every 6 months in urban areas. Measles vaccine is 90% effective if the cold chain is not broken.

Maternal antibodies protect the newborn infant for the first 6 months of life, but thereafter the child becomes readily susceptible to infection with a peak around 1 year. The seroconversion rate is some 76% at the age of 6 months, 88% at 9 months and 100% at 12 months. Giving measles vaccination at 1 year would produce the best conversion, but, by this time in developing countries some 50% of the population would have already had the disease. Giving it at 6 months will be before all but a few have had the disease, however the seroconversion rate is so poor at this time that not many will be protected. The best compromise is a first vaccination at 9 months, with the possibility of a second opportunity through periodic mass campaigns. In condi-

tions of high infectivity, such as during an epidemic, admission to hospital or refugee camp or if the infant has HIV infection, then reducing the age of vaccination to 6 months is justified. In this case, another vaccination should be given at 12–15 months.

In developed countries, vaccination is given at 12–15 months so that the time taken to reduce the incidence in the population will be less, as shown in Fig. 12.1. The greater the coverage the more rapidly this is achieved. For example, 60% coverage will theoretically take 12 years to reduce the incidence to zero if vaccination is given at 12 months, but never be achieved at 9 months. However, 70% coverage will achieve zero incidence with vaccination given at 9 months, which is being achieved by an increasing number of developing countries.

Effective measles vaccination coverage will not only reduce the number of children developing the disease in an epidemic, but will have the secondary benefit of raising the age of developing the disease, as can be seen in Fig. 12.2. Epidemics had occurred in Namanyere, Tanzania, regularly every second year until 1978 when there was only a minor increase, the main epidemic being delayed until 1979. This meant that children born in 1977, who could have expected to become infected in their second year of life (1978), had their measles put off until 1979 when they were beyond the age of maximum mortality.

The chances of a susceptible child developing measles when admitted to hospital is very high as it is already sick with another complaint. It is fortunate that measles vaccine can produce protective immunity quicker than the wild virus (about 8 days for the vaccine and 10 days for the disease), so as long as the child is vaccinated within 48 h of admission, it will be protected. Because of the severity of disease in the debilitated child, there are very few contraindications and the malnourished and those with minor infection should all be vaccinated. HIV infection is not a contraindication

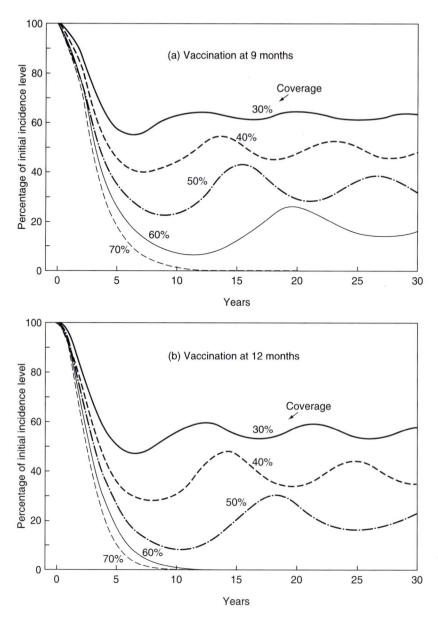

Fig. 12.1. The relative impact of immunization programmes on measles incidence in the age group 0–19 years, according to age at vaccination and population coverage. (Reproduced by permission from Cvetanovic, B., Grab, B. and Dixon, H. (1982) *Bulletin of the World Health Organization*, 60(3), 405–422.)

as the child is more likely to die from measles than from complications of receiving a live vaccine.

The policy in many countries is to give a second measles vaccination at 4–5 years or on school entry. Other countries, especially in South and Central America, give a second measles vaccination using vaccination days or special campaigns. Countries of the western hemisphere have set a target for the cessation of measles transmission by 2007.

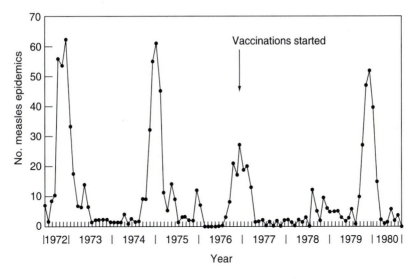

Fig. 12.2.   Prolongation of the time interval between measles epidemics due to vaccination in Namanyere, Tanzania.

As vaccination coverage is increasing, a potential problem could arise because less maternal antibody is produced by mothers who have acquired their immunity from vaccination rather than by having measles. This means that infants of a younger age will become susceptible, so vaccination may need to be given earlier if coverage is not complete.

Measles vaccine is conveniently combined with rubella (MR) or both with rubella and mumps (MMR). Despite adverse publicity given to the MMR vaccine, no complications have been confirmed and the vaccine should continue to be used.

Treatment There is no specific treatment, but supportive therapy with fluids and easily digested foods needs to be given. Vitamin A supplementation should be given to all children with measles. Complications may require additional treatment, such as antibiotics for bacterial chest infections.

Surveillance All cases of measles should be recorded and monthly totals charted to indicate epidemics and estimate when new epidemics will occur (Fig. 12.2). Measles has a seasonal pattern, which can vary markedly from country to country (Fig. 1.7); so this

needs to be determined to work out the best time to supplement routine vaccination programmes. If measles cases are focal, then this may indicate gaps in vaccination coverage (Fig. 3.2). Since all children should be vaccinated, an estimate of vaccine coverage can be made by comparing the number of new vaccinations with the number of children born.

12.3 Rubella

Organism Rubella virus, a member of the Togaviridae family of viruses.

Clinical features Infection in the adult is generally mild, presenting with a maculopapular rash of short duration, fever, conjunctivitis and cervical lymphadenopathy. Some 20–50% of the infections are subclinical. However, if the woman is pregnant, especially in the first 10 weeks of pregnancy, her developing fetus will suffer from congenital rubella syndrome (CRS). The congenital defects are more severe if the infection is acquired earlier in pregnancy, resulting in stillbirth in the first few weeks. Otherwise a range of congenital defects can result, including cataracts, glaucoma, deafness, heart defects and microcephaly. Milder defects will develop between the 11th and the 16th weeks and after the 20th week of pregnancy, there is no further risk.

Diagnosis is by detecting IgM from serum or saliva and is important if infection in a pregnant woman is suspected.

Transmission The virus is transmitted in droplets from the nasopharynx by the airborne route or direct contact. Most infections are acquired from children and adults during an outbreak, but infants with CRS can produce virus from pharyngeal secretions and urine for up to 1 year so are a potent source of infection.

Incubation period 15–20 days.

Period of communicability From 7 days before the onset of the rash to 4 days after. CRS infants continue to shed virus for up to 12 months.

Occurrence and distribution Worldwide distribution, but the importance of rubella in developing countries has not been appreciated until comparatively recently. It occurs in an epidemic form probably due to the number of susceptibles in the population, with children becoming infected when they are 2–8 years of age in urban areas and 6–12 years in rural areas.

Control and prevention The objective is to prevent CRS by vaccination of children and adults. Although adolescent girls and women of childbearing age are the target population, just vaccination of this group will never eliminate rubella; therefore, all children of both sexes should ideally be vaccinated. However, if the vaccination programme is far from complete, the effect will be to postpone the age of infection to older and more dangerous ages in women likely to become pregnant. Developing countries, therefore, need to decide between protecting adolescent girls and women of childbearing age only, with no attempt to eliminate

rubella or to vaccinate all children aged 9–15 months as part of the routine childhood vaccination programme. If the vaccination programme is considered sufficiently efficient to embark on the latter strategy, then an extra campaign to target all women and girls over 12 years of age should be run at the same time for the first few years of introducing rubella vaccination.

If a policy of childhood vaccination is adopted, then rubella vaccine is best administered with measles vaccine as MR or in combination with measles and mumps as MMR (see Sections 12.2 and 12.4).

Surveillance An estimate of the level of CRS can be obtained from hospital records and MCH records of deaf and blind infants. Measles vaccination records and numbers of cases of measles are good indicators of the efficiency of the childhood vaccination programme in deciding which strategy of rubella vaccination to introduce.

12.4 Mumps

Organism Mumps virus is a member of the Paramyxoviridae family of viruses.

Clinical features Mumps is not a true skin infection, but is included here as it shares common means of control with measles and rubella. It is an infection of the salivary glands producing enlargement and pain in the parotid gland, but can lead to orchitis, mastitis, meningitis, pancreatitis and acute respiratory symptoms (see Section 13.1). Commonly an infection of children 2–5 years of age, the more serious manifestations are more likely in adults, especially males.

Diagnosis is made on clinical grounds, but serological confirmation can be made with mumps-specific IgM, a rise in IgG or culture of saliva or urine.

Transmission The virus is transmitted via direct contact or by droplets spread by the airborne route. Any contact of saliva, such as sharing of cutlery, wiping the mouth with a common cloth, or kissing, can result in transmission.

Incubation period 14–24 days.

Period of communicability 6 days before to 6 days after the start of parotitis.

Occurrence and distribution Mumps is probably more common than assumed to be with up to 85% of the population found to have been infected in adult life, although few would have manifested the disease. With such a high proportion of the population meeting the virus, there is a relatively high risk of complications and cost–benefit studies have shown that vaccination produces substantial economic savings.

Control and prevention The reason for including mumps in the routine childhood vaccination programme is similar to that for rubella (Section 12.3). Where there is an efficient programme with the majority of children being vaccinated, it is advantageous to include it with measles and rubella as the MMR vaccine. However, if less than 75% of children are vaccinated, then this could result in an epidemiological shift to older age groups, increasing the likelihood of complications. If mumps vaccination is included, then a second opportunity, either by the routine programme or by catch-up campaigns, should be given unless coverage is over 90%.

Surveillance Comparing the number of children born with those who complete their childhood vaccinations or are vaccinated against measles will give an estimate of the efficiency of the vaccination programme and whether mumps vaccination should be added.

12.5 Streptococcal Skin Infections

Organism *Streptococcus pyogenes,* group A.

Clinical features Streptococcal infections of the skin can present as pyoderma, impetigo,

erysipelas or scarlet fever. Pyoderma and impetigo are superficial skin infections with vesicles, pustules and crusts. Erysipelas is a red, tender, oedematous cellulitis of the infected part of the body, originating from the point of infection. Scarlet fever presents as a generalized rash that blanches on pressure with high fever, strawberry tongue and flushing of the cheeks. In some cases, there is an appreciable mortality or else it can result in otitis media, glomerulonephritis or acute rheumatic fever (ARF, Section 13.10). Although not a skin infection, streptococci can also cause puerperal fever due to post-delivery infection of the female genital tract.

Diagnosis Culture of the organism from the point of infection or pharynx on blood agar.

Transmission is mainly by the respiratory route or direct contact with the lesion or skin (in impetigo). Flies can transfer the organism and are a major means of infecting scratches and wounds in tropical countries. The organism can be carried in the nose, pharynx, anus and vagina or in chronic skin lesions, and is an important cause of hospital infections.

Incubation period 1–3 days.

Period of communicability 10–21 days or until a chronic infection has been treated.

Occurrence and distribution Worldwide, predominantly in children, but scarlet fever is more common in temperate regions. Infected skin lesions either due to streptococci or staphylococci are very common in tropical regions.

Control and prevention Treat all cases promptly and dress infected lesions in a sterile manner. Any person with an infected lesion should not be involved in operations or hospital duties until healed. Personal hygiene, especially the washing of hands after defecation, and the discouragement of nose-picking should be advocated. Use of proper latrines and the control of flies are long-term preventive measures.

Treatment Benzathine penicillin G intramuscular, or penicillin G or V orally.

Surveillance Scarlet fever and puerperal fever are notifiable diseases in some countries.

12.6 Leprosy

Organism *Mycobacterium leprae.*

Clinical features Leprosy illustrates the conflict between the infecting organism and the host more dramatically than any other disease. *M. leprae* is widespread in the environment, yet only a small proportion of people ever show clinical symptoms of the disease and those few who do get the disease respond in different ways to the challenge.

The generation time from inoculation to multiplication of a stable number of *M. leprae* is only 18–24 days, but the development of the disease will take anything from 7 months to in excess of 7 years (mean 3–6 years). The first lesion is described as indeterminate (Fig. 12.3) because at this early stage, it is impossible to decide to which place in the spectrum of disease it will develop. There is either a single ill-defined, slightly hypopigmented macule, commonly seen on the face, trunk or exterior surfaces, or there may be a small anaesthetic patch. The lesion will then develop into a lepromatous or tuberculoid type or oscillate in the transitional state of borderline leprosy between these two extremes.

Lepromatous leprosy (LL) reflects the complete breakdown of the host's immune responses and the maximum infection with *M. leprae*. In the early stages, the signs

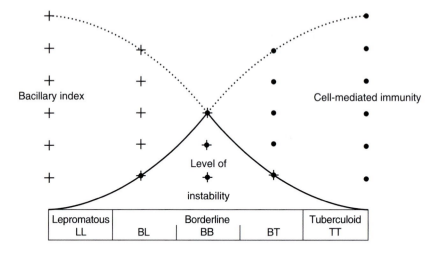

Indeterminate

Fig. 12.3. The spectrum of leprosy illustrating the proportion of bacilli, the cell-mediated immune response and the level of instability, in the different forms of the disease.

of the disease may be very few, but a skin smear will reveal large numbers of mycobacteria (multi-bacillary). Early signs that have been described, but rarely observed, are oedema of the legs and nasal symptoms of stuffiness, crust formation and blood-stained discharge. These are unlikely to be recognized as leprosy and it is generally not until the more obvious skin lesions become apparent that the diagnosis is made.

Leprosy lesions favour the cooler parts of the body, so the buttocks, trunk, exposed limbs and face are the more likely sites. Lesions may be macules, papules or nodules, with or without a colour change and often show lack of sweating when the patient becomes hot. The signs of nerve damage do not appear until much later in LL, with a concurrent thickening of the skin of the forehead, loss of eyebrows and damage to the cartilage of the nose. The eyes are also attacked with an infiltrative keratitis, iritis and eventually leads to blindness.

Tuberculoid leprosy (TT) is at the opposite end of the spectrum, showing the full response of cell-mediated immunity to the attacking organism (Fig. 12.3). *M. leprae* has a predilection for nervous tissue and it is within this nervous tissue that the cell-mediated response takes place, causing early damage to the nerves. The tuberculoid patient, therefore, tends to present early with signs of weakness or loss of sensation. Palpation of the nerves will often demonstrate a thickening with loss of sensation or motor power in the distribution of the affected nerve. The ulna nerve, as it bends over the medial epicondyle at the elbow, or the lateral popliteal nerve, where it curves round the neck of the fibula, are good places to palpate nerves for thickening. Dermal lesions are not raised, often appearing as apparently normal areas of the skin, lacking sensation or sweating when the patient exercises. Occasionally though, they are well-defined and scaly with raised edges, but quite different from the succulent macules and papules of LL. Loss of sensation should be elicited with a pin as well as

light touch. A skin smear in TT is nearly always free of bacilli (pauci-bacillary), so the diagnosis depends upon the detection of nerve damage.

Borderline leprosy, as its name suggests, is on the border between the two extremes of LL and TT. True borderline (BB) is uncommon, with the disease tending to progress to either the lepromatous (BL) or tuberculoid (BT) part of the spectrum. Signs, therefore, vary between the two extremes with features of each, but predominating in one or the other. Borderline leprosy is common, but its instability leads to reaction and nerve damage, which can often be severe.

Where the host response is adequate and cell-mediated immunity high, the disease tends towards the tuberculoid end of the spectrum, where it is low to LL. Simultaneous HIV infection will shift the host response from the tuberculoid towards the lepromatous. Otherwise the host response can vary over the course of the illness producing reactions, which can either be upgrading (towards TT) or downgrading (towards LL). These are type 1 reactions. The nearer the case is to the centre of the spectrum, the more severe is the reaction. Type 1 reactions may affect all tissues, skin and nerves only or produce a generalized systemic reaction.

A different type of reaction (type 2) is found in lepromatous and borderline lepromatous cases and is associated with massive destruction of bacilli. Immune complexes are formed in the tissues and these lead to an increased reaction in existing lesions. The characteristic finding is erythema nodosum leprosum, which appears on the skin as painful red nodules commonly on the face and exterior surfaces.

Diagnosis A skin smear is made from every suspected case of leprosy, collecting dermal tissue without drawing blood. A negative smear does not mean that a case is not leprosy as tuberculoid cases rarely have mycobacteria. Smears are stained with Ziehl–Neelsen stain and the number of mycobacteria counted, giving the *bacterial index*:

6+	Over 1000 bacilli in an average field
5+	100–1000 bacilli in an average field
4+	10–100 bacilli in an average field
3+	1–10 bacilli in an average field
2+	1–10 bacilli in 10 fields
1+	1–10 bacilli in 100 fields

Mycobacteria can also be obtained from nasal scrapings of the inferior turbinate. A skin biopsy is taken from tuberculoid and borderline patients or a nerve biopsy where there is no skin lesion.

Transmission The method of transmission has not been conclusively demonstrated, but several factors, such as prolonged close contact, the finding of large numbers of bacilli in the nasal discharges of lepromatous cases and in the skin, suggest that both airborne and direct skin contact are important. *M. leprae* have been found to survive from 2 to 7 days outside the body in nasal secretions. Individuals vary in their susceptibility and it is possible that repeated doses of bacilli or a large infective dose are required to produce the disease.

Incubation period 1–20 years.

Period of communicability Possibly 1 month to 20–30 years. Treatment with rifampicin renders the patient non-infectious after 3 days.

Occurrence and distribution Leprosy is found mainly in the tropical regions of the world, with poor socio-economic conditions probably being a major factor. LL is more common in Asia and TT more common in Africa. This differing susceptibility might help to explain the response of the peoples of these two continents to BCG. BCG, given at birth, can produce a hypersensitivity and change the cell-mediated immunity from negative to positive, but some people appear to have no natural immunity and remain always susceptible to the lepromatous form of the disease. BCG protected over 80% of school children in Uganda, but only 40% of children under 5 years of age in Myanmar.

Leprosy can occur in an epidemic as well as an endemic pattern, but due to the incredibly protracted life history of the disease, the epidemic form is rarely seen. Between 1921 and 1925, there was an epidemic in the Pacific island of Nauru, with 30% of the population becoming infected and the disease was notably non-focal. All ages were susceptible and most people developed tuberculoid (BT–TT) leprosy, which healed spontaneously.

It has been estimated that as much as 5% of people are susceptible to LL and contact with a lepromatous case increases the risk of infection. Children and young adults are more commonly affected, but the children of leprosy patients do not develop LL any more frequently than the general population. It would seem that leprosy is very similar to tuberculosis in that the organism is more common than assumed to be, asymptomatic infections may occur, but only those who are susceptible will develop the disease.

Due to active control measures and multiple drug therapy, there has been a marked reduction of leprosy in the world, with a global prevalence of one case in a population of 10,000 in 2001. Among 122 countries considered endemic in 1985, 107 have achieved elimination and leprosy remains a public health problem only in Angola, Brazil, Central African Republic, Congo, Côte d'Ivoire, Guinea, India, Liberia, Niger, Madagascar, Mozambique, Myanmar, Nepal, Paraguay and Tanzania. It is diminishing as a disease burden in India, Brazil, Myanmar, Madagascar, Nepal and Mozambique.

Control and prevention The immediate control is a reduction of the leprosy reservoir by case finding, treatment and follow-up, especially those with the lepromatous form of the disease. A small proportion of cases will present themselves, but active search must be made for others concentrating on selective groups. School children should receive priority, as they are likely to contain a quarter of all cases and a higher proportion of new ones. Also contacts of any case should be examined at frequent intervals, as leprosy is more common in those people who have prolonged contact with a leprosy case. All new cases are treated by multiple drug therapy (see below).

BCG vaccination induces hypersensitivity and increased resistance to developing leprosy in some ethnic groups and is valuable in the prevention of leprosy as well as tuberculosis (Section 13.1). *M. leprae*-based vaccines are under trial in several countries with promising results. The long-term reduction of disease will require an improvement in general hygiene, better housing and less overcrowding.

Treatment is determined by the bacterial index of the case.

- *High-risk* (*multi-bacillary*) *LL and BL cases*: A three-drug regime consisting of rifampicin 600 mg once a month supervised, dapsone 100 mg daily self-administered, clofazamine 300 mg once a month supervised, then 50 mg daily self-administered. Treatment should be continued for a minimum of 12 months.
- *Non-bacillary cases BT or TT*: Rifampicin 600 mg once a month supervised, plus dapsone 100 mg daily self-administered, for 6 months or six monthly doses within a 9-month period.

All patients with positive skin smears at the start of treatment should have repeat skin smears at 6 and 12 months. Clofaza-mine has the advantage of being anti-inflammatory as well as bacteriostatic, and, therefore, can be used in the treatment of reactions at a dose of 100 mg three times a week. Steroids and thalidomide are also useful in the treatment of reactions.

Part of any leprosy programme is the development of a rehabilitation service. This not only encourages leprosy patients to present themselves for treatment, but helps them to return as participating members of the community. Much can be done from limited resources, such as making sandals out of old tyres and pieces of wood. The elements of rehabilitation are to protect anaesthetic limbs, actively treat sores and ulcers and provide support (including surgery) to restore function. The eyes are also damaged in leprosy and, supportive treatment can do much to prevent blindness from developing.

Surveillance Dedicated leprosy field workers have been found to be of considerable value in detecting new cases and following up cases under treatment, otherwise a system within the existing health service should be developed. Combining leprosy and tuberculosis surveillance is economically useful.

Initially whole populations should be screened in areas of high endemicity, then concentration made on examining school children and all contacts of cases. All cases should be registered, often managed as a combined programme with tuberculosis. Section 13.1 on follow-up and registration is equally applicable to both diseases.

13

Respiratory Diseases and Other Airborne Transmitted Infections

The vulnerable respiratory apparatus is easily invaded by microorganisms. Breathing is continuous and as respiratory gases are wafted in and out, infecting organisms find free passage deep inside the body. The site of entry is commonly the nasopharynx, but entry can also occur through the oropharynx and the conjunctiva. The lachrymal glands drain into the nasopharynx and experimental studies have shown that this is often a more certain method of infection than directly through the nose. The respiratory system also includes connections to the middle ear, the sinuses and the gastro-intestinal tract.

The ciliated lining and mucus-secreting cells of the respiratory tract can act as non-specific host defence mechanisms entrapping microorganisms and passing them to the exterior. In attempting to expel these secretions from the body by coughing or spitting, organisms may be transmitted to another host. The lymphoid tissues, especially the tonsils and adenoids, guard the respiratory apparatus, but sometimes may themselves become foci of infection.

Respiratory infections are usually transmitted by direct contact between individuals and generally the closer the contact, the greater the chance of spread. As contact

between human beings is a necessary part of life, control becomes more difficult and non-specific. Even so, the respiratory diseases are an enigma, the voluminous quantities of expelled organisms are sufficient to infect the entire population, yet only some individuals manifest disease. It is the infective dose and the host response, which determines whether infection will occur. Environmental factors that increase the infective dose (e.g. overcrowding) or reduce the host resistance (e.g. malnutrition or concomitant infections) can have a marked effect.

This chapter includes airborne transmitted infections that present as diseases of the respiratory system and also includes diseases of other systems of the body that are transmitted by the airborne route. Most of the skin infections, covered in Chapter 12, are also transmitted mainly by the airborne route.

13.1 Tuberculosis

One of the major diseases in the world, tuberculosis poses considerable challenge in developing countries. Not only are a proportion of the population infected with this debilitating and often fatal disease, but the period of infectiousness is prolonged (approximately 5 years in an untreated case), permitting transmission to many other persons. Indeed, in a number of countries, an endemic balance has been achieved whereby the number of cases that resolve spontaneously, are cured by medical treatment or die, are replaced by an equal number of new cases entering the pool of tuberculosis. HIV infection has added to the likelihood of people developing tuberculosis so that it is increasing in sub-Saharan Africa. In the world, 8 million people develop tuberculosis every year and 2 million die from it.

Organism *Mycobacterium tuberculosis,* but infection can also be caused by *M. bovis* (from cattle) or *M. africanum.* There are many mycobacteria occurring naturally, including *M. avium, M. intracellulare* and *M. scrofulaceum,* that can sensitize the individual and interfere with BCG vaccination. In endemic countries, *M. tuberculosis* is widespread, with 1–3% of the population per year being at risk of infection.

Clinical features A productive cough with weight loss, fever and anaemia are the most important signs of tuberculosis. Any chronic cough persisting for 3 weeks or more, especially if there is also weight loss and anaemia, should be regarded as a possible case of tuberculosis and sputum smears taken. Haemoptysis is an important diagnostic sign and may be streaking of the sputum with blood or frank coughing-up of fresh blood.

Tuberculosis infects people in a spectrum of severity depending on the host response, the dose of organisms and the length of time. The first sign of infection is the primary complex in which the organism is localized to an area of the lung with a corresponding enlargement of the hilar lymph nodes. In the majority of people, this heals completely or with a residual scar, and the person develops immunity to further challenge. If healing does not occur, then the focus extends to cause glandular enlarge-

ment, pleural effusion or cavity formation. The third phase of the disease results from complications of the regional nodes. These may be obstructive, leading to collapse and consolidation, cause erosion and bronchial destruction or spread locally. The final stage is one of blood stream spread, disseminating bacilli to all parts of the body where they may produce tuberculous meningitis or miliary infection. Long-term complications are those of bones, joints, renal tract, skin and many other rare sites. These features are illustrated in Fig. 13.1.

The risk of developing local and disseminated lesions decreases over a period of 2 years. If the majority of cases are going to progress, they will do so within 12 months of infection or 6 months from the development of the primary complex. By the end of 2 years, 90% of the complications would have occurred. Bone and other late complications are a very small proportion beyond this time.

Diagnosis Tuberculosis is spread by droplet infection, so sputum-positive cases transmit the disease much more efficiently than those whose sputum is negative on microscopy. The risk to the community is, therefore, from pulmonary tuberculosis and the emphasis should be on finding these cases by taking a sputum smear, ideally confirmed by culture. The comparative costs of diagnostic techniques are:

Smear	0.02
Culture	0.20
Sensitivity	0.40
Full plate X-ray	1.00

Fifty sputum smears can be made for the equivalent cost of one X-ray and this economy can be used for diagnosing cases in the community. Anybody presenting to the health services with a cough for 3 weeks or more should be asked to produce some sputum and a smear made. This is dried and stained with Ziehl–Neelsen for acid-fast bacilli. X-ray examination has a high sensitivity and, therefore, is of more value in countries with a low incidence and plentiful

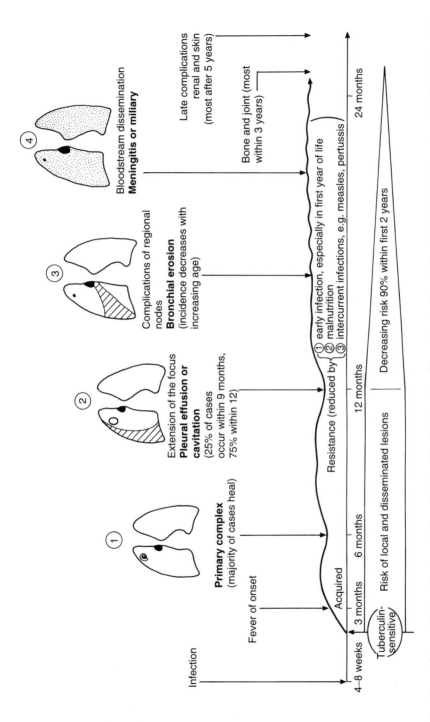

Fig. 13.1. The evolution of untreated primary tuberculosis (modified). (Reproduced by permission from Miller, F.J.W. (1982) *Tuberculosis in Children*, Churchill Livingstone, Edinburgh.)

resources, but sputum microbiology is still necessary to confirm the diagnosis and provide cultures for drug susceptibility testing.

A simpler form of search is made in the village of a newly diagnosed case. The contacts are examined to see if there is anybody with a productive cough or clinical signs, and a smear made. Contacts should be given BCG. Chemoprophylaxis is given to children under 6 years and to contacts positive for HIV, and followed up at regular intervals. This can all be included in the national registration system.

Transmission is by the airborne route, with coughing and spitting being the main modes of disseminating the organism. Many people meet the tubercle bacillus in early life, acquire resistance and are quite unaware of ever having come into contact with it. A proportion, approximately 5%, will manifest the disease in varying levels of severity. It might be nothing more than an enlargement of the primary focus with a few systemic effects, only to resolve spontaneously, while others may have respiratory symptoms or progress rapidly to blood stream spread presenting as a case of miliary or tuberculous meningitis. The type and severity of the disease is determined by the host response, but why one person should develop tuberculosis, and another should not, cannot generally be determined. There is some evidence that susceptibility may be genetically determined as people who have suffered from tuberculosis, even if adequately cured, are more likely to develop a new infection a second time. Some families are particularly susceptible, as with the famous literary family the Bronte sisters, where first the mother died from tuberculosis, followed by nearly all the children, yet the father never succumbed to the disease. The dose of bacilli might also be important because young children in close contact with an active case more commonly develop severe tuberculosis (miliary or meningitis). Factors that are known to reduce resistance are:

- young age, especially the first year of life;
- pregnancy;
- malnutrition;
- intercurrent infections, such as measles, whooping cough and streptococcal infection;
- HIV infection;
- occupations or environments that damage the lung (mining, dust, smoke).

As well as variation amongst individuals, there are also considerable differences in the susceptibility of populations. This can be measured by the annual tuberculosis infection rate, which compares the tuberculin reaction of non-vaccinated subjects of the same age every 5 years. With BCG vaccination at birth, this cannot be done any longer, but data obtained before this became a universal policy is still valid. Another method of estimating incidence is from tuberculosis notifications as seen in Fig. 13.2.

There are also environmental factors and density is as important as susceptibility of the population. The dose of bacilli that the individual will meet is increased by continued contact over a period of time. This dose/time factor is more likely to be found in conditions of poverty and overcrowding. If the dose is sufficiently large and maintained for long enough, even the defences of the immunologically competent individual may be broken down.

The risk of infection is greatest in the young and rises again in the old, so overcrowding increases the opportunity for infection to be acquired at a younger age. Since the young mix extensively, they will have a greater opportunity for passing on infection. At the other end of life, the elderly often form persistent foci in a community, a potent source of infection to the young.

HIV infection has changed the epidemiology and presentation of tuberculosis, especially in Africa, leading to more lower lobe and extrapulmonary disease. (There are estimated to be more than 20 million persons worldwide with dual tuberculosis and HIV, with the majority of these cases in Africa.) Reduced host response has increased susceptibility and allowed reactivation or reinfection to take place as well as increasing the likelihood of new infection

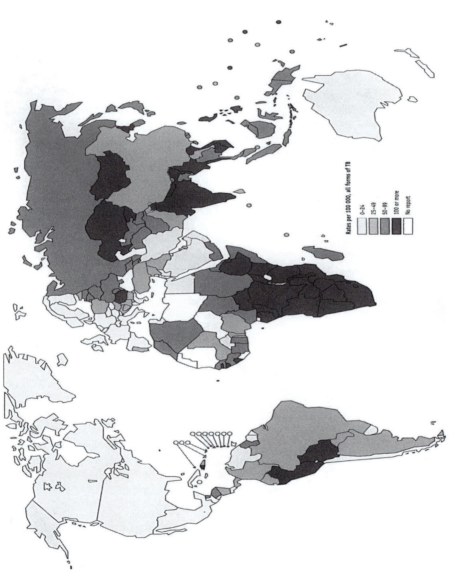

The designations employed and the presentation of material on this map do not imply the expression of any opinion whatsoever on the part of the World Health Organization concerning the legal status of any country, territory, city or area or of its authorities, or concerning the delimitation of its frontiers or boundaries. Dashed lines represent approximate border lines for which there may not yet be full agreement.

Fig. 13.2. Tuberculosis notification rates, 2002. Reproduced by permission of the World Health Organization, Geneva.

from a contact or case; however, there is evidence to suggest that HIV/tuberculosis patients are less infectious. Conversely, tuberculosis patients are more likely to rapidly progress to full-blown acquired immunodeficiency syndrome (AIDS) when infected with the HIV virus. Initially HIV-infected tuberculosis patients commonly present with pulmonary infection similar to the HIV negative case, but as the disease progresses, extrapulmonary tuberculosis predominates and other manifestations of HIV disease, such as chronic diarrhoea, generalized lymphadenopathy, oral thrush and Kaposi's sarcoma, are more common. All HIV-positive cases should, therefore, be investigated for tuberculosis and all tuberculosis cases tested for HIV. Despite the increase in extrapulmonary tuberculosis, it is still the sputum-positive case that is responsible for transmission of infection and this must remain the priority in searching for cases.

Consumption of unpasteurized milk may result in bovine tuberculosis in humans where the disease is present in the animal population. This presents with enlargement and suppuration of the cervical lymph nodes rather than pulmonary disease. It is now less common than before with the testing of cattle and pasteurization of milk, but in developing countries where cattle and their produce are an important part of the diet, such as in Central and South America, bovine tuberculosis is found.

Incubation period The period between infection and development of the primary complex is 4–12 weeks.

Period of communicability A new, untreated case of tuberculosis will normally produce organisms for 12–18 months, but in those that develop a low-grade infection with chronic cough, infection can continue for a considerable period of time (about 5 years). Once treatment has started, the person becomes non-infectious in about 2 weeks.

Occurrence and distribution Tuberculosis is found worldwide (Fig. 13.2) in various levels of severity. Countries of low preva-

lence are defined as those where less than 10% of children under 15 years have a positive tuberculin test. These are largely the countries of Western Europe and North America. Tuberculosis, however, is increasing in Eastern Europe and the former USSR. Nearly the whole of the tropical world has a high prevalence rate with some countries experiencing over 50% of the under 15-year-olds being tuberculin-positive. In addition, urban areas have higher prevalence rates than rural areas. The rates are high in Africa and parts of South America. Asia, India, Myanmar, Thailand and Indonesia all have high tuberculin-positive rates. In the Americas, the indigenous peoples have a much higher rate than the non-indigenous. There is a high susceptibility in Pacific Islands in which tuberculosis was an unknown disease until the arrival of explorers, who introduced the disease.

Control and prevention There are four main strategies for the control and prevention of tuberculosis in the following order of priority:

- search and contact tracing for new cases;
- adequate treatment of all cases, especially the sputum-positive;
- improvement of social and living conditions;
- BCG vaccination.

Vaccination by BCG induces cell-mediated immunity to the mycobacteria and does not generate humoral immunity, as do other vaccines. BCG vaccination, therefore, alerts the body's defences rather than inducing antibody formation. After a BCG vaccination a primary infection will still take place, but the progressive or disseminated infection will be reduced.

Effectiveness of BCG varies considerably in different countries – in Europe, there is a good response, while in India, it is marginal. This is thought to be due to atypical mycobacteria circulating in the environment and, therefore, BCG should be given at birth in developing countries or as soon after as possible. School entry or 10–14 years is the main age for giving BCG in developed countries, while it is likely that some developed countries will move to a selective vaccination policy giving BCG only to high-risk groups, such as immigrants. BCG should be administered to all infants, including those born to mothers with HIV infection. It should not, however, be given to those with symptomatic HIV or pregnant women.

BCG is a freeze-dried vaccine given intra-dermally. Other methods, such as multiple puncture, jet injection or scarification, have been found to be not so satisfactory. The vaccine is sensitive to heat and light and, therefore, must be carefully protected.

Sputum smear examination is a very simple technique for screening populations, especially where there has recently been a case of tuberculosis. All contacts of a case should have several sputum smears taken, concentrating on the young and elderly. If a contact has not been vaccinated, then they should be given BCG. Close contacts under 6 years of age and HIV-positive persons should be given prophylaxis, unless they are suspected of having disease in which case they should be given treatment.

Tuberculosis is particularly a disease of poor social conditions and overcrowding as shown by the remarkable decline of the infection from industrialized countries prior to the advent of chemotherapy. The disease was as bad, if not worse in Europe, at the turn of the century than in many developing countries now, but showed a progressive and continuous reduction of cases as living conditions improved. As standards increased, there was a demand for improved housing with less people sharing the same room so that overcrowding declined. Personal hygiene improved and such practices as spitting disappeared almost completely (see Fig. 13.3).

Treatment and prophylaxis The functions of chemotherapy can be summarized as follows:

- treatment of individual cases to reduce morbidity and mortality;
- reduce the number and period of infectious cases;
- provide a method of disease reduction in developing countries where the

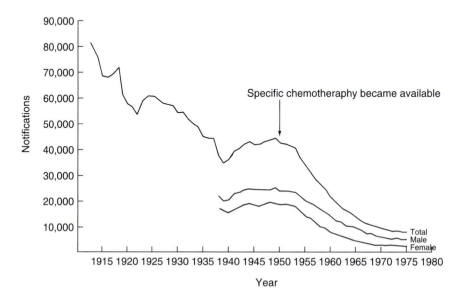

Fig. 13.3. The decline of tuberculosis in England and Wales 1912–1975. (From DHSS (1977) *Annual Report of the Chief Medical Officer, Department of Health and Social Security for 1976,* Her Majesty's Stationary Office, London. Crown copyright, reproduced with the permission of the Controller of HMSO.)

raising of social standards would take some time to achieve;

- prevent the emergence of resistant strains.

All treatment should be directly observed therapy (DOT) to ensure compliance. A newly diagnosed case of tuberculosis should be treated with a four-drug regimen for 2 months consisting of the following:

Isoniazid	300 mg daily
Rifampicin	10 mg/kg up to 600 mg daily
Pyrazinamide	35 mg/kg up to 2 g daily
Ethambutol	25 mg/kg daily or streptomycin 15 mg/kg daily

This is followed by isoniazid and rifampicin taken daily or three times weekly, for a further 4 months. If the taking of treatment cannot be directly observed, then isoniazid plus ethambutol taken daily should be used instead and given for a period of 6 months. Treatment should continue for 9–12 months in those cases of miliary, tuberculosis meningitis or bone/joint disease.

Prophylaxis with isoniazid can be given to close contacts under 35 years of age and to babies (5 mg/kg) born to mothers, who develop tuberculosis shortly before or after delivery.

Surveillance A system to follow-up all diagnosed cases of tuberculosis discharged from hospital or health centre is required on the following lines:

1. Register the case with a central registry on diagnosis.
2. When the patient is discharged, inform the registry, the nearest clinic to the person's home and the supervising doctor.
3. The clinic ensures the patient receives regular follow-up treatment or goes and finds them if they default.
4. The supervising doctor visits on a regular basis to check the clinical records and make sure that the registered patients are receiving treatment.
5. When the full course of treatment is completed and the doctor is satisfied that the patient is cured, the Central Registry is notified. Reminders and double checks can be built into the system, such as the central registry sending out quarterly checks on each patient.

The sophistication of the system depends upon the resources of the country, but lack of resources is never an excuse not to have a system at all. To not follow-up a partially treated patient is a waste of expensive hospital treatment, encourages the development of resistant organisms and increases the risk to the community. Follow-up is always cheaper than re-diagnosis and treatment.

Evaluation of the tuberculosis control programmes is primarily by cohort analysis in which the proportion of new smear-positive cases that are cured or are certified to have completed the treatment, but no smear done, is measured. The WHO target is 85%. Other useful indicators are:

- annual rate of new tuberculosis cases diagnosed;
- rate of sputum-positive cases diagnosed;
- proportion of children under 5 years of age diagnosed;
- proportion of miliary and meningeal tuberculosis;
- rate of sputum smears examined;
- rate of BCG scars, on survey;
- relapse rate;
- rate lost to follow-up.

A decrease in the proportion of children under 5 years of age diagnosed and those with miliary and meningeal tuberculosis will indicate improvement. However, this will need to be confirmed by a sputum smear survey. Nursing staff should be taught to always give the BCG vaccination in the same place, normally the deltoid area or lateral forearm below the elbow of the left arm, so that touring staff, school teachers, etc. can rapidly examine a group of children.

The WHO DOT's strategy is summarized as:

- political commitment;
- secure drug supply;

- diagnosis by smear microscopy of passive case-finding;
- treatment with rifampicin containing DOT for 6–8 months;
- cohort analysis.

13.2 Acute Respiratory Infections (ARI)

The acute respiratory infections (ARI) are the commonest causes of ill health in the world. WHO have estimated that there are 14–15 million deaths a year in children under 5 years of age and one-third of these are due to ARI, yet despite their importance, they are a poorly defined group of diseases. They include the common cold, influenza, pneumonia, bronchitis and a number of other infections. They can be separated by clinical criteria, but it is the differing response of the individual to the organism that determines the clinical severity and management. A mild infection from an upper respiratory tract infection in one person may develop in another to a life-threatening attack of pneumonia. It is, therefore, not only the organism that determines the disease, but also the patient's response to the organism.

Organisms A number of different organisms have been implicated including *Streptococcus pneumoniae*, *Haemophilus influenzae*, *Mycoplasma pneumoniae*, influenza, rhinoviruses, adenoviruses, metapneumovirus and respiratory syncytial virus (RSV). Viruses are of a wide range, with each species having a number of serotypes, with new ones appearing from time to time. However, the most important cause is *S. pneumoniae* or the pneumococcus or *H. influenzae*. The host defends him or herself by producing an appropriate immune response, but because of the large number of serotypes, it is a continuous process. Infection will cause illness in some people, but not in others who have developed an immune response to the specific organism or an antigenically similar serotype. New antigenic mutations, as occur in influenza, can cause epidemic or pandemic spread

because no prior contact with the new variant has been made.

Clinical features ARIs are divided into upper and lower ARIs, the former producing a running nose, sneezing and headache, while the main symptoms of lower respiratory tract infection are cough, shortness of breath and inward drawing of the bony structure of the lower chest wall during inspiration, which is called chest indrawing. Both are generally accompanied by fever. The main pathological feature is pneumonia, which can either be lobar or bronchial. In lobar pneumonia, one or more well-defined lobes of the lung are involved, whereas in bronchial pneumonia the condition is widespread. The causes of pneumonia are listed in Table 13.1.

Diagnosis Identifying the organism by culture of the sputum can be attempted where facilities permit, but in most developing countries, ARI will be diagnosed on clinical criteria.

Transmission is by coughing out a large number of organisms in a fine aerosol of droplets, which are either breathed in, enter via the conjunctiva or are swallowed from fingers or utensils. Susceptibility and response are determined by host factors, some of which are listed below:

1. *Age.* Young children develop obstructive diseases, such as croup (laryngo-tracheo-bronchitis) and bronchiolitis. Tonsillitis is commonest in school age, whereas influenza and pneumonia are important causes of death in the elderly. In young children, mortality is inversely related to age.
2. *Portal of entry.* Volunteers have been more easily infected by some organisms applied to the conjunctiva than through the nasopharynx.
3. *Nutrition.* Low birth weight and malnourished children have a higher morbidity and mortality. Certain nutritional deficiencies, such as deficiencies of vitamin A and zinc, contribute to the development of a more severe disease and higher death rate.

Breast-feeding appears to have a protective effect.

4. *Socio-economic.* ARI is a disease of poverty with higher incidence in lower socio-economic groups and those that live in urban slums. Higher rates of lower respiratory disease have been found with increasing family size. Much of the reason for this increase appears to be due to increased contact and agglomeration as shown by children attending day care facilities or school where infection occurs irrespective of social class.

5. *Air pollution.* A correlation with domestic air pollution has been shown in South Africa and Nepal. Passive smoking may affect pulmonary function and make the child more susceptible to infection as well as influence the child to become a smoker.

6. *Climate.* More respiratory infections are found in the cooler parts of the world or in the higher altitude regions of the tropics. There is a distinct seasonal effect in many countries, with more respiratory infections in the winter. However, cold alone is not a causative factor. 'Cold' derives its name from the belief that becoming chilled or standing in a draught is responsible, but when volunteers are subjected to these stresses and inoculated with rhinoviruses, they develop no more 'colds' than controls.

7. *Other infections.* Any infection, which causes damage to the respiratory mucosa, will allow a mild infecting organism to progress to more serious consequences. The most important of these diseases is measles, with post-measles pneumonia being particularly common.

Incubation period This varies with the organism, but in most cases is 1–3 days.

Period of communicability Variable; for the entire period of any respiratory symptoms.

Occurrence and distribution Worldwide, the most important cause of death in children in developing countries.

Treatment The first line of action is to assess the severity of illness and give treatment. This is supportive therapy for mild infec-

tions and the active administration of antibiotics to the severe case. The mild infection is best treated at home and kept away from sources of other infection, which may cause more serious disease, while the severe case requires early treatment to prevent complications and death. In children, the respiratory rate and chest indrawing are used to decide management:

- Mild cases, with a respiratory rate of less than 40 breaths/min in children of age 2–12 months and 50 breaths/min in the children of age 1–5 years, are treated at home with supportive therapy. The mother should be encouraged to nurse her child, giving it plenty of fluids (breast-feeding or from a cup), regular feeding, cleaning the nose, maintaining it at a comfortable temperature and avoiding contact with others.
- Moderate cases, with a respiratory rate of over 40 breaths/min in under-1-year-olds and 50 breaths/min in children 1–5 years old, but with no chest indrawing, should be given antibiotics (oral cotrimoxazole (4 mg/kg twice daily), oral amoxycillin (15 mg/kg three times a day) or intramuscular penicillin G) and nursed at home.
- Severe cases, with chest indrawing, cyanosis or too sick to feed, must be admitted as in-patients and given active support as well as treatment with antibiotics.

Control and prevention The first step in management of a child with ARI is to separate the mild from the moderate and to treat the moderate and severe. The essence is speed and active treatment. This can easily be taught at the primary health care level. The mother can be educated on the management of her child with a mild infection and when to refer. It is the delay in referral and treatment that will allow a moderate case to become severe and the severe to die.

The village health worker can identify and treat the mild or moderate case of ARI using simple diagnostic criteria and a standard treatment protocol. Measuring the respiratory rate and knowing which action to take are the most important aspects. Training and supervision of primary health care workers is a priority in the management of ARI.

Preventive actions that can be undertaken are listed below:

- *Reduce contact.* ARIs are just as common in industrialized countries as they are in developing countries, but infant deaths from respiratory infections in the former have declined. The reason would appear to be due to smaller families and greater birth intervals, permitting increased individual care of children and better nutrition. The child is reared at home and does not need to be carried round where it is exposed at a very young age to infecting organisms.
- *Good nutrition.* Well-nourished children are in a stronger position to defend themselves against any infection. Encourage breast-feeding, especially during early stages of illness. Providing additional nutritional support to children with measles can prevent them developing post-measles pneumonia.
- *Health education.* Teach people to cough away from others, cover the mouth when coughing, not to spit or smoke and provide proper ventilation for smoke and fumes.
- *Vaccination of childhood infections.* The danger of developing pneumonia after measles is a serious problem, so prevention of measles will reduce the severe forms of ARI. Indeed, measles vaccination is perhaps the single most effective preventive method (Section 12.2). Vaccination for *H. influenzae* is now recommended by WHO in routine childhood immunization programmes. Pertussis, diphtheria and BCG vaccination should also be encouraged.
- *Other vaccines.* Influenza vaccine is prepared annually according to the expected strain of influenza and should be given to those at risk (e.g. immunocompromised and those with chronic respiratory infections) if facilities allow. The polysaccharide pneumococcal vaccine is not recommended in routine childhood vaccination programmes, but could be used in special circumstances, such as for sple-

nectomized children and the immuno-deficient. However, the new conjugate pneumococcal vaccine shows promise in children under 2 years of age and is likely to be included in childhood vaccination programmes if sufficient supplies can be made available. Vaccines against RSV, parainfluenza and the adenoviruses are in preparation.

Surveillance Measles generally occurs as seasonal epidemics, which can be forecasted and top-up vaccination given (Section 12.2). Influenza is normally pandemic with warning given of strain of organism and vaccine composition, allowing sufficient time for persons at risk to be protected.

13.3 Influenza

Organism There are three types of influenza viruses A, B and C with H antigen (15 subtypes) and N antigen (9 subtypes), so that the virus is designated as H1N1, H1N2,..., H3N2. In addition, the site of isolation, culture number and year of isolation are used (e.g. A/Beijing/262/95) (H1N1). So far a major antigenic shift to H4 or N3 in human infection has not yet occurred. Antigenic drift in both A and B viruses, producing new strains occurs at infrequent intervals and is responsible for most epidemics.

Clinical features Influenza presents with fever, malaise, muscle aches and upper respiratory symptoms of sudden onset. There is initially a dry cough, which can sometimes be severe and often leads to secondary infection, with the production of sputum. It is a serious infection in the elderly with high death rates. When a major antigenic shift occurs as it did in 1918, all ages are susceptible and the number of deaths can be enormous (an estimated 50 million).

Diagnosis is on clinical grounds taking care to differentiate influenza (occurring seasonally or in epidemics) from other causes of respiratory infections, especially the common cold. Direct immunofluorescence (DIF) or virus isolation from throat or nasal swabs can be made in specialist centres.

Transmission is via the airborne route through sneezing or coughing, but can also be by direct contact with mucus. Influenza is highly infectious and spreads throughout whole communities, potentiated by overcrowding and frequent social contact, such as at the work place.

Influenza also occurs in birds and pigs and these may well be the reservoir from which human infection originates. The close association of humans with domestic birds and animals, particularly in South China, is thought to be how new variants arise.

Incubation period 1–5 days with a mean of 2 days.

Period of communicability 2 days before onset of symptoms to 5 days after.

Occurrence and distribution Influenza A is responsible for pandemics and regular seasonal outbreaks, B for smaller localized outbreaks and C produces mild infections. In the tropics, epidemics tend to occur in the rainy season, while in temperate climates, influenza is nearly always a disease of the winter months. Pandemics have occurred in 1889, 1918, 1957, 1968 and 1977.

Control and prevention As influenza is highly infectious, the majority of the population becomes infected during an epidemic, but any reduction of social contact, particularly in crowded places, can reduce this likelihood. Spitting should be outlawed and people encouraged not to cough directly at people. The wearing of masks, as practised in China and Japan, is probably more effective in preventing spread from an infected person wearing a mask than in protecting the non-infected. Once the cloth mask becomes damp through exhaled breath, it ceases to be effective, but tight-fitting masks with changeable filters should offer reasonable protection.

Influenza vaccine is available for protecting at-risk persons, such as people over 65 years of age, those with chronic chest or kidney disease and the immunocompromised. The difficulty of producing a vaccine is that a new one has to be produced each year, containing the expected composition of antigenic sub-units. The WHO collaboration centres, with reference laboratories throughout the world, provide advance warning to assist countries in producing vaccine, but new techniques, such as virus manipulation to anticipate natural change in the virus, could allow banks of virus to be kept in store.

Surveillance Sentinel reporting centres with an agreed case definition probably provide a better idea of the influenza situation than collecting data of variable quality from every clinic and hospital. This can be compared with laboratory-confirmed cases where facilities permit. WHO reports on the global situation in the Weekly Epidemiological Record (WER) from a worldwide network of reporting centres.

13.4 Whooping Cough (Pertussis)

Organism *Bordetella pertussis. B. parapertussis* produces a milder disease.

Clinical features Illness commences with upper respiratory symptoms, fever and cough, which becomes paroxysmal with the characteristic whoop, or sometimes ends in vomiting. The classic 'whooping' disease is not seen in children under 3 months of age, when instead, they have attacks of cyanosis and stop breathing. Whooping cough is a serious disease if it occurs at a young age, the severity being inversely proportional to age. A mild infection in the older child, it becomes an important cause of death in the very young.

Diagnosis is mainly on clinical criteria, but culture of the organism from a nose or throat swab can be attempted, although the organism is difficult to grow. Serology is useful.

Transmission is via airborne spread of droplets particularly during the early stage of illness. Older children and adults may have such a mild infection that their importance as a source of infection is not realized. Vaccinated individuals can have subclinical infection in which organisms are disseminated.

Incubation period 7–10 days.

Period of communicability 4 weeks from the first symptoms, being most infectious in the first week, before the paroxysms start.

Occurrence and distribution Whooping cough is a serious disease in tropical countries contributing to high rates of infant mortality. Vaccination programmes have markedly reduced the disease in the temperate regions of the world, but where the vaccination programme has decreased or been abandoned, it has rapidly returned as a major health problem.

Where the young infant is always carried around by its mother, there is an increased opportunity for exposure, coming into close contact with other children who might be infectious.

Control and prevention Isolation of cases, especially of young children and infants, should be instituted. Infective children should be kept away from school, markets and any place where young children are likely to congregate. Known contacts of a case of whooping cough (e.g. in the extended family of a case) should be given a booster vaccination if they have been vaccinated before, otherwise they should receive prophylactic erythromycin and vaccine.

The median age for the disease is 2 years, but because of its severity, vaccination should be started at 1–2 months. Three doses of vaccine are given, normally combined with tetanus and diphtheria as triple vaccine.

Treatment Erythromycin is only effective when given in the first week of the disease.

Fluid loss is an important cause of mortality so mothers should be encouraged to give extra fluids and breast-feed immediately after a coughing bout.

Surveillance In many countries, whooping cough is a notifiable disease.

13.5 Diphtheria

Organism *Corynebacterium diphtheriae* and rarely *C. ulcerans*.

Clinical features Diphtheria produces both local and systemic effects. The organism can infect the tonsils, pharynx, larynx, nose or skin, forming a pale grey membrane and local inflammation. Symptoms are fever, sore throat and enlarged cervical lymph nodes in the pharyngeal form, blood-stained discharge in the nasal form and skin ulcers in the cutaneous form. The inflammatory reaction produced in the respiratory tract can lead to swelling of the neck and respiratory obstruction. From the primary site, exotoxin is produced, which can cause myocarditis or neuropathy, especially cranial nerve palsies.

Diagnosis Throat, nose or skin swab of the exudate. A culture of the organism should be sent to a reference laboratory if possible.

Transmission Diphtheria can be transmitted by:

- airborne transmission of droplets;
- direct contact with lesions and exudates;
- indirect through articles soiled with discharges;
- ingestion of contaminated milk.

In an unimmunized population, there is a high incidence of carriers and a low incidence of cases in a ratio of approximately 19:1. Between 6% and 40% of children are infected every year so that by 5 years, some 75% have been infected and by 15 years, nearly all the children are infected. This means that by 15 years of age, the majority of children have developed immunity either by a sub-clinical infection or one in which clinical symptoms were revealed.

Incubation period 2–5 days.

Period of communicability About 2 weeks.

Occurrence and distribution Commonly a disease of children, diphtheria can occur in non-immunized adults with serious results. Outbreaks of the disease are seen, but it is probably a much more frequent disease than realised, as sub-clinical transmission through skin and possibly nasal lesions, maintains immunity. This was probably the situation in many tropical countries, but now universal childhood vaccination programmes are protecting young children. A breakdown of these programmes, or remaining pockets of unvaccinated adults, leads to serious disease.

Control and prevention Diphtheria is prevented by vaccination of all children with three doses of diphtheria toxoid. This is normally combined with pertussis and tetanus as triple vaccine commencing in the first or second month of life. Ideally, a booster dose should be given at 18 months to 4 years of age. As with polio and rubella vaccination, diphtheria immunization shifts the likelihood of disease to an older and more dangerous age so complete coverage of all children is imperative. Adults visiting an endemic country from one in which the vaccination status is good, should have an adult-type booster (adult Td) in which the concentration of the toxoid is reduced. Ideally, adults, particularly travellers, should have booster doses of adult Td every 10 years.

In the event of an outbreak, previously vaccinated contacts should be given tetanus and diphtheria toxoids and those not vaccinated the toxoid and an antibiotic (erythromycin or penicillin).

Treatment If diphtheria antitoxin is available, it should be given to cases following a test dose for hypersensitivity. Erythromycin or procaine penicillin G should be used for specific treatment.

Surveillance Diphtheria is a notifiable disease in most countries.

13.6 Meningococcal Meningitis

Organism *Neisseria meningitidis.* Many serogroups and sub-groups have been identified, but of these A, B, C and Y are the most important in producing disease, while A and C predominate in epidemics. W135 has recently been responsible for some outbreaks.

Clinical features Fever, headache, vomiting, neck stiffness and progressive loss of consciousness. A petechial rash, which does not blanch, is an important sign. Infants show floppiness and high-pitched crying, while children may present with convulsions.

Diagnosis is by lumbar puncture, but should not delay early treatment, which can be given straight away and lumbar puncture done afterwards if necessary. A Gram stain is only reliable in some 50% of cases, so culture should be attempted wherever possible and sensitivity obtained. Blood should also be taken for culture and polymerase chain reaction (PCR). Smears from petechiae can also be examined by Gram stain.

Transmission is by airborne spread of droplets and from direct contact with secretions from the nose or throat. The organism is found commonly in the nasopharynx so other factors must also be responsible for meningitis to occur.

Epidemic meningitis was first studied in cooler climates and an association found with overcrowding, especially in military institutions. The organism when introduced into an overcrowded environment produced both cases and carriers (nasal). As the number of carriers increased, the number of cases of meningitis did so likewise.

However, in the African (Sahel) epidemic form, the heat makes people spend much of their time out of doors and overcrowding is not a phenomenon at this time of year (Fig. 13.4). Although overcrowding seems to increase the number of carriers and the potential for more cases, it does not explain the mechanism for causing meningitis.

The organism inhabits the nasal mucosa within which it is anatomically very close to the meninges, although separated by formidable barriers of bone and membrane. The generally accepted theory is that the organism passes from this site into the blood stream, crosses the blood–brain barrier and enters the cerebrospinal fluid (CSF). Experimental evidence does not substantiate this route unless there has been some trauma to the meninges. Difficult though the direct route may seem, it has been shown that minute passages through the bone of the skull do occur and transmission of organisms along this route is a possibility. Furthermore, if organisms are introduced directly into the sub-arachnoid space, infection will only occur if a critical level is exceeded (10^3 organisms in dogs), suggesting that this route could frequently be invaded, but only when there is excessive infection does meningitis develop. An alter-native explanation is that transmission is directly from the nose through the skull and any traumatic insult to the nasal mucosa, such as the intense drying out during the Sahel hot season, or upper respiratory tract infection in colder climates, potentiates a greater number of organisms to pass along these minute channels and overcome the defences of the meninges.

Incubation period 2–10 days.

Period of communicability Once effective treatment has started, the patient ceases to be infective within 24 h, but any carrier will continue to produce organisms for between 2 weeks and 10 months.

Occurrence and distribution Meningococcal meningitis occurs in epidemics, especially in the Sahel part of Africa in a band stretching from Senegal to Ethiopia. The epidemics are markedly seasonal occurring in the early part of the year when the temperature is hottest and relative humidity at its lowest. With the arrival of the rains, the epidemic abates (Fig. 13.4). The amount of rainfall (1100 mm) delineates the southern boundary of the meningitis belt, whereas

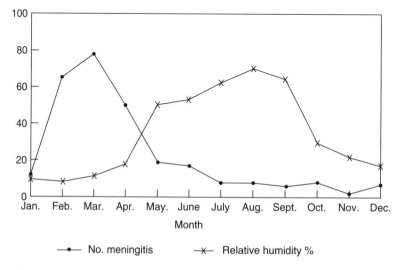

Fig. 13.4. The seasonal variation of meningococcal meningitis in relation to relative humidity in the Sahel region of Africa.

the northern boundary is the desert. Within this area, major epidemics, mainly of group A, occur at 7–14-year intervals, with lesser ones in between.

In addition to the meningitis epidemic belt in Africa, there have also been epidemics of group A organisms in India and Nepal, and group B in the Americas, Europe and Pacific Island Nations.

Epidemic meningitis is commonest in the age group of 5–15 years, with males more frequently affected than females. Only about one in 500 persons infected with the organism will develop meningitis. Large, poor families and other conditions where there is overcrowding, such as religious and social gatherings, refugee camps and labour lines, make meningitis more likely.

Control and prevention Overcrowding encourages the transfer of the infecting organism and the carrier state, as well as increasing the dose of bacteria that may be transmitted. All efforts should be made to reduce overcrowding. It may be necessary to close schools and reduce congregation of people, such as in markets and religious gatherings. In the long term, improvement of housing and family planning will have an effect.

Chemoprophylaxis should be given to close contacts, such as all family members, school friends and anyone sharing in a large communal sleeping place (such as a dormitory). Rifampicin 10 mg/kg twice daily for 2 days, or if still sensitive to sulphonamides, sulphadiazine 150 mg/kg for 2 days can be used. Chemoprophylaxis is not recommended in large epidemics.

There are several vaccines containing either A and C, or A, C, Y and W135. Unfortunately, the very young and those with acute malaria develop reduced immunity. There is also a genetic variation with some ethnic groups having a poor response. Due to these different factors, duration of immunity varies from 3 years or less in young children and must be measured for each community when formulating a vaccination programme. Vaccine can be used to immunize those most at risk concentrating on the 2–20-year age group and household contacts of cases. When there is an epidemic, mass vaccination should be given to communities in the affected area, including vaccinating children below 2 years of age. It has been suggested that an incidence of 15 cases per 100,000 in a well-defined population for 2 consecutive weeks heralds the beginning of an epidemic and the need to start mass vaccination.

A conjugated C vaccine has been found to be effective in all age groups, especially young children, and in countries where group C meningococcal disease is an important health problem it could be included in the national childhood vaccination programme. If an epidemic is found to be due to group C, then this vaccine should be used.

Treatment may need to be organized on a massive scale when an epidemic occurs by using dispensers, school teachers or other educated people to care for isolated communities. Temporary treatment centres (schools, churches, warehouses, etc.) may need to be set up, rather than bring people into hospital. Benzyl penicillin or chloramphenicol should be used, but in many countries, resistance to these antibiotics will require the use of cephalosporins. If the organism is unknown, use chloramphenicol. In epidemics, long-acting chloramphenicol in oil preparations, given as a single injection, avoids the problem of repeat injections. Dehydration is common and intravenous fluids may be required initially, followed by frequent drinks administered by an attending adult.

Surveillance The regular epidemics that occur in Africa can be forecast and a state of preparedness put into action. When there is a case of meningitis, all contacts should be examined with nasal–pharyngeal swabs. Subtyping of the organism can assist in mapping out epidemics.

13.7 *Haemophilus influenzae* (Meningitis and Pneumonia)

Organism *Haemophilus influenzae*, commonly serotype b (Hib).

Clinical features Fever, vomiting, stiff neck and rigid back in older children, bulging fontanelle in infants. A common cause of secondary infection in measles and other respiratory infections, resulting in pneumonia (see Section 13.2). *H. influenzae* can also cause epiglottitis, cellulitis, septic arthritis, osteomyelitis, empyema and pericarditis.

Diagnosis The CSF is often purulent, but this can occur in other causes of meningitis; hence culture of CSF or blood should be made. Serological tests are also of value.

Transmission Airborne transmission of droplets and direct contact with nasal–pharyngeal secretions. The organism is carried asymptomatically in the nose of carriers who are often the source of infection to infants.

Incubation period 2–4 days.

Period of communicability Chronic nasal infection can remain for a prolonged period.

Occurrence and distribution *H. influenzae* is the commonest cause of meningitis in infants and young children under 5 years of age, mainly 4–18 months of age. At present, it is a serious problem in developing countries, but with the advent of universal Hib vaccination, the incidence is likely to decline considerably, as has been the case in developed countries.

Control and prevention Routine vaccination of all children with Hib vaccine is now recommended. Vaccine should be given at the same time as DTP or as a combination vaccine (DTP/Hib). National vaccination programmes may include a booster dose at 12–18 months, but in most developing countries *H. influenzae* infection occurs before this age. Where vaccination programmes are starting or catch-up vaccination of adults and children over 18 months is to be done, a single dose of vaccine is sufficient. Hib can safely be given at the same time as meningococcal vaccine.

In the event of an outbreak of several cases of meningitis, vaccination should be given to all children under 5 years of age within the area. Contacts of all ages in households or close communities where there are unvaccinated children should be given prophylaxis with rifampicin (see also Section 13.6).

Treatment is with ampicillin or chloramphenicol.

Surveillance All family and contacts of a case of meningitis should be investigated by nose swabs. Children under 5 years of age, who have been in contact with a case, should be followed-up and treatment started if they develop early signs, such as fever.

13.8 Pneumococcal Disease

The pneumococcus causes a variety of diseases, including ARI (Section 13.2), pneumonia (Table 13.1), meningitis (Table 13.2) and otitis media (Section 13.9), which are more conveniently covered under the various diseases they cause, but in view of the availability of a vaccine, its possible use in preventing these diseases will be discussed here.

Organism *Streptococcus pneumoniae* the pneumococcus.

Clinical features *S. pneumoniae* is the commonest cause of ARI and pneumonia, presenting with cough, fever and rusty coloured sputum (from blood staining). Both bronchopneumonia and lobar pneumonia result, leading to a high mortality in

Table 13.1. The causes of pneumonia.

Organism	Clinical indicators	Occurrence
Streptococcus pneumoniae	Fever, cough, rusty sputum	Infants, elderly
Haemophilus influenzae	Slow onset, purulent sputum	Secondary infection
Influenza A and B	Fever, muscle pains	Epidemic
Morbillivirus	Measles	Seasonal epidemics
RSV	Wheezing, croup	Seasonal winter peak
Adenoviruses	Sore throat, conjunctivitis	Children, winter months
Metapneumovirus	Asthma, bronchiolitis	Children
Coronavirus – SARS	Respiratory distress	Close contact, animals?
Parainfluenza	Croup, wheezing	Children, immunodeficient
Mycoplasma pneumoniae	Slow onset, malaise	Epidemic, young adults
Chlamydia pneumoniae	Slow onset, malaise	Young adults

Staphylococcus aureus,
  Streptococcus pyogenes,
  Klebsiella pneumoniae
	Abscess formation	Secondary infection, particularly of
		  influenza

Legionella pneumophila	Increasing fever, anorexia	Air conditioners, males
Chlamydia psittaci	Fever, unproductive cough	Associated with birds
Coxiella burnetti	Fever, weight loss	Associated with sheep
Pneumocystis carinii	Progressive dyspnoea	Immunosuppressed, HIV
Cryptoccus neoformans	Mycosis, disseminated	Immunosuppressed, HIV
Nocardia asteroides	Chronic, disseminated	Immunosuppressed, HIV

Table 13.2. The causes of meningitis.

Organism	Clinical indicators	Occurrence
Neisseria meningitidis	Fever, headache, rash	Epidemic, African meningitis belt, children and adults
Haemophilus influenzae	Fever, vomiting, lethargy	Infants
Streptococcus pneumoniae	Fever, purulent CSF	Infants, elderly
Mycobacterium tuberculosis	Fever, cough, haemoptysis	Children, young adults
Staphylococci	Secondary infection	Unsterilized instruments
Escherichia coli	Floppy infant, not feeding	Following delivery
Group B streptococci	Floppy infant, not feeding	Following delivery
Listeria monocytogenes	Neonates, following birth	Infection in the mother from domestic animals or cheese
Campylobacter jejuni	Diarrhoeal illness	All ages (Section 9.2)
Echoviruses	Clear CSF, rash	Epidemic and seasonal
Coxsackieviruses	Clear CSF, rash	Epidemic and seasonal
Arboviruses	Clear CSF, encephalitis	Epidemic (Section 15.2)
Influenza A or B	Reye syndrome	Children given salicylates
Herpes zoster	Reye syndrome	Children given salicylates
Mumps virus	Parotid swelling, encephalitis	(Section 12.4)
Rubella virus	Rash, encephalitis	Neonates (Section 12.3)
Polio virus	Flaccid paralysis	Children (Section 8.10)
Herpes simplex type 1 and 2	Primary sore or genital infection	Neonates, children or adults
Treponema pallidum	Secondary or latent syphilis	Adults (Section 14.4)
Cryptococcus neoformans	Fungal infection	Tropics, males
Leptospira interrogans	Fever, myalgia, rash	Infection from rat urine
Lymphocytic choriomeningitis virus	Influenza-like symptoms	Associated with mice
Angiostrongylus cantonensis	Nematode worm	Eating snails and slugs
Borrelia burgdorfi	Lyme disease	Deer ticks (Section 16.8)
Negleria and *Acanthamoeba*	Amoebic meningoencephalitis	Swimming pools, immunocompromised

infants and the elderly. *S. pneumoniae* is also the commonest cause of otitis media, causing fever and pain in the ear. If untreated, this can lead to bacteremia and fulminant meningitis, with a high fatality rate. There is a high fever, lethargy and the patient rapidly descends into coma. *S. pneumoniae* is also a common cause of conjunctivitis.

Diagnosis is by culture of sputum, blood, eye discharges or CSF. Gram stain of the characteristic blue staining diplococci provides a rapid indication of the likely infecting organism.

Transmission is normally airborne spread of droplets during sneezing or coughing from infected persons or healthy carriers. Some 25% of persons carry *S. pneumoniae* in their nasopharynx, although these might not all be the disease-producing serotypes. Transmission can also be by direct contact or through articles soiled with secretions, such as handkerchiefs or clothes used to wipe the eye in conjunctivitis.

Incubation period 1–3 days.

Period of communicability is as long as secretions are produced in the clinical case, but the importance of healthy carriers is unclear, with some possibly responsible for producing infection in the young or elderly over considerable periods of time. Adequate treatment should render the case or carrier non-infectious within 2 days.

Occurrence and distribution Worldwide distribution, especially in developing countries, with ARI being a major cause of mortality in children. It is one of the commonest causes of terminal pneumonia in the elderly in the developed world. Overcrowding and deprived socio-economic conditions favour the disease. Miners and people living in smoke-filled huts, such as in Papua New Guinea, have an increased incidence.

Control and prevention Active management and treatment of cases of ARI and pneumonia should be carried out as outlined in

Section 13.2 and in the same way as for otitis media in Section 13.9. Family planning and the reduction of overcrowding should be advocated; smoking and having open fires in the main living part of the house should be discouraged. Hand-washing and the careful disposal of discharges from nose, throat and the infected eye should be practised.

A polysaccharide vaccine provides approximately 65% efficacy in adults and can be used in high-risk patients, such as healthy elderly adults living in institutions, patients with chronic organ failure, those with immunodeficiencies, splenectomized children and those with sickle cell disease. Unfortunately, the vaccine has limited efficacy in children under 2 years of age and, therefore, cannot be included in the routine childhood vaccination programme, and is not currently used in developing countries where a suitable vaccine would be of most value. However, a conjugate vaccine was introduced into general use in USA in June 2000 for all children 23 months old and younger, and for children 24–59 months of age who are at high risk of serious pneumococcal disease. The vaccine has been shown to be highly efficacious against invasive pneumococcal disease, but only moderately efficacious against pneumonia and otitis media. At present, demand is outstripping supply, but depending on the results experienced in USA and supply problems, it is likely that this vaccine will soon be included in routine childhood vaccination programmes in other countries, including the developing world. An alternative strategy may be to vaccinate pregnant women so that maternal antibodies are passed on to the newborn child.

Treatment Penicillin G or erythromycin are effective in the majority of cases, but where resistant strains are found or the child is seriously ill, cotrimoxazole, amoxicillin or ampicillin should be used.

Surveillance for ARI will be found in Section 13.2 and for otitis media in Section 13.9.

13.9 Otitis Media

Acute ear infections are a common problem in children and are responsible for considerable morbidity (Table 1.1). Acute middle ear infection or otitis media is the main disease, but this can lead to chronic otitis media or mastoiditis (chronic infection of the bony air cells below the ear) or meningitis.

The ear is joined to the nasopharynx by the eustachian tube through which infecting organisms pass, so ear infections are generally associated with respiratory infections.

Organism S. pneumoniae and H. influenzae are the most common causative organisms, but various viruses may initiate infection and Pseudomonas aeruginosa and Staphylococcus aureus are common in the discharges of chronic otitis media.

Clinical features Fever and pain in the ear are the main presenting symptoms, but in the young child, crying and irritability will be more prominent. The eardrum is red and bulges outwards, rapidly leading to perforation and the appearance of pus. There will be deafness in the ear until the perforation has healed, or permanent deafness if the condition remains untreated.

Diagnosis is on clinical grounds and the infecting organism can be cultured if the eardrum has ruptured.

Transmission is secondary to an upper respiratory infection, such as a sore throat or tonsillitis.

Incubation period 1–4 days.

Period of communicability Not normally transmitted from person to person, except as an upper respiratory infection.

Occurrence and distribution This is a very common condition throughout the world and many children develop ear infections during the course of their childhood.

Where the drum has ruptured, deafness will result, leading to problems at school, so what started off as a seemingly insignificant problem can lead to poor development and disability throughout the life of the individual. Otitis media and deafness occurring in the first 2–3 years of life can interfere with spoken language acquisition, leading to difficulties in communication, understanding and a barrier to education.

There is a particularly high level of otitis media in Australian aboriginals and the Inuit people of the Arctic with Pacific Islanders and native North Americans next in order of magnitude. This may be due to these people having larger eustachian tubes, which offer lower resistance to the passage of organisms.

Control and prevention Upper respiratory infections should be adequately treated and the eardrum always examined for redness and bulging. The same risk factors that cause ARI (Section 13.2) predispose to otitis media, so relevant preventive action can be instituted.

The conjugate pneumococcal vaccine has been shown to be moderately efficacious against otitis media and once it becomes more universally available, it can be anticipated to contribute to a reduction of this infection.

The child with deafness should be examined and if found to have a discharging ear should be treated as below: if the eardrum does not heal, then corrective surgery can be performed.

Treatment In acute otitis media, penicillin G or erythromycin given systemically for 5 days may be sufficient, but if there is poor response or perforation has occurred, then cotrimoxazole twice a day or amoxicillin three times a day for 5 days should be used. In the chronically discharging ear, it is imperative to dry the ear out with wicking, which the mother can be taught to do. Clean tissue paper is twisted into a point and placed in the ear, replacing it as soon as it becomes wet and repeating until the ear remains dry. The child should not swim or water allowed to enter the ear when washing. Boric acid in spirit ear drops can be instilled to help in drying the ear.

Surveillance Surveys of deaf and partially deaf children will give an indication of the amount of otitis media leading to perforation of the eardrum. Where finances permit, this is best done by typanometry, but a simple test using the spoken voice can give a rough estimate:

- responds to a whisper – no deafness;
- responds only to the normal voice – moderate hearing impairment;
- responds only to a loud voice – severe deafness.

13.10 Acute Rheumatic Fever

Organism Group A β-haemolytic streptococcus (GAβHS). The M-protein in the wall of the streptococcus is responsible for its virulence and certain predominant serotypes, 1, 3, 5, 6, 14, 18, 19, 24, 27 and 29, have a much greater rheumatogenic potential.

Clinical features ARF is a delayed non-suppurative sequel of upper respiratory tract infection or scarlet fever with GAβHS. ARF is important because it can lead to rheumatic heart disease (RHD), the resulting cardiac damage producing considerable morbidity and mortality.

Diagnosis of ARF is based on major and minor clinical criteria and a rising serum antibody titre of a recent streptococcal infection by the antistreptolysin-O titre (ASOT), antihyaluronidase or anti-DNase B tests.

Transmission ARF results from an interaction of the bacterial agent, human host and environment. GAβHS are transmitted from person to person through relatively large droplets, up to a distance of 3 m. ARF develops at a fairly constant rate of 3% following untreated epidemics of streptococcal pharyngitis. The attack rate is much

lower (<1%) following endemic or sporadic streptococcal infections. Healthy primary school children are commonly found to be carriers of GAβHS. Cutaneous streptococcal infection is a frequent precursor of acute nephritis, but has not been shown to cause ARF. Scarlet fever, however, is associated with ARF.

Why only a small percentage of the youthful population develop ARF remains a mystery. ARF patients, as a group, show a higher antibody level to group A streptococcal antigens suggesting that repeated exposure to GAβHS may precipitate illness. Susceptibility is due to the immunological status of the host, including both humoral and cell-mediated immunity, with a 2% familial incidence of ARF. A larger proportion of children born to rheumatic parents contract the disease. The carditis of RHD might be the result of an autoimmune mechanism developing between group A streptococcal somatic components and myocardial and valvular components.

Incubation period of the initial streptococcal infection is 1–3 days and 19 days for ARF.

Period of communicability 10–21 days of an acute, untreated streptococcal infection.

Occurrence and distribution ARF/RHD is the commonest form of heart disease in children and young adults in most tropical and developing countries. The peak incidence is 5–15 years, but both primary and recurrent cases can occur in adults. There is neither a sex predilection nor a racial predisposition.

ARF is a disease of lower socioeconomic groups, particularly those massed in the densely populated areas of urban metropolitan centres. It is widespread with a high incidence in South Asia, Pacific Islands, North and South Africa and urban Latin America. It has been estimated that RHD causes 25–40% of all cardiovascular diseases in the developing world.

Control and prevention There is no permanent cure for RHD and the cumulative expense of repeated hospitalization for supportive medical care is a considerable drain on the meagre health resources of developing countries. The only reasonable solution is the prevention of rheumatic fever. ARF is now a rare condition in developed countries due to improved housing, reduction of overcrowding and the provision of adequate health services, so this should be the long-term aim.

Prevention of the first attack (primary prevention) is by proper identification and antibiotic treatment of streptococcal infections. The individual, who has suffered an attack of ARF, is inordinately susceptible to recurrences following subsequent streptococcal infection and needs protection (secondary prevention). While primary prevention is preferable, the incidence of ARF as a sequel of streptococcal sore throat is never greater than 3%, even in epidemics. A vast number of infections would need to be treated in order to achieve any meaningful reduction of the total number of sore throats and streptococci are responsible for only 10–20% of them.

Most cases of severe RHD would be prevented by adequate prevention of recurrences of ARF. No matter how mild the first attack of ARF, secondary prevention with intramuscular long-acting benzathine penicillin G 1.2 million units should be given at monthly intervals. Penicillin V or sulphadiazine may be used for oral prophylaxis. Regular taking of prophylaxis is essential and compliance is a major problem. Patients with no evidence of cardiac involvement should receive prophylaxis for a minimum of 5 years after the last attack of ARF, while those with carditis should continue until they are 25 years old. Prophylaxis should be continued with penicillin in the pregnant woman.

The emphasis of a prevention programme should be on health education, early diagnosis and treatment of sore throats and the provision of treatment facilities at primary level.

Surveillance In developing strategies, baseline data on streptococcal epidemiology and ARF/RHD prevalence in high-risk groups should be collected. A fully established programme centre would operate a central register, coordinate case-finding surveys, run a system of secondary prophylaxis (especially follow-up) and promote health education. Community control of ARF and RHD is viable only if it is firmly based on existing health services, which are an integral part of the primary health care activities in the country. It is especially relevant to school health services, by screening children and supporting those on secondary prophylaxis.

14

Diseases Transmitted Via Body Fluids

This category includes infections transmitted from one human to another by the physiological fluids of the body: blood, serum, saliva, seminal fluid, etc. Transmission is normally direct, but indirect transmission via fomites or flies can occur in some cases. It includes the treponematoses, both the sexually and non-sexually transmitted. Sexual transmission accounts for the largest number of persons affected by these diseases.

These are the diseases of close personal contact, either thriving in conditions of poor hygiene, or in the most intimate contact of all – by sexual intercourse. They are, therefore, social diseases, determined by the habits and attitude of people and it is only by effecting change in these values that any permanent improvement will occur.

14.1 Yaws

Organism *Treponema pallidum* subspecies *pertenue*.

Clinical features Yaws is a non-venereal treponemal disease affecting both the skin and bone. It commences as a primary papule that starts to heal, but after a period, varying from a few weeks to several months, it is followed by generalized lesions, multiple rounded papules, scattered all over the body. These lesions exude serum, which is highly infectious. There is also a mild periostitis in focal bony sites, but these and the skin lesions normally heal with little residual damage. It is the tertiary stage that appears after an asymptomatic period and some 5 years after initial infection that results in gross damage to skin and bone, leading to hideous deformities. The opposite ends of the body are affected with destructive lesions of the nasal bones (gangoza) and scarring, and deformity of the lower limbs (sabre tibia).

Diagnosis is by finding *T. p. pertenue* in the exudates of lesions. In the motile state, the spirochete can be seen by dark ground microscopy or stained by Giemsa or silver salts. The serological tests for syphilis (Section 14.4) are positive.

Transmission Yaws is a disease of poor hygiene, with close bodily contact being the manner in which infection is commonly transmitted. Flies may be involved in transmission from clothing and dressings that have become contaminated by fluid from sores. The spirochete cannot penetrate unbroken skin, but requires a minor skin abrasion or cut by which to enter.

Incubation period 2–8 weeks.

Period of communicability can be as long as moist lesions persist in the untreated case, which can be several years.

Occurrence and distribution Yaws is predominantly an infection of children, with the mother becoming infected if she did not acquire her infection in childhood. The large overcrowded family with a poor standard of hygiene is the characteristic environment in which yaws so readily spreads. The need to stay indoors and keep close together for warmth in the rainy season might be the reason why the disease is more common at this time of year.

Yaws is restricted to the moist tropical areas of the world in a band that passes through the Caribbean, South America, Africa, Southeast Asia and the Pacific Islands (Fig. 14.1). A resurgence of cases has occurred in West Africa, India, Southeast Asia, Pacific Islands, South America and the Caribbean.

Control and prevention Yaws with its rapid response to a single injection of penicillin has been the subject of successful mass treatment campaigns in the endemic parts of the world. Treatment in a mass campaign is to:

- all those with clinical signs of yaws;
- household, school and other close contacts;
- any person suspected of incubating the disease.

The campaign is preceded by health education encouraging all people to come forward with any suspicious lesions. Each village is visited in turn, everyone examined and treatment given to cases, contacts or suspects. A follow-up surveillance service treats missed cases or new infections. This can readily be done by an effective rural health service.

The success of the WHO mass campaigns against yaws resulted in the virtual disappearance of the disease from many areas, but unfortunately, there is now a resurgence. Newly trained health personnel are unaware of the disease and penicillin has been replaced by other antibiotics in the treatment of common infections.

In the long term, improvements in the level of hygiene and socio-economic status will reduce the conditions in which yaws thrives.

Treatment is a single injection of benzathine penicillin G (1.2 million units for an adult, 0.6 million units for a child). Response is very satisfactory and lesions heal within 2–3 weeks.

Surveillance Due to the possible appearance of new cases, a continuing awareness of the disease needs to be kept, with the taking of smears from any suspicious lesions. It is likely that search will discover more cases, so treat cases and contacts along the same lines as in the eradication campaigns.

14.2 Pinta

Organism Treponema carateum.

Clinical features The disease has many similarities to yaws, commencing as a primary, painless papule. Secondary lesions, which develop in 3–12 months, are flat and erythematous, but cover large areas of the body. Tertiary lesions result in pigmentary changes often with large patches of leucoderma. Only the skin is involved in pinta with lesions commonly on the face and extremities.

Diagnosis is made on clinical grounds with supporting evidence from positive serological tests for syphilis. *T. carateum* can be found in the serous exudates from lesions by dark ground microscopy.

Transmission Direct contact or carriage by flies has been suggested as the means of transmission. Trauma, especially to the

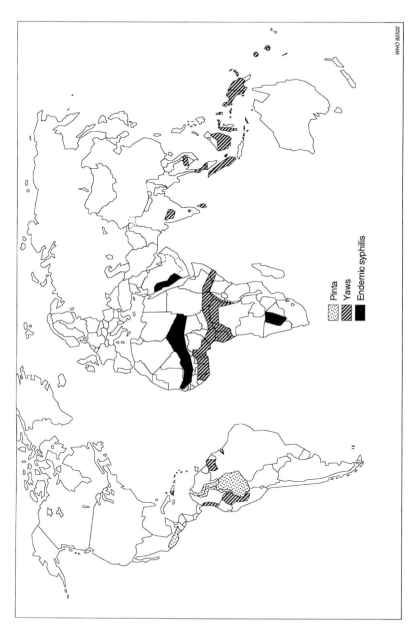

Fig. 14.1. Distribution of the endemic treponematoses. (Reproduced by permission from *Weekly Epidemiological Record*, World Health Organization, Geneva.)

lower limbs, might facilitate entry of organisms.

Incubation period 1–3 weeks.

Period of communicability is probably several years, while secondary lesions are present.

Occurrence and distribution Pinta is restricted to moist tropical areas of Central and South America (Fig. 14.1), occurring in communities with poor hygiene, such as in the Amazon and Orinoco basins. Adults and adolescents are mostly involved. Recent surveys found the disease to be naturally dying out.

Control and prevention Mass treatment with penicillin in the same manner as for yaws (see above).

14.3 Endemic Syphilis

Organism *Treponema pallidum* subspecies *endemicum*, which is indistinguishable from the *T. pallidum* that causes venereal syphilis.

Clinical features The primary lesion is commonly found at the angle of the mouth, appearing as a raised mucous plaque. A more florid skin infection follows with moist papules under the arms and between the buttocks and a maculo-papular rash on the trunk and limbs, resembling venereal syphilis. Destructive tertiary signs in the skin, nasopharynx and bones develop after months or years, but the nervous and cardiovascular systems are rarely involved.

Diagnosis is made on clinical grounds in endemic areas and by detecting the organism with dark ground microscopy. Serological tests for syphilis are positive and remain so for many years.

Transmission Because of the site of the primary lesion on the mouth, transmission by shared drinking vessels and eating utensils is considered the most likely route. Direct contact with lesions is also a likely method of spread. It resembles venereal syphilis in many of its features except that it is not spread venereally.

Incubation period 2 weeks to 3 months.

Period of communicability is for as long as moist lesions are present, generally several months.

Occurrence and distribution The non-venereal form of syphilis is found in localized foci in Africa and the Arabian peninsula (Fig. 14.1), where it is known locally as Bejel or Njovera. Predominantly an infection of childhood, it thrives in conditions of poverty, overcrowding and where there is limited sanitation.

Control and prevention It is a disease of low personal hygiene where crowding together and contact with lesions readily occurs. Cross-immunity is shared with venereal syphilis, therefore, eradication of the disease by mass treatment generally means a replacement by the more serious and devastating venereal syphilis. Family planning, better housing, education and improving the general standard of hygiene might be a preferable control strategy in such situations.

Treatment is with penicillin in the same manner as yaws.

14.4 Venereal Syphilis

Organism *Treponema pallidum* subspecies *pallidum*.

Clinical features. The primary lesion of syphilis is the chancre (a painless ulcer with a serous discharge) normally found on the genitalia of males and females, but can occur in the mouth, on the breast or in the ano-rectal region. A regional lymph node often enlarges to form a bubo. The primary lesion heals spontaneously after a few weeks, but 6 weeks to 6 months later, the signs of secondary syphilis appear. This may take several forms, but the commonest is a maculo-papular rash and mucocutaneous condylomata around the genitalia and anus. As the infection is systemic, a generalized lymphadenopathy and splenomegaly can occur, often accompanied by fever. Following the period of secondary syphilis, there is a latent phase after which the destructive cardiovascular (aortic aneurysm) and central nervous symptoms (meningitis, paresis or tabes dorsalis) occur, often many years later. Should a woman be pregnant while she has syphilis, her fetus may be seriously affected. If she is pregnant during early syphilis, then the child is likely to be stillborn, while the later stages of the disease are more likely to produce a live-born child suffering from congenital defects (deafness, sabre tibia, Hutchinson teeth and CNS involvement).

Diagnosis is confirmed by finding *T. p. pallidum* in the serous exudate from a chancre or by gland puncture. This can be examined by dark ground microscopy or immunofluorescent staining. Serological tests can assist in the diagnosis or be used in epidemiological studies. The rapid plasma reagin (RPR) is a sensitive test, while specific tests, such as the fluorescent treponemal antibody absorbed (FTA-Abs) test or *T. pallidum* haemagglutination antibody (TPHA), are more difficult and expensive to perform. Cross-reaction between the *Treponema* of yaws, pinta and endemic syphilis negate the differential diagnosis of these diseases. All patients with syphilis should be encouraged to have an HIV test because of the high frequency of dual infection.

Transmission Syphilis is transmitted by direct contact with an infectious lesion or its discharge during sexual intercourse. Transmission can also occur congenitally or from blood transfusion if the donor is in the early stages of syphilis. Kissing can more rarely transmit the spirochete.

Because of the almost identical nature of the *T. pallidum* of endemic syphilis and venereal syphilis, it has been considered that venereal syphilis developed from this more benign form. Once a venereal method of transmission had been developed, the disease was able to extend its boundaries from the tropics to the Arctic.

Infection with *T. p. endemicum* confers immunity to venereal syphilis and infection with *T. p. pallidum* gives immunity to the other treponem infections and from contracting venereal syphilis again, but this is reduced by HIV infection. There is also some innate resistance or inadequacy of the transmission mechanism as only some 30% of contacts of a known infected source become infected.

Incubation period 9–90 days (usually 3 weeks).

Period of communicability Up to 1 year after the primary lesion first appears.

Occurrence and distribution The venereal diseases are totally cosmopolitan, taking no account of climate, ethnic group or social class; wherever sexual contact occurs, venereal diseases can occur also. It is estimated that there are some 12 million cases in the world today, with a large proportion of these in the tropics. The highest incidence is amongst the 20–24-year age group, followed by those 25–29 years old.

Syphilis is predominantly a disease of urban areas and in conditions of sexual imbalance, such as mines, military establishments and amongst seamen. With the rapid urbanization that has occurred in the developing world and large movements of migrant labour, syphilis has been on the increase in the tropics. When the migrant workers return to their homes and families, they bring venereal disease back with them. The main reservoir of infection is generally in commercial sex workers or deserted women forced into prostitution to support their children. Due to the prolonged incubation period, the hidden site of the primary lesion within the vagina, and the latent period of the disease, syphilis is either not suspected or purposely hidden. A large number of contacting males can be infected by a single female.

Control and prevention Contact tracing and the adequate treatment of all cases is the main method of control, but in developing countries, it is largely an impossible task. In restricted communities, such as mines or plantations, it can be used to considerable value, but in the vast, sprawling urban slums where people come and go and address is not known, it is a hopeless task. The prohibition of commercial sex workers only drives the practice underground and is generally not acceptable in developing countries where they form a recognized segment of society in many cultures. A preferable answer is to try and examine known commercial sex workers at regular intervals and encourage them to bring in others for check-ups. A commercial sex worker aware of the damage that can be caused by the disease, once converted, can be a greater proponent of health education than any trained worker.

Health education should start at school, encouraging delay of first sexual experience and the benefits of a monogamous relationship. Programmes should also be targeted at high-risk groups, such as miners, truck drivers and the commercial sex industry, encouraging safe sex and the use of condoms. The likelihood of contracting a sexually transmitted infection (STI) is proportional to the number of sexual partners.

Diagnostic and treatment facilities need to be widely available on a walk-in basis. It is preferable to provide special clinics as well as the routine health services. Unfortunately, many private practitioners, often not even medically qualified, offer inadequate treatment, so encouraging resistant organisms to develop as syphilis is often contracted at the same time as other STIs.

All pregnant women should be tested for syphilis, preferably both in early and late pregnancy. All blood donors should be screened (see also Box 14.1).

Treatment is with benzathine penicillin 2.4 million units as a single dose (but often given intramuscularly at two different sites). Alternatively, tetracycline 500 mg four times a day or doxycycline 100 mg twice daily, both for 14 days can be given, especially in the patient allergic to penicillin and not pregnant.

Surveillance Antenatal and family planning clinics provide an important opportunity to examine a large number of women and also prevent cases of congenital syphilis. Routine RPRs should be performed and all positive cases fully investigated and treated.

14.5 Gonorrhoea

Organism Gonorrhoea is a bacterial disease caused by *Neisseria gonorrhoeae* (the gonococcus).

Clinical features In the male, infection commences as a mucoid urethral secretion, which soon changes to a profuse, purulent discharge (as opposed to NGU where it is scanty, white, mucoid or serous). The discharge is best seen first thing in the morning (dew drop) and a smear should be made from this before the patient urinates. The main symptom is pain on micturition, but the degree of discomfort is very variable. In the female, the infection generally passes unnoticed, but may present with urethritis or acute salpingitis. It is this latter presentation of the disease that can lead, in an acute or chronic form of pelvic inflammatory disease, to sterility in the female. This is a serious problem in the unmarried woman and a cause of divorce in the married. In the male, untreated or improperly treated infection can result in urethral stricture, while generalized symptoms of arthritis, dermatitis or meningitis can rarely occur in either sex. In the pregnant woman, there is a danger of the newborn infant developing gonococcal conjunctivitis at the time of delivery. The discovery of this infection in the newborn infant may be the manner in which the infection is found in the woman.

There has been a considerable increase in STI with new STIs appearing or their relative importance changing. Some of the reasons for these changes are:

- increasing world population, especially of younger age groups;
- urbanization and migrant labour;
- increasing travel and mixing of populations;
- alteration of social values and increasing promiscuity;
- development of contraceptive practice;
- ignorance of STI and lack of sex education;
- vulnerability of women biologically, culturally and socio-economically;
- inadequate treatment and development of resistant organisms.

International travel has allowed a mixing of cultural groups that would otherwise have remained isolated, potentiating the spread of different types and strains of STI. The development of resistant strains has posed a problem of imported cases to the developed world, but has left the developing world with an intolerable situation that they are economically unable to deal with.

STIs are more prevalent in young people, yet with an increasing world population, it is predominantly these younger age groups that are expanding at a more rapid rate than others. This increase in the youth of the world has thrown a greater strain on the education services so that health education, especially of STIs, is neglected.

Change has occurred in the social structure whereby traditional values and the monogamous married couple are no longer regarded as the norm. The development of contraceptives has freed the woman from the risk of unwanted pregnancy, but at the same time, increased the opportunity for developing an STI. Married women are particularly vulnerable when they are abandoned or their husbands have to find work away from the confines of the family. STIs are often asymptomatic in women so they do not seek treatment, putting their lives and those of any future children at greater risk.

Generally, the risk of developing an STI is more recognized, rather than the shock that previously led to concealment or recourse to treatment from a medical quack. Also contraceptive practice should not be discouraged for it is the problem of the rapidly expanding young population that is a major contributory factor. The key is health education with a combined approach of contraceptive advice and STI information. If this is to succeed there must be a considerable increase in treatment facilities, especially in urban areas. Standard treatment regimes should be decided by specialists and administered by primary healthcare workers. Improved treatment facilities, contact tracing, training of health workers and more effective drugs will not only reduce the prevalence and seriousness of STIs, but also of HIV infection.

Diagnosis Due to the similarity in presentation of gonococcal and non-gonocococcal urithritis, the emphasis is on making a diagnosis syndromically of a urethral discharge. A smear should be made and stained with Gram stain, the finding of Gram-negative intracellular diplococci indicating gonococcal infection. Where facilities permit, the discharge should be cultured, but as the organism is very sensitive, it must be inoculated on to a culture plate or placed in transport medium (less satisfactory) as soon as possible.

Transmission is by sexual intercourse or with contact of the infected mucous exudate. *N. gonorrhoeae* is unable to penetrate stratified epithelium, but has a predilection for mucous membranes where it produces an accumulation of polymorphonuclear leucocytes and outpouring of serum to give the characteristic discharge.

Important factors in the transmission of gonorrhoea are:

- the short incubation period;
- the often asymptomatic disease in women (estimated to be 80%);
- promiscuous sexual intercourse;
- urbanization and changing social values;
- use of contraceptives;
- inadequate treatment.

The combination of a short incubation period and promiscuous sexual activity means that a large number of people can become infected in rapid succession. Since women are often largely unaware of their infection they serve as a continuous reservoir of the disease. Urbanization changes the social balance that occurs in the village, traditional values and taboos are lost and promiscuity develops. Contraceptives allow increased opportunity for sexual intercourse although the condom provides limited protection. The contraceptive pill by reducing the acidity of genital secretions removes some of the natural defences, while the intra-uterine contraceptive device encourages mechanical spread of infection to the uterus and tubes. Improper treatment both by doctors and quacks, usually with grossly inadequate doses of antibiotics, has led to chronic infections and the development of resistant organisms.

Incubation period 2–7 days (average 3 days).

Period of communicability can be months in untreated cases, especially hidden infections in women.

Occurrence and distribution The number of cases of gonorrhoea in the world today is estimated to be some 62 million. Under-reporting, illegal treatment and the protection of contacts make any standard methods of case treatment and contact tracing quite inadequate in most developing countries. Gonorrhoea is not so much found as a reservoir in commercial sex workers as more widely distributed amongst the promiscuous under-25-year-olds.

Control and prevention Where possible, cases presenting at STI clinics should be encouraged to bring their partners (or provide information so that they can be traced) for counselling and treatment. Alternatively, contact cards can be sent anonymously to all contacts of a case, recommending them to present at a clinic. Condoms can be given out at the same time as a person presents at a clinic. Health education concentrating on the dangers of STIs is the main preventive action (see also under syphilis above and Box 14.1). The eyes of babies as they are being born should be wiped and a 1% aqueous solution of silver nitrate instilled (Section 7.7).

Treatment which used to be a simple matter with penicillin, is now fraught with problems of resistance not only to this antibiotic, but to many others that have subsequently been tried. Any recommended treatment regime may be ineffective in certain parts of the world and local expertise must be consulted to develop routines that are compatible with the resistance patterns and available resources. Recommended regimens are:

- ciprofloxacin 500 mg as a single oral dose (but not in pregnant women or children), or
- azithromycin 2 g orally as a single dose, or
- ceftriaxone 125 mg by single intramuscular injection, or
- cefixine 400 mg as a single oral dose, or
- spectinomycin 2 g by single intramuscular injection.

Patients diagnosed with gonorrhoea often have *Chlamydia* infection as well, so treatment for this condition should be combined as a routine (see below).

Surveillance Strains of the gonococcus resistant to the standard treatment regime in the country are likely to be imported from time to time, so sensitivity should be regularly tested and the treatment regime modified accordingly.

14.6 Non-gonococcal Urethritis (NGU)

Organism A number of organisms have been found to be responsible for urethritis not caused by the gonococcus, including *Chlamydia trachomatis*, *Ureaplasma urealyticum*, *Trichomonas vaginalis* and *Mycoplasma hominis*.

Clinical features A low-grade urethritis with mucoid rather than purulent discharge in the male, in which intracellular diplococci are not found in the smear, suggests NGU. Infection is a low-grade discharge in the female or is often asymptomatic so that a reservoir of infection can occur if simultaneous treatment to both sexual partners is not given. Sterility in women can result if the infection is not treated. In areas where gonococcal urethritis is common, the prevalence of NGU is also high so treatment should be given for both conditions.

Diagnosis This differs markedly in different parts of the world with developing countries adopting a syndromic approach (see above under gonorrhoea), while developed countries specifically test for *Chlamydia.* Where possible, diagnosis should be made by smear and culture, the absence of intracellular diplococci indicating NGU. The nucleic acid amplification test (NAAT) or IF test with monoclonal antibody can be used on urethral or cervical swabs.

Transmission is by sexual intercourse. *C. trachomatis* and *T. vaginalis* are risk factors for HIV infection in the female.

Incubation period 1–2 weeks.

Period of communicability In the asymptomatic case, infection can continue for a considerable period of time.

Occurrence and distribution NGU is more common than gonorrhoea and is found all over the world with high levels in the sexually promiscuous.

Control and prevention is the same as for gonorrhoea and syphilis (see above).

Treatment is with azithromycin 1 g orally in a single dose, doxycycline 100 mg orally twice daily for 7 days, erythromycin 500 mg orally four times a day for 7 days or tetracycline 500 mg orally four times daily for 7 days. Sexual intercourse must be avoided until both partners are free of signs. While cases of gonorrhoea should always be treated for NGU, if gonorrhoea has been excluded, then cases of NGU do not also need to be treated for gonorrhoea. If a low-grade offensive discharge with some staining persists in the female, or irritation in the male, this is probably *Trichomonas* infection, which is effectively treated with metronidazole 2 g orally or tinidazole 2 g orally in a single dose.

Surveillance Several STIs can occur together, hence NGU is an indicator of possible syphilis and gonorrhoea, which should always be looked for.

14.7 Lymphogranuloma Venereum

Organism *Chlamydia trachomatis.*

Clinical features Lymphogranuloma venereum is a chronic infection presenting as a small painless papule, vesicle or ulcer on the genitalia that often goes unnoticed, lymphadenitis being the clinical sign. The lymph nodes become grossly enlarged and generally suppurate with fistulas and fibrosis developing, especially in the rectal area if treatment is delayed.

Diagnosis is by finding the organism in lymph node aspirate with immunofluorescence or DNA probe.

Transmission Although sexual intercourse is considered the main means of transmission, infection can also happen by direct contact with open lesions.

Incubation period 3–30 days.

Period of communicability is for as long as there are active lesions, which may be for several years.

Occurrence and distribution Although it occurs worldwide, lymphogranuloma venereum is commoner in the tropics, especially in sub-Saharan Africa and parts of Asia.

Control and prevention Treatment should be commenced as soon as the diagnosis has been made, the patient being advised to refrain from sexual intercourse and close contact with others until all lesions have healed. Other methods of control are the same as for syphilis and gonorrhoea above.

Treatment is with doxycycline 100 mg daily for 14 days, erythromycin 500 mg four times daily for 14 days or tetracycline 500 mg four times daily for 14 days.

14.8 Granuloma Inguinale

Organism *Calymmatobacterium granulomatis.*

Clinical features Granuloma inguinale is a chronic, progressive, ulcerating disease of the ano-genital area without regional lymphadonopathy. An initial lesion on the genitalia becomes eroded and ulcerated with new nodules forming at the margins as the lesion extends. The lesions readily bleed on contact and ulceration can continue to produce extensive destruction. Carcinoma of the vulva has been reported to be associated with granuloma inguinale.

Diagnosis is made from smears or scrapings of the lesions stained with Giemsa, in which intracellular rod-shaped organisms (Donavan bodies) are found.

Transmission The disease is transmitted by direct contact with lesions either via sexual intercourse or other methods. It is frequently associated with anal intercourse.

Incubation period 1–16 weeks.

Period of communicability is while open lesions are present, which can be for a considerable period of time in the untreated patient.

Occurrence and distribution Mainly in the tropical regions of the world, especially in southern India and Irian Jaya/Papua New Guinea and amongst the aboriginal people of Australia. It is less commonly found in Africa and people of African origin, such as in the Caribbean and the northern part of South America. It is a disease of the sexually active 20–40-year age group, in males more than females, but children under 5 years also contract the disease (presumably from contact with their parents).

Control and prevention Control is the same as for syphilis and gonorrhoea above. Care should be taken to prevent transmission from open lesions to others and other parts of the body.

Treatment is with azithromycin 1 g orally on the first day followed by 500 mg daily for a maximum of 14 days, doxycycline 100 mg twice daily for 14 days, erythromycin 500 mg orally four times a day for 14 days or tetracycline 500 mg four times daily for 14 days.

Surveillance As with all STIs, it is possible that more than one STI is present.

14.9 Chancroid

Organism *Haemophilus ducreyi.*

Clinical features An acute venereal infection characterized by a soft chancre on the external genitalia and regional lymphadenopathy. The lesion has an indurated base of the chancre, which differentiates it from syphilis. Chancroid is a predisposing cause of HIV infection with which it is frequently associated.

Diagnosis The organism can be identified with Gram-stain from the exudate of lesions, but this is often difficult due to secondary infection.

Transmission is by sexual intercourse or direct contact with lesions.

Incubation period 3–14 days.

Period of communicability is as long as lesions continue to discharge, which can be months in the untreated case.

Occurrence and distribution Predominantly found in the tropical regions of the world where it is common in men who probably obtain their infection from a commercial sex worker.

Control and prevention See syphilis above.

Treatment Chancroid can be treated with one of the following regimes:

- azithromycin 1 g orally as a single dose, or
- ceftriaxone 250 mg intramuscularly as a single dose, or
- ciprofloxacin 500 mg orally twice daily for 3 days, or
- erythromycin 500 mg orally four times daily for 7 days.

14.10 Genital Herpes

Organism Herpesvirus simplex type 2 (HSV2); less commonly type 1 (HSV1).

Clinical features Painful vesicles develop on the genitalia or surrounding area, which can subsequently ulcerate. Healing occurs after initial infection only to recur at frequent intervals, often precipitated by stress or menstruation. Infection of the neonate can occur during delivery resulting in encephalitis, liver damage or lesions in the eye, mouth or skin. Infection with HSV2 carries an increased risk of developing HIV infection.

Diagnosis is made on clinical presentation and by scrapings of the lesions where characteristic multi-nucleated giant cells with intranuclear bodies are seen on microscopy.

Transmission is by sexual intercourse or direct contact, such as oral–genital, or to the infant during delivery.

Incubation period 2–12 days.

Period of communicability 2–7 weeks during the initial clinical infection and 5 days during a recurrence.

Occurrence and distribution A worldwide and increasing problem amongst the sexually active. As the infection is difficult to treat there is a recurrent reservoir of infection with each clinical attack and if one of these should occur during delivery, then neonatal death or disability will result.

Control and prevention The same as with gonorrhoea and syphilis (see above). Infected persons should be warned of the increased risk of developing HIV infection.

Treatment There is no cure, but acyclovir 200 mg orally five times daily for 7 days or acyclovir 400 mg orally three times a day for 7 days, or other analogues will reduce the formation of new lesions, pain and the period of healing, but not recurrent attacks.

14.11 Human Papilloma Virus (HPV)

Organism Human papilloma virus (HPV).

Clinical features The main clinical presentation is genital warts on the external genitalia or within the vagina, but a large proportion of infected persons show no clinical signs. When cellular immunity is depressed condylomata acuminata, large fleshy growths in moist areas of the perineum develop. However, the most serious consequence of HPV infection is the development of carcinoma, particularly of the cervix, but the anus and penis can also be involved.

Diagnosis Cervical smears stained by the Papanicolau method can detect precancerous changes.

Transmission is by sexual intercourse, but direct contact, as with other warts, is possible.

Incubation period 2–3 months.

Period of communicability Probably for a considerable period of time as cancer of the cervix appears to be associated with the cumulative number of sexual encounters.

Occurrence and distribution It has been estimated that between 9% and 13% of the world population is infected with HPV, which is some 630 million people. Seventy percent of these infections are sub-clinical with only a proportion developing genital warts and some 28–40 million the pre-malignant condition. The prevalence of chronic persistent infection is about 15% in developing countries and 7% in developed. Eighty per cent of the worldwide incidence of cervical cancer is in developing countries.

Control and prevention The usual methods of reducing STI, such as delaying the age of first intercourse, monogamous relationship and the use of condoms will all assist in decreasing the likelihood of developing HPV infection. The promotion of cervical smear testing in developed countries has allowed detection of pre- and early cervical cancer amenable to surgical treatment, but few if any developing countries are able to afford such a service.

Three HPV vaccines are currently under trial and offer considerable hope that either the non-infected can be protected or that a therapeutic vaccine can be used in the already infected.

Treatment of the warts is by cryotherapy, podophyllin or with trichloroacetic acid, but HPV infection will remain.

Surveillance Cytological services for screening women at regular intervals have been shown to be cost-effective in reducing cervical cancer and should be set up wherever resources permit.

14.12 Human Immunodeficiency Virus (HIV)

Organism Human immunodeficiency virus (HIV) either type 1 (HIV-1) or type 2 (HIV-2), HIV-1 being more pathogenic.

Clinical features HIV infection leads to a disruption of the helper T4 cell-mediated immune mechanisms, resulting in an increased susceptibility to opportunistic infections. This breakdown of the body's defence system and the range of symptoms produced is called acquired immunodeficiency syndrome (AIDS). Presentation is generally by the symptoms of the opportunistic infection, so can be many and varied.

Initially, there may be an acute retroviral infection with fever, sweating and myalgia, but after this subsides, there is a dormant period for months or years, after which symptoms of an opportunistic infection occur. The opportunistic infections are:

- oral, vulvovaginal candidiasis, or of the oesophagus, trachea, bronchi or lung;
- pulmonary or extrapulmonary tuberculosis (Section 13.1);
- atypical disseminated mycobacteriosis;
- severe bacterial infections, such as pneumonia (Table 13.1) or pyomyocitis;
- *Pneumocystis carinii* pneumonia (Table 13.1);
- non-typhoid *Salmonella* septicaemia;
- oral hairy leucoplakia;
- reactivated varicella (Section 12.1);
- cytomegalovirus of an organ other than liver, spleen or lymph nodes;
- herpes simplex, visceral or not resolving mucocutaneous;
- disseminated mycosis, such as histoplasmosis, coccidioidomycosis or penicilium;
- cryptococcosis, extrapulmonary;
- cryptosporidiosis with diarrhoea (Section 8.2);
- isosporiasis or microsporidiosis with diarrhoea;

- toxoplasmosis of the brain (Section 17.5);
- intractable scabies not responding to treatment (Section 7.1);
- disseminated *Strongyloides* (Section 10.4);
- florid Chagas' disease with acute myocarditis or meningoencephalitis (Section 15.11);
- reactivated leishmaniasis (Section 15.12);
- lymphoma (Section 1.1);
- Kaposi's sarcoma (Section 1.1);
- HIV encephalopathy;
- progressive multifocal leucoencephalopathy.

Any process that stresses the immune mechanism, such as repeat infections, will accelerate progression to AIDS. Tuberculosis and leprosy are affected by the disruption of the immune process. Any person with tuberculosis who contracts HIV infection will progress more rapidly, while tuberculoid leprosy cases can convert to lepromatous.

Diagnosis and AIDS case definition With such a range of possible symptoms and lack of resources in developing countries to perform serological confirmation, various attempts have been made to formulate a case definition for AIDS. The one most widely followed is the 1985 Bangui definition, updated in 1994 by WHO, which is as follows:

> An adult or adolescent (>12 years of age) is considered to have AIDS if at least two of the following major signs are present in combination with at least one of the minor signs listed below, if these signs are not known to be due to a condition unrelated to HIV infection.
>
> *Major signs*
> - weight loss ≥ 10% of body weight;
> - chronic diarrhoea for more than 1 month;
> - prolonged fever for more than 1 month (intermittent or constant);
>
> *Minor signs*
> - persistent cough for more than 1 month;
> - generalized pruritis dermatitis;
> - history of herpes zoster;

- oropharyngeal candidiasis;
- chronic progressive or disseminated herpes simplex infection;
- generalized lymphadenopathy;

The presence of either generalized Kaposi sarcoma or cryptococcal meningitis is sufficient for the diagnosis of AIDS.

If a test for HIV antibody in an adult or adolescent (>12 years old) is positive then the person is considered to have AIDS if one or more of the following conditions are present:

- ≥10% body weight loss or cachexia, with diarrhoea or fever, or both, intermittent or constant, for at least 1 month, not known to be due to a condition unrelated to HIV infection;
- cryptococcal meningitis;
- pulmonary or extra pulmonary tuberculosis;
- Kaposi sarcoma;
- neurological impairment that is sufficient to prevent independent daily activities, not known to be due to a condition unrelated to HIV infection;
- candidiasis of the oesophagus;
- clinically diagnosed life-threatening or recurrent episodes of pneumonia, with or without aetiological confirmation;
- invasive cervical cancer.

Where full diagnostic facilities are available, the Centres for Disease Control and Prevention (CDC) definition of infection (2000) can be used:

In adults or adolescents (≥18 months), a reportable case of HIV infection must meet one of the following criteria:

1. Positive result on a screening test for HIV antibody (e.g. repeatedly reactive enzyme immunoassay), followed by a positive result on a confirmatory test for HIV antibody (e.g. Western blot or immunofluorescence antibody test)

or

2. Positive result of a detectable quantity on any of the following HIV virologic tests:

- HIV nucleic acid detection (e.g. DNA polymerase chain reaction);

- HIV p24 antigen test, including neutralization assay;
- HIV isolation (viral culture).

Transmission is by:

- sexual contact with an infected person;
- inoculation with infected blood or blood products (including unsterile needles and syringes);
- from an infected mother to child before, during delivery or for up to 2 years after if breast-fed;
- from tissue transplants (rare).

Sexual contact is the commonest method of transmission, with both heterosexual and homosexual practice. The important epidemiological factor is number of sexual contacts so that prostitutes or promiscuous homosexuals with hundreds, if not thousands of new contacts annually are at greatest risk. However, one contact with an infected person is able to produce infection. Anal intercourse carries a higher risk of infection than vaginal. There is no evidence of increased risk during menstruation and circumcision is protective in the male. There is an association with other STIs, particularly genital herpes simplex virus type 2 and ulcerating conditions, such as chancroid. Other STIs may potentiate infection.

Blood transfusion of infected blood will almost always transmit HIV. Pooled blood, such as for producing factor VIII for the treatment of haemophilia, is particularly dangerous because it contains donations from many people, any of which could be infected. Syringes and needles, if they are not properly cleaned and sterilized, can contain small quantities of blood sufficient to transmit infection. This method may be responsible for many infections in developing countries and is an important way of transmitting infection amongst drug abusers. Transmission by needle stick injury can occur, but is uncommon.

The infected mother can pass on infection to her child. Infection can be transmitted congenitally, but it is more likely to occur from a mixing of the mother's and infant's blood at the time of delivery. HIV is found in breast milk with about a 25% chance of it being transmitted to the infant.

Serological tests may not become positive for up to 3 months after the person became infected, so it is possible for a person to transmit infection before they are shown to be positive.

Incubation period to full-blown AIDS ranges from 1 to 18 years with a mean of 10 years. In perinatal infection, the incubation period is often shorter than 12 months. With such a long incubation period the epidemic will last for about 100 years if an effective intervention is not found.

Period of communicability Infectiousness is highest during initial infection, probably extending throughout the life of the individual, increasing again as immunity becomes suppressed. With the extension of life of the treated individual the period of communicability is also increased, although virus shedding is diminished.

Occurrence and distribution HIV infection has now spread to most parts of the world, but is particularly prevalent in Africa, the Americas, Europe (including Russia), South and Southeast Asia and an increasing problem in China. Some 25 million people have so far died from AIDS and 40 million are infected, comprising 36.8 million adults, 18.3 million of which are women, and 3.1 million children under 15 years of age (at 2003). Sixty-four per cent of all cases of AIDS are in Africa with southern Africa being the worst affected part of the continent. Nearly 40% of women of age 15–24 years attending ante-natal clinic in Swaziland were HIV-positive, with only slightly lower rates for Botswana and Zimbabwe. In contrast though there has been a reduction in prevalence in East Africa where the epidemic first started.

Initial spread in East Africa was along transport routes, where lorry drivers made use of local bar-girls at each of their stops. In South Africa, HIV infection was introduced into the mining communities in which it spread rapidly via prostitutes. Sadly many infections in developing countries have been due to the use of poorly sterilized needles when people have attended at clinics for other illnesses.

Parts of South America and some Caribbean islands have very high incidence rates due to the general attitude towards promiscuity. Prostitution and injecting drug use are responsible for very high rates in parts of Thailand and India, from which spread is being encouraged through illegal networks. Girls from Yunnan in China sent to work in brothels in Thailand returned infected with HIV and disseminated it to other parts of the country. However, both Thailand and Cambodia have now shown sustained reductions in the past 4–5 years.

A worrying trend has been the unchanged incidence in Western countries, with an increasing rate in Europe, despite the availability of antiretroviral (ARV) therapy. Indeed this suggests that treatment, by prolonging the life of HIV-infected persons, is increasing transmission, or the availability of treatment is reducing the fear of infection and allowing more risky behaviour. It is hoped that ARV therapy will reduce the stigma of AIDS and allow preventive programmes to work in developing countries, so both strategies must proceed at the same time.

HIV-1 is common in the Americas, Europe, Asia, Central and East Africa, whereas HIV-2 is found in West Africa or in people that acquired their infection there.

Control and prevention Methods of control and prevention are aimed at the three routes of transmission – sexual, blood and perinatal. Several vaccines are under trial including a prime boost technique using a DNA vaccine followed by HIV in a modified vaccinia virus, but the problem with all the vaccine candidates so far developed is the rapid rate at which the HIV virus alters its antigenic makeup. A live, attenuated vaccine has been developed, which seems to be effective, but because of the ability of the retrovirus to alter itself so rapidly, it is likely to be too dangerous. Until a vaccine is

developed, other control measures are required.

To prevent **sexual** spread:

- limit the number of sexual partners, encouraging monogamous relationships;
- avoid sexual contact with persons at high risk, such as commercial sex workers, bisexuals and homosexuals;
- encourage male and female condom use;
- provide adequate facilities for the detection and treatment of STIs;
- provide counselling and HIV testing;
- provide general education for girls and sex education to both boys and girls;
- provide lifestyle training (how to say 'no').

To prevent **blood** spread:

- screen all blood for transfusions;
- test donors before they give blood;
- only use blood transfusions when essential;
- discontinue paid blood donors;
- use disposable syringes, needles, giving sets, lancets, etc. or ensure they are properly sterilized;
- injecting drug users should be discouraged from sharing equipment, preferably using needle exchange schemes;
- medical workers should wear gloves when dealing with possible infected blood (e.g. at delivery and in the laboratory).

To prevent **perinatal** spread:

- advise infected mothers about the possible risk to their infant and themselves if they become pregnant;
- good obstetric practice, especially reducing trauma in procedures, such as artificial rupture of membranes and fetal scalp monitoring, and only cutting the cord when it has stopped pulsating;
- priority ARV therapy should be given to HIV-positive pregnant women and to the newborn infant (nevirapine has been shown to be effective in Uganda, but zidovudine and lamivudine can also be used);

- provide information on breast-feeding to allow each mother to decide.

Caesarean section should not be encouraged in developing countries as the risk to the mother in subsequent pregnancies is considerably increased, but might be the strategy of choice in developed countries. WHO recommends that no change should be made in vaccination programme to mothers and children even though they may be infected with HIV, except in the child with clinical AIDS who should not be given BCG.

HIV is **not** spread by:

- mosquitoes;
- casual contact such as shaking hands, or lavatory seats;
- through food, water or the respiratory route.

CONTROL PROGRAMMES   The main method of control is health promotion and should involve community leaders, religious organizations and NGOs. This can be to the general public to supply them with the correct information or to specific groups. The most cost-effective health education will be to high-risk groups, such as commercial sex workers, homosexuals, single workers, etc. However, they are difficult to motivate and it is probably better to concentrate effort on school children. Girls should have equal opportunity for education, whereas sex education should be an integral part of the school curriculum. Counselling and testing facilities need to be readily available as well as programmes on mother-to-child transmission. Improved diagnosis and treatment facilities for STIs need to be made available, providing early and adequate treatment. Condoms can be dispensed at clinics, markets or at any suitable social marketing opportunity (see Box 14.1).

All persons with HIV infection, including those under treatment, are at risk of passing on infection to others and should be counselled about preventive measures to be taken.

Treatment is largely unavailable in most developing countries, but efforts are being made to rectify the situation. Individual treatment is a highly specialized subject, but will probably consist of two nucleoside analogues, a non-nucleoside reverse transcriptase inhibitor and/or a protease inhibitor, a three- or four-drug regime being found to be more effective than a two-drug regime. A second-line regimen should be available in case of toxicity or treatment failure. Any opportunistic infection must receive specific treatment for the condition.

Surveillance The prevalence of HIV infection can be estimated by testing anonymously blood that has been obtained for other purposes, such as in ante-natal or STI clinics. Population-based surveys have been conducted in Zambia, South Africa and some other countries. Numbers of cases of AIDS are reported to WHO using the case definitions outlined above.

14.13 Hepatitis B (HBV)

Organism Hepatitis B virus (HBV).

Clinical features In many parts of the developing world, HBV infection is common, but only about 30% show any symptoms. However, these symptomatic cases present as a more severe disease than hepatitis A, with a persistent jaundice, often resulting in liver damage.

After an insidious onset with anorexia, nausea and abdominal discomfort, jaundice then develops, from which the patient either recovers or goes on to develop chronic active disease. Low-grade infection continues with periods of jaundice alternating with remissions, but invariably cirrhosis develops. The disease is more serious in those over 40 years of age, in pregnant women and newborn infants. Hepatocellular carcinoma is associated with chronic hepatitis B infection.

Diagnosis can be made by finding the surface antigens (HBs Ag). There are four subtypes adw, ayw, adr and ayr, which vary in their geographical distribution providing useful epidemiological markers. A further antigen e (HBe Ag) is a marker of increased infectivity as well as indicating active viral replication in hepatocytes (which may result in liver damage).

Transmission can occur from blood, serum, saliva and seminal fluid. It is a hazard of blood transfusions, renal dialysis, injections and tattooing. It can be transmitted by sexual intercourse and during delivery. The virus has been found in some blood-sucking insects (e.g. bed bugs), but transmission by this means has not been shown to occur.

Certain people are more infectious than others resulting in a carrier state, with the period of communicability being considerable. The risk of an infant becoming infected from a carrier mother can be 50–70% in some ethnic groups. There is a greater likelihood of the mother passing on the infection if she has acute hepatitis B in the second or third trimester or up to 2 months after delivery. A high titre of surface e antigen or a history of transmission to previous children increases the risk of a mother infecting her infant. The carrier state is more common in males and in those that acquired their infection in childhood.

Incubation period 6 weeks to 6 months (usually 9–12 weeks), a larger inoculum of virus probably resulting in a shorter incubation period.

Period of communicability From several weeks before the onset of symptoms, continuing until the end of clinical disease, unless the person becomes a carrier in which case it is life long.

Occurrence and distribution The carrier state has been estimated to be present in over 350 million people with varying rates in different parts of the world: Western Europe, 1%; South and Central America 2–7%; and Africa, Asia and Western Pacific, >8%. Infection is thought to occur commonly in infancy or early childhood in the more endemic areas.

Control and prevention Hepatitis B vaccine can be given to those at risk and as part of the EPI programme. If given before infection, it prevents the development of disease and the carrier state. Ideally, Hepatitis B vaccine is given at the same time as DTP, but in countries where perinatal transmission is common, such as in Southeast Asia, a dose at birth is recommended. Immunity is thought to last for at least 15 years in the fully vaccinated. There is convincing evidence that reduction of carriers can prevent the development of primary liver cell cancer.

Preventive methods are strict aseptic precautions in giving blood transfusions, injections and the handling of blood. All blood donors should be screened with contributions to pooled blood being particularly scrutinized. The control of STIs has been covered above. Homosexual practice is particularly liable to lead to HBV infection. Persons at risk should be vaccinated.

Treatment There is no specific treatment, but alpha-interferon and lamivudine have a limited effect in some people, particularly in the early stage of infection. Long-term treatment may also be of value.

Surveillance As with HIV infection, blood obtained in antenatal clinics, STI clinics or for other purposes can be anonymously tested for HbsAg. Surveys in developing countries demonstrated the high levels of carriers, so with the implementation of routine vaccination, follow-up surveys will monitor the effectiveness of the vaccination programmes.

14.14 Hepatitis C (HCV)

Organism Hepatitis C virus (HCV).

Clinical features Similar in many respects to hepatitis B, HCV produces a milder disease, but as many as 10–20% will progress to cirrhosis and 1% to liver cancer in later life.

Diagnosis is difficult, dependent upon detecting antibodies to HCV and confirming by a recombinant immunoblot assay (RIBA). PCR is now commonly used.

Transmission is due to the use of poorly sterilized needles, giving-sets and other methods of parental administration and so is common in developing countries and in those who abuse drugs in developed countries. Sexual or perinatal transmission probably only occurs rarely.

Incubation period 2 weeks to 6 months (usually 6–9 weeks).

Period of communicability Weeks before the start of clinical symptoms to lifelong.

Occurrence and distribution Infection is found worldwide in the general population in developing countries and mainly in drug users sharing equipment in developed countries. However, there are probably many more cases than present figures suggest and WHO estimates that there are 200 million people infected, which amounts to 3% of the world's population. This means that there are about 170 million chronic carriers who could go on to develop cirrhosis or liver cancer.

Control and prevention There is no vaccine for HCV, so all precautions need to be taken to prevent further spread by rigorous adherence to sterilization of needles and instruments.

Treatment and surveillance See hepatitis B above.

14.15 Hepatitis Delta (HDV)

Organism Hepatitis delta virus (HDV) is dependent on HBV infection of the person. Either both viruses can infect at the same time or HDV infects an already infected HBV carrier.

Clinical features With coinfection (both viruses infecting at the same time), there is

normally a self-limiting infection with only about 5% continuing into the chronic form of HDV. However, with super-infection (HDV infection of an already HBV-infected person), there is a severe acute hepatitis with 80% continuing to chronic active hepatitis, often progressing to cirrhosis. Hepatocellular carcinoma due to HDV occurs with about the same frequency as with HBV. The mortality due to HDV is between 2% and 20% making it some ten times greater than for HBV alone.

Diagnosis is made by detecting antibody to HDV using a serological assay.

Transmission is the same as for HBV with the main route of transmission via infected blood and blood products. Super-infection produces the greatest amount of virus and chance of HDV transmission.

Incubation period 2–8 weeks.

Period of communicability It is probably most infectious in the weeks prior to symptoms, becoming negligible once disease is manifest.

Occurrence and distribution Areas of high prevalence are the Mediterranean, Southwest and Central Asia, West Africa and certain Pacific Islands. In the Amazon Basin, there is a particularly fulminant genotype (III), which carries a high mortality rate. In Western Europe and North America, infection is endemic in the drug addict community. Worldwide WHO estimates that more than 10 million people are infected.

Control and prevention Since HDV is dependent on HBV infection, the main strategy of control is to reduce HBV by vaccination. However, once chronically infected with HBV, vaccination offers no protection. This makes all the other methods for the control of HBV relevant.

Treatment and surveillance See hepatitis B above.

14.16 Ebola Haemorrhagic Fever

Organism Virus of the *Filoviridae* group of organisms.

Clinical features Illness presents with sudden onset of fever, headache, muscle pains, sore throat and profound weakness. This progresses to vomiting, diarrhoea and signs of internal and external bleeding, generally with the occurrence of liver and kidney damage. Mortality is 50–90%.

Diagnosis is by ELISA for specific IgG and IgM antibody or by PCR, but should only be carried out in laboratories with maximum facilities for protecting staff.

Transmission is by person-to-person contact via blood, secretions, semen or tissues of an infected person. Infected blood, especially via syringes, causes the most serious infections, while transmission has occurred via semen up to 7 weeks after clinical recovery.

Infection has also occurred through handling ill or dead chimpanzees, but it is thought that like humans, they are susceptible to the infection rather than being a reservoir.

Incubation period 2–21 days.

Period of communicability From start of symptoms and for up to 10 weeks for seminal fluid. Healthcare workers are particularly liable to become infected, especially during the phase of vomiting and diarrhoea. Contact with blood is invariably fatal.

Occurrence and distribution The main focus of infection is the rain forest of Central Africa, outbreaks having occurred in Sudan, Congo (formerly Zaire), Gabon and Uganda. Another focus of an Ebola-related virus has been found in monkeys in the Philippines exported for experimental purposes. The focal nature suggests a zoonosis, but despite extensive search, no reservoir has been found. Bats have been infected experimentally, but do not die, so might be responsible for maintaining the virus in the wild.

Control and prevention The strictest level of barrier nursing is required taking particular care to avoid contact with blood and all secretions. Patients who die must be buried or cremated immediately using the same precautions, with relatives being forbidden to take the body away for burial. Patients who recover must be counselled about the dangers of sexual intercourse and the infective nature of semen.

All contacts of a case and accidental contacts by healthcare workers must be quarantined and the temperature checked twice a day. Surveillance should continue for 3 weeks from the date of contact.

Treatment There is no specific therapy and hyper-immune serum does not offer any long-term protection.

Surveillance Outbreaks should be reported to WHO, neighbouring countries and those with air connections so that surveillance can be mounted on travellers.

14.17 Marburg Haemorrhagic Fever

A closely related virus infection, first identified from laboratory monkeys in Marburg, Germany, produces a similar illness to Ebola haemorrhagic fever, but with a mortality of about 25%. Cases have occurred in Uganda, Kenya, Zimbabwe and Congo (Zaire). In all other respects, it is similar to Ebola haemorrhagic fever to which reference should be made above.

14.18 Lassa and Crimea–Congo Haemorrhagic Fevers

Lassa and Crimea–Congo haemorrhagic fevers have similar presentations to Ebola and Marburg disease and are highly infectious through blood, urine and other body fluids, but as they are both primarily zoonoses, they are covered in Sections 17.9 and 16.9.2, respectively.

15

Insect-borne Diseases

By adopting a more specific means of transmission, some parasitic organisms have
become dependent on vectors for carriage
to a new host. Several vectors may be used
by some infecting organisms, such as arboviruses, but often a parasite is restricted to
only one kind of vector. This may appear to
reduce the chance of infection, but compared with the haphazard method of scatter-
ing large numbers of organisms into the
environment, in the hope that one of them
will find a new victim, using a vector can
have a greater chance of success. The parasite is carried right to the new host and in
many cases introduced directly into it.
Often, a development stage takes place in
the vector and the infective stage continues
for the rest of the vector's life. However,
transmission depends on the vector being
able to find a new host, often within a
limited period of time, at a vulnerable stage
in the life cycle, where control methods are
most likely to succeed.

Vector transmission is one of the commonest methods of spreading disease and
many of the infections transmitted this way
are of major importance, so large sections
need to be devoted to them. Such is the
importance that vector-transmitted diseases
are discussed in two chapters – this chapter,
which includes all the vectors that use
flight, such as mosquitoes and tsetse flies,

and the next chapter on ectoparasites, which
attach to the host, such as fleas and lice.
Since the vector is all-important in transmission, the diseases transmitted by them are
grouped according to the vector.

15.1 Mosquito-borne Diseases

The mosquito is the most important vector
of disease, because it is abundant, lives in
close proximity to humans and needs to feed
on blood (the female must have a blood meal
for the development of its eggs). Incredibly it
is a very delicate insect, being easily blown
by the wind, is a weak and slow flier, and
susceptible to climatic change. Its success
lies in its opportunism and rapid developmental cycle, allowing large numbers to be
produced in a short period of time. Once a
suitable breeding place appears, be it a few
puddles after a rainstorm or a man-made
water storage tank, mosquitoes will quickly
lay their eggs. These develop within a short
period of time into a large number of adults.
Each may become a vector, and although
many will die, there will be a sufficient
number left to seek out suitable blood
meals and transmit infection.

Some parasites are specific to certain
types of mosquitoes (e.g. malaria and
the anophelines), while others, like the

© R. Webber 2005. *Communicable Disease Epidemiology and Control,* 2nd edition (Roger Webber)

arboviruses, are less selective and utilize many different species. Different kinds of mosquitoes may be required in a complex transmission cycle such as yellow fever.

Development of the parasite within the mosquito may be morphological without multiplication (as with filaria), asexual (arbovirus) or sexual reproduction (malaria). Each of these methods confer advantages and disadvantages, such as the sheer number of organisms produced by asexual reproduction, or the opportunity to produce strains of varying type with sexual reproduction, but if the mosquito does not live long enough for these developmental stages to take place, then all is lost.

There are two main groups of mosquitoes – the anophelines and the culicines (which includes *Aedes*), separated by characteristics found in all of the development stages (Fig. 15.1). The adult *Anopheles* mosquito raises its hind legs away from the surface, easily remembered by its stance being like one side of a letter 'A', while the lava lies horizontal to the surface. The eggs are laid singly and have little floats on each side. In contrast, culicine mosquitoes rest horizontal to the surface, their larvae hang down from a single siphon and their eggs have no floats and are often laid in rafts. It is better to try and differentiate an adult male, with bushy antennae, from a female before subsequently separating anophelines from culicines by the length of the palps. More precise species identification is required to identify which mosquitoes are principal vectors, but this needs entomological help.

Mosquitoes differ in their habits, some preferring to take blood meals on humans (*anthropophilic*) or on animals (*zoophilic*) or are non-specific depending on which is most readily available. They also have particular biting times, either only indoors, only outdoors or a mixture of the two. The biting period can be mainly during the night or predominantly in the daytime. All these different parameters need to be measured in determining the importance of each type of mosquito as a vector.

15.2 Arboviruses

Arthropod-borne virus (arbovirus) infections occur in an epidemic form in different parts of the world. Many viruses have been identified (see Table 15.1 and Chapter 19) and are grouped into three-symptom complexes.

(a) Those producing mainly fever and/or arthritis

15.2.1 Chikungunya, Onyong-nyong, West Nile, Orungo, Oropouche and Ross River

This group of infections are summarized in Table 15.1. They present as a dengue-like disease (see below) with headache, fever, malaise, arthralgia or myalgia, lasting for a week or less. Rashes are common in Chikungunya, Onyong-nyong and West Nile. Chikungunya may present as a haemorrhagic fever in India and Southeast Asia (see below), and West Nile and Oropouche as encephalitides. Ross River predominantly presents as a polyarthritis and rash. There are many other arbovirus infections presenting as fever, listed in Chapter 19.

Diagnosis of all the arbovirus infections is generally made on clinical grounds, once the initial cases have been identified by virus isolation in a specialist laboratory. A rise in specific IgM in serum or CSF is useful, if available.

Incubation period 2–15 days.

Period of communicability of all the arbovirus infections is as long as there are still infected mosquitoes remaining.

Susceptibility is general, but infection leads to immunity, probably life-long. In endemic areas, they are diseases of children, otherwise they are epidemic, affecting all age groups and both sexes. In 2002, there were epidemics of West Nile virus in Israel,

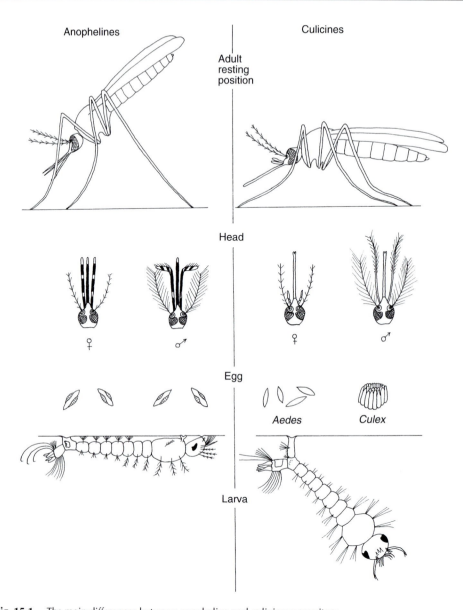

Fig. 15.1. The main differences between anopheline and culicine mosquitoes.

Canada and the USA (resulting in 3231 cases and 176 deaths in the USA), countries where this infection had not occurred before. While most people suffered minor illness, individuals with weakened immune systems, such as people with chronic diseases, those on chemotherapy or the elderly suffered more serious effects, including meningitis and encephalitis.

(b) Those presenting as fever and encephalitis

15.2.2 Western equine, Eastern equine, St Louis, Venezuelan, Japanese, Murray Valley and Rocio

This group of diseases present with a high fever of acute onset, headache, meningeal

Table 15.1. The important arbovirus infections of humans.

Virus	Distribution	Vectors	Reservoir
Mainly fever or arthritis			
Chikungunya	Africa, South and Southeast Asia	*Aedes aegypti, Ae. africanus, Ae. leuteocephalus*	Baboons, bats, rodents, monkeys
Onyong-nyong	E. Africa, Senegal	*Anopheles gambiae, A. funestus*	Mosquito?
West Nile	Africa, Asia, Europe, USA	*Culex pipens molestus, C. modestus, C. univittatus*	Birds?
Oropuche	Trinidad, South America	Mosquitoes, possibly *Culicoides*	Monkeys, sloths, birds
Orungo	W. Africa, Uganda	*Ae. dentatus, Anopheles* spp.	
Ross River	Australia, New Zealand, Pacific Islands	*C. annulirostris, Ae. vigilax, Ae. polynesiensis*	Mosquito
Fever and encephalitis			
Western Equine	Americas	*C. tarsalis, Culista melanura*	Birds
Eastern Equine	Americas, Caribbean	*C. melanura, Aedes* and *Coquillettidia* spp.	Birds, rodents
St Louis	Americas, Caribbean	*C. tarsalis, C. nigripalpus, C. quinquefasciatus*	Birds
Venezuelan Equine	Central/South America, Caribbean, parts of USA	*C. tarsalis* and other *Culex, Aedes, Mansonia, Sabethes, Psorophora, Anopheles, Haemagogus*	Rodents
Japanese	East, South and Southeast Asia	*C. tritaeniorhynchus, C. gelidus, C. fuscocephala*	Birds, pigs
Murray Valley	New Guinea, Australia	*C. annulirostris*	Birds
Rocio	Brazil	Probably mosquitoes	Birds? Rodents
Haemorrhagic fevers			
Yellow fever	South America and Africa	*Ae. aegypti, Ae. africanus, Ae. simpsoni, Ae. furcifer/ taylori, Ae. luteocephalus, Haemagogus* spp.	Monkeys, mosquitoes
Dengue 1, 2, 3 and 4	Asia, Pacific, Caribbean, Africa, Americas	*Ae. aegypti, Ae. albopictus, Ae. scutellaris* group, *Ae. niveus, Ochlerotatus*	Human/mosquito, (Monkeys in jungle cycle)
Rift Valley	Africa, Southwest Asia	*Ae. caballus, C. theileri, C. quinquefasciatus* and other *Culex* and *Aedes*	Sheep, cattle, etc. Mosquito
Kyasanur forest	South India	*Haemaphysalis* (hard ticks)	Rodents, monkeys
Crimean–Congo haemorrhagic fever	Europe, Africa, Asia	*Hyalomma* spp. (hard ticks)	Domestic animals

irritation, stupor, disorientation, coma, spasticity and tremors. Fatality rates are variable with up to 30% in Japanese, Eastern equine and Murray Valley. Their distribution, vectors and reservoirs are summarized in Table 15.1. Japanese encephalitis is covered in more detail below.

From the reservoir bird or animal, the organism is often first transmitted to another host, such as horses in the equine arbovirus infections. Humans are then mainly infected from mosquitoes feeding on the horses.

Incubation period is 5–15 days. Susceptibility is highest in the very young and old, with inapparent infection occurring at other age groups.

(c) Haemorrhagic fevers

15.2.3 Yellow fever, dengue, Rift Valley, Kyasanur forest disease, Crimean–Congo and Chikungunya

Apart from yellow fever, which will be covered in more detail below, a group of generally mild viral fevers including dengue, Rift Valley, Kyasanur forest disease (KFD) and Chikungunya, which at certain places and occasions take on a severe form resulting in vascular permeability, hypovolaemia and abnormal blood clotting. Infection commences as an acute fever, malaise, headache, nausea or vomiting with petechial rashes, severe bruising, epistaxis and bleeding from various sites. After a few days, sudden circulatory failure and shock may occur producing a mortality of up to 40%.

Rift Valley Fever is normally a disease of cattle, sheep, camels and goats, in which high mortality can cause considerable economic loss, but spread to humans also occurs. A large number of unexplained abortions in livestock is often the first sign of an impending epidemic. The disease was normally restricted to Africa, but in 2000, it spread to Saudi Arabia and Yemen, raising the fear that it could infect other parts of Asia and Europe.

Some arbovirus infections can also be spread by non-mosquito arthropods, such as KFD and Crimea–Congo fever (see Section 16.9.2).

Control and prevention of arbovirus infections The main method of control is the destruction of vector mosquitoes and breeding places. The most important are *Culex* and *Aedes* mosquitoes, which live in collections of water close to the home. Search is made for larvae and all breeding places destroyed. A simple method is to use school children, making it a game or giving a reward for the number of breeding places found. Water tanks, blocked drains, discarded tin cans or old tyres are favourite breeding places. Large breeding areas (such as water tanks) can be covered, screened, treated with insecticides or natural predators introduced (e.g. fish or dragonfly larvae). An improvement on covering water pots and containers is to use an insecticide-treated pot cover rather than place the insecticide in the container.

Where there is an epidemic in a compact area such as a town, the quickest and simplest (although expensive) method of bringing the epidemic to an end is to use fogging or ULV aerial spraying. Compared with working hours lost, this can be a cost-effective procedure.

Personal prevention with repellents (see malaria) can protect the individual. The infected case should be nursed under a mosquito net so as not to infect other mosquitoes. A vaccine is available for Venezuelan, Eastern and Western equine encephalitis, which can be used both for humans and horses.

Where an animal reservoir is involved, some restriction of animals or reduction of rodents can help. In Rift Valley fever, special precautions should be taken in handling domestic animals and their products by wearing gloves and protective clothing. Blood and other body fluids of patients are also infectious, so barrier nursing should be instituted. All animals should be vaccinated. A vaccine for use in humans is under trial.

Treatment There is no specific treatment, supportive therapy being given (Ribavirin may be of value).

Surveillance Regular checks should be made on mosquito-breeding places and control methods instituted where mosquitoes are found. People can be taught to regularly search their home areas for mosquito breeding. (See further under yellow fever below.)

15.3 Japanese Encephalitis (JE)

Organism The Japanese encephalitis virus (JEV) is a member of the flavivirus family, the same group of viruses as West Nile and St Louis encephalitis.

Clinical features Japanese encephalitis presents as a sudden onset of fever, headache, body aches and pains. Mild cases recover completely, but a high proportion develop encephalitis and progressive coma. Children under 10 years of age may present with gastro-intestinal symptoms and convulsions, rapidly leading to death. Those who survive the severe disease may have residual neurological or psychiatric disabilities.

Diagnosis is by finding the specific IgM in CSF or serum. The virus can be cultured in specialist laboratories.

Transmission The main vectors are *Culex tritaeniorhynchus, C. gelidus* and *C. fuscocephala,* mosquitoes that predominantly breed in rice fields. The reservoir of infection is probably wading birds, but domestic pigs also harbour the virus, from which it is transferred to humans. The mosquito breeds when the rice fields are flooded and the first green shoots appear, dying off when the rice grows and shades the water, thereby displaying a marked seasonality, with a peak period of July and August in Thailand, August in China, and September and November in India and Nepal. In irrigated areas, mosquito breeding can occur throughout the year, while outbreaks have occurred in urban areas, where suitable stagnant water permits the breeding of vector mosquitoes.

Incubation period 4–14 days.

Period of communicability As long as there are infected mosquitoes continuing to bite people. Mosquitoes can also become infected by feeding on a clinical case any time during the illness.

Occurrence and distribution Serological surveys indicate that most people living in endemic areas contract sub-clinical infection before the age of 15 years. However, young children and adults, who have not been infected as children (including visitors), may get clinical disease and possibly severe disease, with 20–30% mortality. There are about 50,000 cases and 10,000 deaths reported annually.

The endemic area is South and Southeast Asia, particularly Cambodia, Laos, Vietnam, Thailand, Malaysia, Myanmar, Indonesia, Philippines, the Indian subcontinent, Russia and a decreasing incidence in China, Japan and Korea. A small outbreak in Torres Strait islands is a worrying sign that the infection might spread into northern Australia. Risk within any of these countries is greatest during the rice-growing season and when an epidemic is ongoing.

Control and prevention Agricultural methods, such as drying out rice fields when no crop is growing or decreasing the number of crops, can reduce the period of risk. Personal protection with long sleeved clothing, the wearing of trousers and use of repellents can reduce mosquito biting. The mosquito bites during the daytime, so babies and young children should be made to sleep under insecticide-treated mosquito nets. The main method of prevention is the use of vaccination to all children in endemic areas, after the age of 1 year, so as not to interfere with remaining maternal antibodies. However, allergic reactions to the vaccine are reasonably frequent, so caution should be exercised especially in allergic persons. Repeat booster doses are necessary as the period of protection has not been fully worked out and there is some suggestion of a shift in the age group contracting the disease, in areas where vaccination has been used for some years.

Treatment There is no treatment.

Surveillance Notification of cases should be reported to WHO, so that neighbouring countries and visitors can take precautions.

15.4 Dengue

Organism Dengue virus has four serotypes (1, 2, 3 and 4).

Clinical features Dengue presents as a sudden onset of fever, retro-orbital headache, joint and muscle pains. A maculo-papular or scarlatina-form rash usually appears after 3–4 days. Depression and prolonged fatigue often occur following the acute manifestations. Dengue haemorrhagic fever (DHF), in which there is profound bleeding into skin and tissues, is now a serious feature of many epidemics.

DHF is probably due to a sensitization with a previous dengue serotype, either acquired at birth or from a previous infection, type 2 being the most potent and types 3, 4 and 1 being responsible in decreasing importance. Differential effect on racial groups suggests that host factors may also have a role, as well as the geographical origin of the dengue strain.

Diagnosis Virus can be isolated from the blood in acute cases or a rising antibody level may assist in diagnosis.

Transmission Mosquitoes of the *Aedes* group, especially *Ae. aegypti*, *Ae. albopictus* or a member of the *Ae. scutellaris* group are responsible for transmission. These mosquitoes are more easily identifiable than most by their black colour, with distinctive white markings (Fig. 15.2). They like to breed close to humans, taking advantage

of any water containers, old tyres, empty tins or other small collections of water in which they can breed. They are daytime biters and can be found in large numbers in urban and peri-urban areas. *Ae. albopictus* has comparatively recently become established in the USA, Central America and the Caribbean due to the trade in used tyres.

Virus is maintained in a human/mosquito cycle in many parts of the world, but in Africa and Southeast Asia, a monkey/mosquito cycle is involved.

Incubation period 3–15 days (commonly 4–6 days).

Period of communicability The mosquito is able to transmit infection for 8–12 days after taking an infective blood meal and remains so for the rest of its life. Humans and monkeys are infectious during and just before the febrile period.

Occurrence and distribution Dengue is now endemic in many parts of the world, South and Central America, sub-Saharan Africa, South and Southeast Asia. In more isolated communities, large epidemics have occurred, especially in the island countries of the Caribbean and Pacific with devastating effect. The epidemic can be so massive as to immobilize large segments of the population, disrupt the work force and cause a breakdown in organization. The development of DHF has been variable, producing a number of deaths. It is estimated that there are about 50 million cases of dengue, 0.5 million cases of DHF and 12,000 deaths due to dengue every year. Children are the main sufferers of both dengue and DHF.

Control and prevention The main method of control is to reduce mosquito breeding, especially of the *Aedes* mosquito, by depriving it of collections of water or covering them so that mosquitoes cannot enter. All water tanks, pots or other containers must be covered at all times, a recent improvement being to treat these covers with insecticides as it is often difficult to get a perfect fit.

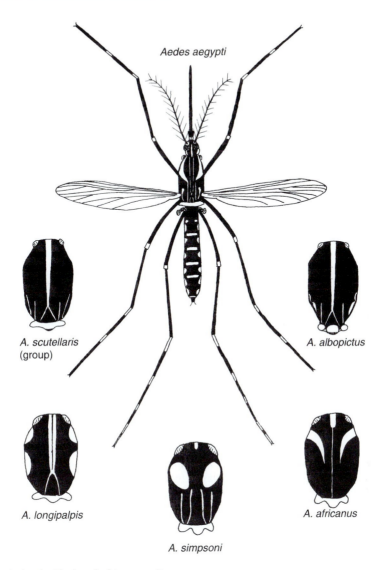

Aedes aegypti

A. scutellaris
(group)

A. albopictus

A. longipalpis

A. simpsoni

A. africanus

Fig. 15.2. *Aedes,* the black and white mosquitoes.

Guttering around the roof can also allow pools of water to collect, so these should be of sufficient slope and cleaned out regularly so that water cannot collect. Old tyres should have holes cut in them or removed altogether (one answer to the disposal problem is to weight them and bury them at sea to form artificial reefs).

People should check their gardens and immediate vicinity at regular intervals to remove any cans, coconut shells or other temporary collections of water. Children are very effective at doing this and can be encouraged with a marks or reward scheme.

Screening of houses and mosquito nets are of little use because people are often outside their houses when the mosquito bites, but are of value for young children. ULV spraying, either by fogging or by aircraft, is of value in the presence of an epidemic, but only adult mosquitoes are killed and are soon replaced by young adults unless simultaneous larval control is also in operation.

Treatment There is no specific treatment, but hypovolaemic shock must be treated with rapid fluid replacement and oxygen therapy.

Surveillance Regular checks should be made on mosquito breeding, especially of *Ae. aegypti*. Samples should be taken and the number of larvae breeding counted to give an indication of the risk of transmission. Further details will be found under yellow fever.

15.5 Yellow Fever

Organism The yellow fever virus is a *Flavivirus*.

Clinical features One of the haemorrhagic group of arbovirus infections, yellow fever presents with a sudden onset of fever, headache, backache, prostration and vomiting. Jaundice commences mildly at first and intensifies as the disease progresses. Albuminuria and leucopenia are found on examination, while haemorrhagic symptoms of epistaxis, haematemesis, melena and bleeding from the gums can all occur. In endemic areas, the fatality rate is low except in the non-indigenous areas. The death rate may reach 50% during epidemics.

Diagnosis is made on clinical grounds after initial identification of an outbreak. Virus can be isolated from the blood in specialist laboratories. Specific IgM in early sera or a rise in titre in paired serum can be of value, but cross-reactions can occur with other flaviviruses.

Transmission Yellow fever is a disease of the forest, maintained in the monkey population by *Haemagogus*, *Sabethes* and *Aedes* mosquitoes in America, and *Aedes* in Africa. The monkeys are generally not affected by the disease, but occasionally start dying, indicating that spread to the human population may soon begin. In South America, it may be a reduction in the monkey population that will make

the canopy mosquito look for another blood meal and perhaps feed on humans. More commonly, it is the person who goes into the forest to cut wood or hunt and is bitten incidentally. When they return to their village or town, they are fed on by *Ae. aegypti* and an urban yellow fever transmission cycle is set up (see Fig. 15.3). In Africa, three different kinds of mosquitoes are involved. *Ae. africanus* remains in the jungle canopy rarely feeding on humans, but should the monkey descend to the forest floor or even enter areas of human habitation, it is fed on by *Ae. simpsoni*, *Ae. furcifer-taylori* or *Ae. luteocephalus*. The mosquito then bites a person on the edge of the forest, who returns to the village soon to suffer from yellow fever. Fed upon by the peri-domestic mosquito *Ae. aegypti*, an urban cycle is started (Fig. 15.3). The extrinsic cycle of infection takes 5–30 days in the mosquito depending on temperature and type of mosquito. Trans-ovarian infection can also occur.

Incubation period 3–6 days.

Period of communicability is from before the fever commences to 5 days after, so the patient should be nursed under a mosquito net to prevent new mosquitoes from becoming infected.

Occurrence and distribution Yellow fever nearly always presents as an epidemic in humans, affecting all ages and both sexes, although adults (particularly males) who go into the forest are likely to be the first to contract the disease. There are estimated to be 200,000 cases and 30,000 deaths annually from yellow fever, most of them in Africa. Most cases have been reported from Nigeria in recent times. Yellow fever is restricted to the areas of Africa and South America, and Panama in Central America, shown in Fig. 5.1.

Control and prevention The most important part of the complex mosquito transmission cycle is *Ae. aegypti*. With its proximity to humans, it is capable of infecting a large

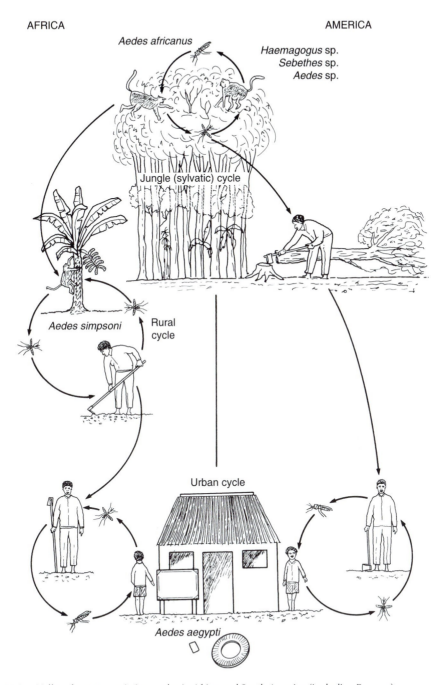

AFRICA

AMERICA

Aedes africanus

Haemagogus sp.
Sebethes sp.
Aedes sp.

Jungle (sylvatic) cycle

Aedes simpsoni Rural cycle

Urban cycle

Aedes aegypti

Fig. 15.3. Yellow fever transmission cycles in Africa and South America (including Panama).

number of people as well as being the most easy to control. It breeds in small collections of water near people's houses, so a careful search for larvae and the destruction of breeding places can do much to reduce the danger. Simple clearance is the most effective method of reducing the mosquito population (see under dengue above), but insecticides such as temephos (Abate) can be used where collections of water cannot be destroyed. In the event of an epidemic, emergency reduction by fogging or ULV spray from aircraft will rapidly destroy the adult population (but not the larvae).

One attack of yellow fever confers immunity for life if the person survives the disease. Inapparent infections can also occur. A very effective vaccine has been developed which provides immunity for at least 10 years and probably longer, so all those at risk in the known endemic areas should be vaccinated (Fig. 5.1). This has been attempted by offering vaccination at markets and meetings or systematically to school children. WHO has now recommended that yellow fever vaccination be included in the childhood vaccination programme in the 33 countries of Africa in the yellow fever zone, to be given at the same time as measles vaccine. In the event of an epidemic, ring vaccination can be performed; the epidemic is surrounded by a circle of vaccinated persons, progressively closing in on the centre of the outbreak. Areas of Africa and South America have been designated as yellow fever areas (Fig. 5.1) and all visitors to this zone require vaccination.

In these days of rapid air transport it has always been surprising that yellow fever has not been transported to Asia, where there are the vectors and conditions for transmission. A suggested reason is that there is some cross-immunity with other Group B viruses and the level of such induced immunity may be sufficient to prevent epidemic spread. A precaution is to spray all aircraft coming from a yellow fever area.

Treatment There is no specific treatment, but supportive therapy is given to combat shock and renal failure.

Surveillance All cases of suspected or confirmed yellow fever must be reported to WHO. The prevalence of the urban vector can be measured by the *Ae. aegypti* index. This is the number of houses found with *Ae. aegypti* breeding within a specified area of 100 houses. Alternatively, the Breteau index can be used, which is the number of containers in which larvae are found out of 100 samples. If these are kept below 5% or preferably 1%, then the danger of an epidemic is minimized.

15.6 Malaria

Organism There are four human malaria parasites, *Plasmodium falciparum*, *P. vivax*, *P. malariae* and *P. ovale*. *P. falciparum* causes the most serious disease and is the commonest parasite in tropical regions, but differs from *P. vivax* and *P. ovale* in having no persistent stage (the hypnozoite), from which repeat blood stage parasites are produced. *P. vivax* has the widest geographical range, being found in temperate and sub-tropical zones as well as the tropics. *P. vivax* infection will lead to relapses if a schizonticidal drug only is used for treatment and some strains, e.g. the Chesson strain in New Guinea (Papua New Guinea and Irian Jaya) and Solomon Islands requires a more prolonged radical treatment. *P. malariae* produces a milder infection, but is distinguished from the other three by paroxysms of fever every fourth day. *P. malariae* can persist as an asymptomatic low-grade parasitaemia for many years, to multiply at a future date as a clinical infection. *P. ovale* is the rarest of the parasites and is suppressed by infections with the other species.

The malaria parasite reproduces asexually in humans and sexually in the mosquito (Fig. 15.4). A merozoite attacks a RBC, divides asexually, rupturing the cell, each newformed merozoite attacking another RBC. Toxins are liberated when the cell ruptures, producing the clinical paroxysms. After several asexual cycles, male and female gametes are produced, which are ingested when a mosquito takes a blood meal. These go through a complex developmental cycle in the stomach wall of the mosquito, culminating in the production of sporozoites, which migrate to the salivary glands ready to enter another person when the mosquito next takes a blood meal.

The sporozoite enters a liver cell in which development to a schizont takes place. This ruptures, liberating merozoites, which attack RBCs, thereby starting an erythrocytic cycle. In *P. vivax* and *P. ovale*, a persistent liver stage, the hypnozoite is formed, meaning that if parasites are cleared from the blood, relapses can occur, often continuing for many years unless radical treatment is given.

Clinical features Infection commences with fever and headache, soon developing into an alternating pattern of peaks of fever followed by sweating and profound chills. Classically, these take on a pattern of either 3 days (tertiary malaria) or 4 days (quaternary malaria). However, falciparum malaria can present in many different forms including cerebral malaria (encephalopathy and coma) as acute shock, haematuria (blackwater fever) and jaundice.

Diagnosis is with a thick blood smear (to detect parasites) and a thin smear (to determine species) (Fig. 15.5). A dipstick method for *P. falciparum* has made the diagnosis of malaria simpler, but is still too expensive for routine use in many countries. It is particularly useful for surveys. A similar dipstick method for the other malaria parasites has been developed, but is not sufficiently sensitive or specific to replace blood slides.

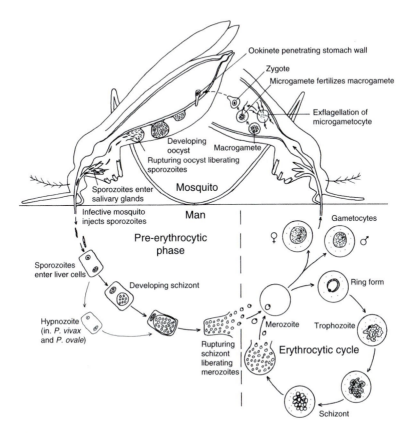

Fig. 15.4. The malaria life cycle.

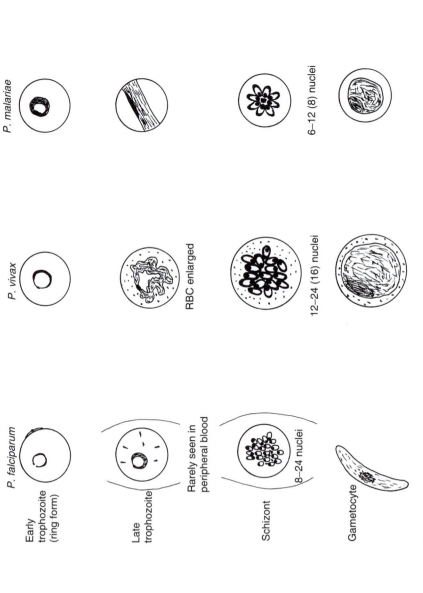

Fig. 15.5. Differential diagnosis of *Plasmodium* spp. RBC, red blood cell.

Table 15.2. The main malaria vectors and their behaviour in relation to control.

Geographical area	Anopheles species	Behaviour in relation to control
More arid areas of sub-Saharan Africa and Western Arabia	*Anopheles arabiensis*	Feeds on animals and humans depending on availability. Some exit after feeding
More humid parts of sub-Saharan Africa	*A. gambiae* s.s.	Bites humans in the middle of the night. Rests indoors after feeding. Breeds in temporary puddles, increasing considerably in wet season and declining in dry
Sub-Saharan Africa, including highlands	*A. funestus*	Bites humans in the middle of the night. Rests indoors after feeding. Breeds in more permanent water bodies, remaining a constant vector throughout the year
Rural areas of Indian sub-continent and Southwest Asia	*A. culicifacies,* species A, C, D and E	Feeds predominantly on animals, but bites humans sufficiently to be the main rural vector in India and Sri Lanka. Tends to bite early in the night. Breeds in water tanks and pools, but not rice fields
Urban areas of Indian sub-continent and Southwest Asia	*A. stephensi*	Feeds on humans and animals throughout night, except in cold weather, when biting is early. Breeds in wells and water tanks
Indian sub-continent	*A. fluviatilis* species S	Bites humans and rests indoors. Associated with hill streams
South and Southeast Asia	*A. sundaicus*	Mainly bites cattle, but also humans sufficiently to be a vector. Breeds in salt-water lagoons
Southeast Asia (including northeast India and southwest China)	*A. minimus*	Feeds on humans and rests indoors, but due to prolonged insecticide spraying has changed to outdoor resting and animal biting in some areas
Southeast Asia	*A. dirus*	Bites humans indoors, but then exits. Associated with forests
	A. aconitus	Lives indoors. Breeds in rice fields
Nepal, Malaysia, Indonesia	*A. maculatus*	Bites humans indoors. Breeds in rice fields
Indonesia	*A. leucosphyrus*	Bites humans and rests indoors
Philippines	*A. flavirostris*	Bites humans and rests indoors
China	*A. sinensis*	Mainly bites animals, inefficient vector
	A. anthropophagus	Bites humans, efficient vector. Both breed in rice fields
Melanesia	*A. farauti*	Bites humans indoors and rests indoors
	A. punctulatus, A. koliensis	Breeds in temporary rainwater pools
Central America, western South America and Haiti	*A. albimanus*	Bites outside and early in the night. More abundant during rainy season
Central and northern South America	*A. pseudopunctipennis*	Bites humans indoors
North urban South America	*A. darlingi*	Bites humans and rests indoors. Biting time variable in different parts of its range. More abundant during rainy season
Northern South America	*A. nuñeztovari*	Bites humans indoors, but exits during night
	A. aquasalis	Bites outside and early in the night. Breeds in brackish water
South America	*A. albitarsis* complex (*A. marajoara*)	Bites humans outdoors. Associated with gold mining
Turkey, Central Asia, Afghanistan	*A. sacharovi, A. superpictus*	Bites humans indoors

Transmission is by *Anopheles* mosquitoes (Table 15.2). The efficiency of the vector will depend upon the species of *Anopheles*, its feeding habits and the environmental conditions. This varies widely, with *A. gambiae* being the most efficient of all malaria vectors, to a species such as *Anopheles culicifacies*, which is comparatively inefficient. This is determined by a number of factors, such as the preferred food source (humans or animals), the time of biting (easier in the middle of the night when people are sleeping) and whether it lives inside the house or outside, but the most important is the mosquito's length of life. Only a few *A. culicifacies* will survive longer than 12 days and so become infective (dying before completion of the extrinsic cycle), whereas 50% of a population of *A. gambiae* will live longer than 12 days. Longer living mosquitoes are better vectors. A female mosquito must have a blood meal before it can complete its gonotrophic cycle and lay a batch of eggs. The gonotrophic cycle is normally about 2–3 days, but varies with temperature, species and locality. Long-living mosquitoes will be able to lay several batches of eggs and this is used to estimate the longevity of a mosquito species.

Another factor is mosquito density. A large number of mosquitoes have greater transmission potential than a few. Some mosquitoes produce large numbers at certain favourable times of the year, while others maintain more constant populations. The environment largely determines mosquito density.

The most important environmental factors are temperature and humidity, with wind, phases of the moon and human activity having lesser effect. Temperature determines the length of development cycle of the parasite and the survival of the mosquito vector. This means that in temperate climates, malaria can only be transmitted in brief periods of warm weather when the right conditions are available. In tropical regions, altitude alters the temperature and highland areas will have less (although possibly epidemic) malaria.

Water is essential for the mosquito to breed. In arid desert countries, the mosquito cannot survive, but water in the wells and that used for irrigation have allowed mosquitoes to breed and malaria to appear. Rainfall generally increases the number of breeding places for mosquitoes, so there is more malaria in the wet season. However, if the rainfall is so heavy as to wash out breeding places, this results in a decrease of mosquitoes.

The mosquito, being a fragile flyer, is easily blown by the wind, sometimes to its advantage, but generally to its disadvantage. On windy evenings, mosquito biting may decrease considerably.

Nocturnal mosquitoes are sensitive to light; so on a moonlit night, there is a reduction in numbers. Measurements of mosquito density must be made on several nights, or ideally over a period of months.

When the mosquito species is mainly zoophilic (feeds on animals), keeping domestic animals in proximity to the household will encourage mosquitoes to feed on them, instead of on the human occupants. It is these environmental factors which determine whether malaria is *endemic* or *epidemic*. Where conditions of temperature and moisture permit all-year-round breeding of mosquitoes, endemic malaria occurs, but if there is a marked dry season or reduction in temperature, then conditions for transmission may only be suitable during a part of the year, resulting in seasonal malaria. If conditions are marginal and only favourable every few years, then epidemic malaria can result. Epidemic malaria is devastating, as large numbers of people who have no immunity are attacked. Endemic and epidemic malaria call for entirely different strategies of control.

Malaria can also be transmitted by blood transfusion, from needles and syringes, and rarely congenitally.

Incubation period depends upon the species and strain of the parasite:

P. falciparum	9–14 days
P. vivax	12–17 days, but in temperate climates, it can be 6–9 months
P. malariae	18–40 days
P. ovale	16–18 days

Period of communicability is as long as there are infective mosquitoes. For a mosquito to become infective, it must live long enough for the parasite to complete the developmental cycle (the extrinsic cycle), which depends upon the temperature and species. *P. vivax* completes this more quickly than *P. falciparum*.

Species of parasite	Development time (days) at mean ambient temperature		
	30°C	24°C	20°C
P. vivax	7	9	16
P. falciparum	9	11	20
P. malariae	15	21	30

At 19°C, *P. falciparum* takes in excess of 30 days (beyond the life expectancy of an average mosquito), whereas *P. vivax* can still complete its cycle in less than 20 days. The absolute minimum temperature for *P. vivax* is 17°C, but the extrinsic cycle is longer than the lifetime of the mosquito.

Occurrence and distribution In a non-immune population, children and adults of both sexes are affected equally. In areas of continuous infection with *P. falciparum*, malaria is predominantly an infection of children in whom mortality can be considerable. The survivors acquire immunity, which is only preserved by the maintenance of parasites in the body, due to re-infection. Should the individual leave an area of continuous malaria, immunity may be reduced. Immunity is also reduced during pregnancy, severe malaria can occur in a pregnant woman, even if she has lived in an endemic area. This is worse in the first pregnancy than subsequently.

The body responds to malaria by an enlargement of the spleen. The degree of enlargement and the proportion of the population with palpable spleens have been used as a measure of endemicity:

- *Hypoendemic*. Spleen rate in children (2–9 years of age) not exceeding 10%.
- *Mesoendemic*. Spleen rate in children between 11% and 50%.

- *Hyperendemic*. Spleen rate in children constantly over 50%. Spleen rate in adults also high (over 25%).
- *Holoendemic*. Spleen rate in children constantly over 75%, but spleen rate in adults low.

In endemic areas, the gametocyte rate is highest in the very young, but in epidemic malaria or areas where transmission has been considerably reduced, gametocytes occur at all ages.

Malaria is found in the tropics and subtropics of the world (Fig. 15.6 and Table 15.2), mostly *P. falciparum*, but *P. vivax* is the predominant species in the Indian subcontinent. It used to be more extensive with seasonal malaria in temperate regions, but extensive control programmes have confined it to its present limits. However, increase in population and the development of resistance, both by the parasite and the mosquito, means that malaria is still the most important parasitic disease in the world. Each year, there are some 300 million cases out of which over a million die.

Global climatic change has resulted in an increase in epidemic malaria (infecting new or infrequently involved areas) and the development of endemic malaria in highland areas, which were normally protected by their lower temperatures (see also Section 1.4.7).

Control and prevention Mathematical models were introduced in Section 2.4, malaria being one of the best examples in which they can be used to work out the strategy for control. The parasite life cycle was described above and illustrated in Fig. 15.4, while each of these stages can be represented mathematically as schematically shown in Fig 15.7. The stages and values for each of the places where the life cycle can be interrupted are given below:

1. In *humans*

- reduction of the duration of infection $(1/r)$ by chemotherapy;
- prevention of infections with gametocytes (b) by chemoprophylaxis and vaccination.

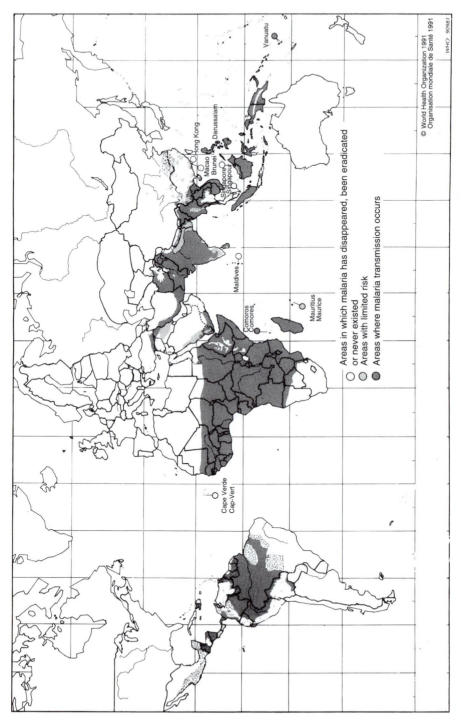

Fig. 15.6. The occurrence of malaria in the world. (Reproduced by permission of the World Health Organization, Geneva.)

2. In *mosquitoes*

- prevention of human biting ($a \times a = a^2$) by personal protection and mosquito nets;
- decreasing mosquito density (m) with larviciding and biological control;
- reduction of the proportion surviving to infectivity (p^n) by residual insecticides and treated mosquito nets;
- reduction of the mosquito expectation of life ($1/-l_n p$) by knock-down and residual insecticides.

(p is the probability of a mosquito surviving through 1 day, n the time taken to complete the extrinsic cycle, and l_n the natural logarithm.)

The complete formula becomes

$$z_0 = \frac{ma^2 bp^n}{-r(l_n p)}$$

where z_0 is the basic reproductive rate (see Section 2.2.3).

Each of the parameters can be given values that have been measured in the field so that the level of control required to interrupt transmission can be calculated (reduce the basic reproductive rate below 1).

Some useful modifications of the formula are the

$$\text{Vectorial capacity} = \frac{ma^2 p^n}{-r(l_n p)}$$

and the critical density of mosquitoes below which the infection will die out given by

$$\frac{-r(l_n p)}{a^2 bp^n}$$

More complex models have been developed to overcome some of the shortcomings of this model, such as the development of immunity, but even in this limited form, it is very valuable.

The effectiveness of any potential strategy can be estimated from the algebraic

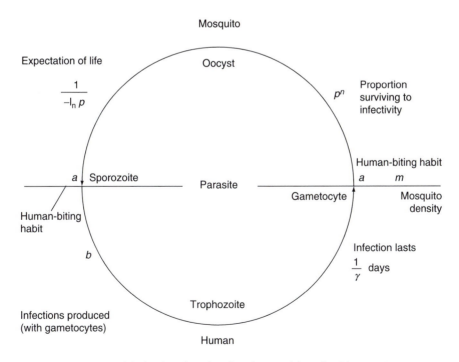

Fig. 15.7. Mathematical model of malaria based on the schematic life cycle of the parasite.

expression given to each part of the formula without making any calculations:

- $1/r$ – the duration of infection reduced by chemotherapy, demonstrates the small effect of just treating malaria cases, and that control efforts, such as MDA used in malaria eradication programmes, need to be total, covering every single person, virtually impossible to achieve.
- b – this is actually a notation normally applied to mosquitoes, being the proportion that ingest gametocytes so that the parasite sexual cycle can take place, but can be applied to the human part of the cycle as any method which prevents the production of gametocytes. This can either be by preventing infection in the first place with vaccination or chemoprophylaxis, the use of gametocidal drugs, or preventing the mosquito feeding on a malaria case by keeping them under a mosquito net. However, b is only a unitary factor, so all of these methods will need to be nearly perfect to work.
- a – the number of bites that need to be made by the mosquito. One bite is needed to introduce infection and another to take up gametocytes, so the interruption of mosquito biting could be quite an effective strategy. Therefore, personal protection with clothing, repellents and mosquito nets is a valuable method of control.
- m – the density of mosquitoes is only a unitary factor demonstrating the poor results of larviciding and biological methods in malaria control.
- p – mosquito survival consists of two factors, its expectation of life (short-lived vectors are poor transmitters) and the number of mosquitoes living long enough to complete the extrinsic cycle. In this p is raised to the nth power showing that reducing the length of life of the mosquito (mainly by the use of insecticides) is the best control strategy.

PERSONAL PROTECTION   Methods of personal protection have been covered in Section 3.4.1. They include clothing, mosquito nets and repellents. Items of clothing, such as socks and shawls, can be treated with repellents, which retain activity for some time, or repellents can be applied directly to the skin. Some naturally occurring plants have repellent properties, such as African marigolds (*Tagetes minuta*).

Mosquito nets are most effective if used properly. Providing subsidized mosquito nets can help in malaria control, especially for mothers and children, who are liable to go to bed early (before mosquito biting starts). This can be improved by treating the nets with synthetic pyrethroid insecticides (such as permethrin, deltamethrin, alpha-cypermethrin or lambda-cyhalothrin). This repels mosquitoes and kills those which come into contact with the net. When used on a community scale, the concentration of insecticide-treated mosquito nets (ITMN) can produce a mass effect reducing the mosquito population and the sporozoite rate. The method of treating mosquito nets will be found in Section 3.4.1. A recently introduced technology is the manufacture of mosquito nets with the insecticide already in the net, known as long-lasting insecticidal nets (LLIN). These retain activity for at least 4 years, so the regular re-treating of nets can be avoided; hence this holds considerable potential as the main method of malaria control.

Mosquito bed nets are more effective and cheaper to maintain than screening the whole house, which is only recommended for people with a high standard of living. A small hole in the netting can render it ineffective. A knock-down spray can be used to kill mosquitoes that have entered a screened house.

The use of smoke from mosquito coils or vaporizing mats can be surprisingly effective and has the advantage that it is a cheaper option for personal protection. Coils are easily manufactured locally and naturally occurring substances, such as pyrethrum, are incorporated. People often sit around fires in the evening and by the addition of certain plants, a repellent smoke can be produced.

Mosquitoes can be deviated to bite other animals if they are the preferred blood meal;

however, if the animals are taken away, such as to market, then the mosquitoes may be forced to take their blood meal from humans. The habits of the malaria vectors will need to be known before encouraging this practice.

RESIDUAL INSECTICIDES   The use of residual insecticides has been covered in Section 3.4. These are applied to the inside surface of houses so that the resting mosquito (after it has taken its blood meal) absorbs a lethal dose of insecticide and dies before the parasites it has taken up in the blood can complete development. This was the main method of the malaria eradication programmes used in many countries of the world. Unfortunately, insecticidal resistance, organizational breakdown and reluctance by people to have their houses sprayed, resulted in an abandonment of the goal of eradication. This has been replaced by a policy of malaria control in which house spraying may be a component.

LARVICIDING AND BIOLOGICAL CONTROL   The number of larvae determines the density of mosquitoes, so any method which reduces the larval numbers inadvertently reduces the potential number of adults. The larvae can be attacked by several different methods:

- using insecticides and larvicidal substances;
- modification of the environment;
- biological control.

Larvicidal substances can be oils that spread over the surface and asphyxiate the larvae or have insecticidal properties. The size and flow of the body of water will determine which is the preferred method to use. Modification of the environment by drainage or filling-in is the most permanent and effective, but is an expensive undertaking. It is worth spending money on engineering methods in areas of dense population, such as towns, while in rural areas, much can be achieved by using self-help schemes. The considerable advantage of this method is

that once done, it lasts for a long period of time, if not permanently, and in these days of resistant mosquitoes, it is seen as an economical proposition in some circumstances (see also Section 3.4.1).

Biological control with fish or bacilli (*Bacillus thuringiensis* or *B. sphaericus*) will reduce mosquito larvae to a certain extent, but a balance, as with much of nature, often results. Biological control can also be used directly against adult mosquitoes with the sterile male technique. This has not been successful with mosquitoes because of the very large numbers involved and their short period of life. Another method that is being considered is species competition whereby a non-malarial mosquito from another part of the world is introduced to compete with the resident vector. This has not met with any great success.

In epidemic malaria, using a fogging machine or ULV spray from aircraft can rapidly reduce adult mosquito density. This will cut short the epidemic by killing off flying adults, but needs to be repeated regularly as new adults will continually be produced from larvae that are not affected by the knock-down sprays.

CHEMOPROPHYLAXIS   Attempts to use chemoprophylaxis on a large scale on pregnant women and young children have not met with much success, but could be given to persons at particular risk, such as non-immune immigrants or migrant workers. Chloroquine 300 mg (two tablets) weekly can be used where chloroquine resistance is not a major problem, but local advice should be sought. It is preferable to give pregnant women and young children priority in the distribution of ITMN or LLIN, or to use chemoprophylaxis in combination with them.

REDUCING THE NUMBER OF GAMETOCYTE   Quinine, chloroquine and amodiaquine are active against the gametocytes of *P. vivax* and *P. malariae*, but not against the more important *P. falciparum*. Proguanil and pyrimethamine act on the development of gametocytes within the mosquito on all four parasites. Primaquine has a highly active and rapid action on gametocytes of all species, whether in the blood or mosquito and is used in combination with treatment in the individual. It has also been proposed as a method of reducing the level of gametocytes within the population, but would require an almost perfect mass treatment as well as the danger of toxicity (especially with G-6-P-D deficient individuals), and therefore, is not considered a suitable method of malaria control.

Any person found to have malaria should, where possible, be protected by a mosquito net so as not to infect new mosquitoes. This is a particularly important measure during eradication and control campaigns, especially when endemicity is brought to a low level.

VACCINES   Attempts to produce a vaccine against malaria have been in progress since 1910. A vaccine made from killed sporozoites by irradiating mosquitoes is reasonably effective, but cannot be produced on a large scale. Easier to produce are vaccines made by isolating the DNA fragments of the circumsporozoite antigen and cloning them through bacteria or yeasts. This has allowed large quantities of pure antigen to be produced and trials of candidate vaccines. Unfortunately, the response has been limited, so current research is to use a prime-boost technique similar to that for HIV. However, even if a vaccine is developed, all the problems of vaccination programmes, such as coverage, administrative difficulties and response of the public (see Section 3.2) will remain.

PROSPECTS FOR MALARIA CONTROL   Malaria attracts the wonder cure – first, it was the eradication programme, now all hope is pinned on the vaccine, but it is more likely to be controlled by simple, non-dramatic methods where care to detail is applied. It is the encouragement of simple protective methods that everybody can follow like ITMN (or LLIN) or community action to modify the environment to make it unsuitable for mosquitoes to breed (see Table 15.2 for the main vectors). A multiplicity of simple methods carried out by many responsible people is likely to be more successful in the long term than more complex methods.

Treatment of the uncomplicated case of *P. vivax*, *P. malariae* and *P. ovale* malaria is with chloroquine:

- 600 mg of chloroquine base as an initial dose;
- 6 h later, 300 mg chloroquine base, followed by
- 300 mg chloroquine base for 3 or more days.

Chloroquine-resistant *P. vivax* has been reported from Western Pacific Islands, including the island of New Guinea, as well as Guyana in South America.

P. falciparum is resistant to chloroquine and many other anti-malarial drugs, so individual countries will have their own treatment schedules depending on the resistance pattern and the drugs available. Quinine, mefloquine, artemether, artesunate, artemotil, chlorproguanil/dapsone (LAPDAP) and artemesin-based combination therapies (ACTs), such as artemether/lumefantrine are available. Artesunate in single-dose rectal suppositories is a new approach to treating malaria in children, who are not able to take medicines orally.

In *P. vivax*, chloroquine will only clear parasites from the blood, and to effect radical cure, primaquine is administered in a dose of 15 mg base daily for 14 days (except in the island of New Guinea and other Western Pacific Islands, where more prolonged treatment is required).

Case finding and treatment is an effective strategy where there is a low level of malaria, so it needs to be used in combination with other methods of malaria control.

Surveillance In all areas where malaria is found, a blood slide should be taken from anyone with a fever. Where attempts are being made to eradicate or reduce the level of malaria, then an active system of surveillance may be instituted as described in Section 4.5.2.

Where a control method is in operation, regular checks should be made, such as the proportion of houses with ITMN and the number of people sleeping under them. More will be found on malaria programmes in Sections 4.3–4.5.

15.7 Lymphatic Filariasis

Organism *Wuchereria bancrofti*, *Brugia malayi* and *B. timori*, nematode worms. Microfilariae, the larval form present in the peripheral blood, are taken into the mosquito's stomach when it feeds on humans (or animal reservoir in *B. malayi*). The larva loses its sheath inside the mosquito, migrates through the stomach wall and burrows into the muscles of the thorax. It becomes shorter and fatter, commonly described as sausage-shaped. Developmental changes take place and it elongates to a third stage – infective larva. Leaving the thoracic muscles, it migrates to the proboscis where it waits for the mosquito to feed. Forcing its way out of the proboscis, it falls on to the skin, finding a way into the tissues, generally through the wound made by the mosquito (Fig. 15.8). (It is important to realize that the infective larvae are *not* injected like the malaria parasite.) This developmental stage in the mosquito – from the time of the blood meal until re-infection – takes 11–21 days (average 15 days) at an optimum temperature of 26–27°C (extremes are 17–32°C), a very similar length of time to the development of *Plasmodium*.

When the larva breaks out of the mosquito to enter the skin, it is a very precarious time for the parasite and only 20–40% are successful. No multiplication takes place in the mosquito, so the single larva that was taken up in the blood meal becomes a single adult in the human. However, many larvae are lost with only about one in 700 succeeding. Since there are male and female worms, it is necessary for the two sexes to meet if the female is to be fertilized. Many are unsuccessful as a result of competition between males, so the intensity of infection will determine the outcome. Once fertilized, microfilariae are liberated into the lymphatic stream, reaching blood vessels via the thoracic duct.

The parasite times its production of microfilariae to coincide with the biting time of the vector mosquito, a phenomenon called periodicity. Mostly this is a nocturnal cycle, with a peak at around midnight, but can also be diurnal, or in the Central and Eastern Pacific Islands, it is aperiodic with similar levels of microfilariae being found throughout the 24 h period.

Microfilariae live for about 6 months and adult worms for 7–12 years although they probably only produce microfilariae for 2–3 years.

Clinical features In the body, the larva reaches the lymphatics and settles down in a lymphatic node to develop into an adult. It is the obstruction of the lymphatic drainage system by the adult worms, especially the fibrotic reaction when they die, that causes the series of disease manifestations. A range of conditions result, including fever, lymphangitis, lymphoedema, hydrocele, elephantiasis and chyluria. Night sweats are a common early indication of infection, with high eosinophilia count found in the blood. An allergic reaction, tropical pulmonary eosinophilia syndrome can also result. Although the signs and symptoms are diverse and variable, in an endemic area, they are often known and a blood sample will soon confirm the diagnosis.

Diagnosis used to be by finding microfilariae in a measured sample of blood using a thick blood smear, counting chamber or filtration technique, taken during the peak microfilarial output, which generally means collecting samples at night time. These laborious methods have now largely been replaced by circulating filarial antigen (CFA) detection, either based on ELISA or an immunochromatographic card. However, the card test only diagnoses positive or negative, while the ELISA is semi-quantitative, so where full quantitative measures are required, measured blood sample methods will still need to be used. This will be the case in assessing control programmes, as a

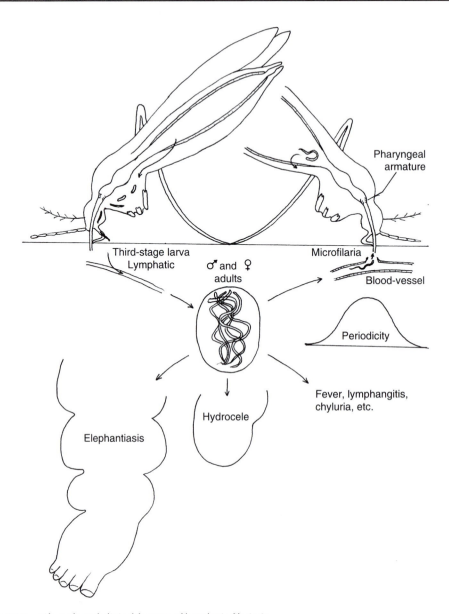

Fig. 15.8. Life cycle and clinical features of lymphatic filariasis.

decrease in the number of microfilariae occurs before conversion to negativity. CFA detection is also not available for *B. malayi* or *B. timori*. Different microfilariae need to be differentiated as seen in Fig. 15.9, as several filarial infections may be present in the same locality.

Transmission is by both culicine and anopheline mosquitoes producing different pat-

terns of infection and as a result, different strategies for control (Table 15.3). If *Anopheles* mosquitoes are the vectors, they are nearly always the same vectors as those that transmit malaria, so the mosquito might well have a double infection or its expectation of life affected by being parasitized by filariasis and/or malaria.

As the microfilaria is quite large and causes damage to the mosquito when it

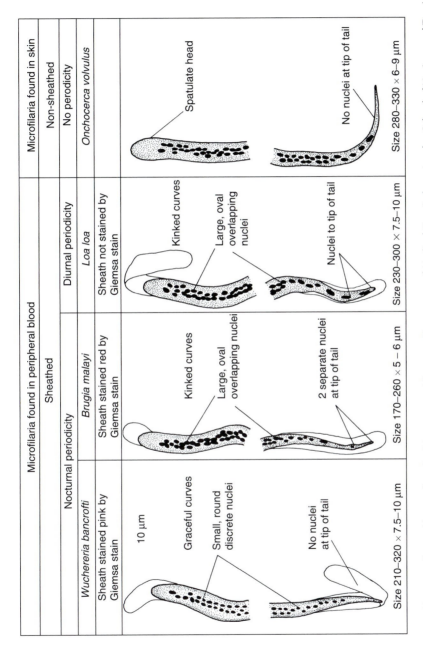

Fig. 15.9. Differential features of microfilariae of medical importance. (Courtesy: Department of Medical Parasitology, London School of Hygiene and Tropical Medicine.)

bores into the thoracic muscles, the more microfilariae it ingests the more likely it is to be killed by a heavy infection. (In *Culex* and *Aedes* mosquitoes, this occurs when the microfilarial density exceeds 50 per 20 mm^3 of blood.) This is seen in Fig. 15.10 at point E for both culicine mosquitoes (upper figure) and anopheline mosquitoes (lower figure). The line P represents the equilibrium level (basic reproductive level of 1), whereby above the line, transmissions will increase and below it, infection will die out; so when infection is excessively heavy, mosquito mortality occurs and the infection dies out. In reality, the number of microfilariae will decrease below E, mosquitoes will survive sufficiently to transmit again and the level will approach E, or the level of equilibrium, again. This is always the case with culicine transmission, but in the bottom figure, it will be observed that there is also a lower point I below which transmission is not sustained for anopheline mosquitoes. In other words, at low levels of microfilariae, the anopheline mosquito seems to be able to prevent itself from becoming infected. This is probably due to the pharyngeal armature in anopheline mosqui-

Table 15.3. The vectors of lymphatic filariasis. (*A.*, *Anopheles*; *Ae.*, *Aedes*; *C.*, *Culex*; *M.*, *Mansonia*; *O.*, *Ochlerotatus*.)

Geographical area	Species transmitting *W. bancrofti*	Species transmitting *B. malayi*
West Africa, rural East Africa, Madagascar	*A. gambiae*, *A. funestus*, *A. arabiensis*, *A. melas*, *A. merus*	
Urban East Africa	*C. quinquefasciatus*	
Egypt	*C. pipiens molestus*	
India, Sri Lanka and Maldive Islands	*C. quinquefasciatus*, *A. minimus*, *Ae. niveus*, *O. harinasutai*	*M. amulifera*, *M. indiana*, *M. uniformis*, *M. annulata*, *M. bonneae*, *M. dives*
China	*Ae. togoi*, *A. sinensis*, *A. anthrapophagus*	*Ae. togoi*, *A. lesteri*, *A. sinensis*, *A. anthrapophagus*
Vietnam	*A. jeyporiensis*	
Rural Thailand	*O. hariniasutai*	*M. annulata*, *M. bonneae*, *M. uniformis*, *M. indiana*
Malaysia	*A. letifer*, *A. whartoni*, *A. maculatus*, *A. dirus*, *A. donaldi*, *A. letifer*, *A. maculatus*	*M. annulata*, *M. annulifera*, *M. bonneae*, *M. dives*, *M. uniformis*, *A. campestris*, *A. donaldi*
Indonesia	*A. balabacensis*, *A. leucosphyrus*, *A. maculatus*	*M. annulata*, *M. bonneae*, *M. dives*, *A. barbirostris* (*B. timori*)
Philippines		*M. dives*
New Guinea (PNG and Irian Jaya)	*A. farauti*, *A. punctulatus*, *A. koliensis*, *C. annulinostris*, *C. bitaneniorhynchus*, *M. uniformis*	
New Caledonia	*Ae. vigilax*	
Fiji	*Ae. polynesiensis*, *Ae. fijiensis*, *Ae. pseudoscutellaris*, *Ae. oceanicus*	
Polynesian Islands	*Ae. polynesiensis*, *Ae. samoanus*, *Ae. upolensis*, *Ae. kesseli*, *Ae. tutuilae*, *Ae. tabu*, *Ae. cooki*	
Northeast Brazil	*C. quinquefasciatus*	

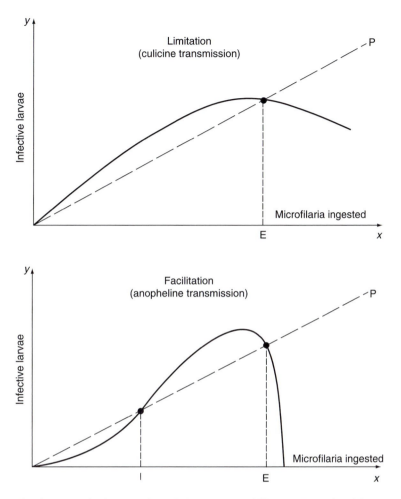

Fig. 15.10. The dynamics of culicine- and anopheline-transmitted filariasis. (Reproduced, by permission, from Pichon, G., Perrault, G. and Laigret, J. (1975) *Rendement parasitaire chez les vecteurs de filarioses.* (WHO/FIL/75.132), World Health Organization, Geneva.)

toes which damages microfilariae. When there are many microfilariae ingested by the mosquito, a sufficient quantity will remain undamaged to produce infection, but at low microfilariae levels, every microfilaria will be damaged. This applies to both *W. bancrofti* and *B. malayi*, so for control, the type of mosquito is more important than the species of parasite.

Filarial infection is determined by the number of infected bites, which can either be the result of a high intensity over a short period of time or constant bites over a long period of time. Mosquito mortality occurs

when density of microfilariae is excessive, so the chronic, long-term pattern is more common.

Incubation period From infection to the development of adult worms is about 1 year, but the first symptoms may not occur until microfilariae are produced (fever) or worms die (lymphatic obstruction).

Period of communicability Since many infective bites are required to produce infection in humans, there will need to be a continuous supply of infected mosquitoes.

The development cycle in the mosquito is 11–21 days (mean 15 days). The infected person can continue to produce microfilariae for more than 10 years, although the maximum output is in the first 3 years.

Occurrence and distribution Only humans are infected with *W. bancrofti*, but an animal reservoir exists for *B. malayi* in monkeys, cats and several other animals. All races, both sexes and all ages of persons are equally susceptible to infection. (There are marked differences between individuals developing elephantiasis, but these are immunological rather than ethnic.)

Three types of filariasis are seen – *rural* filariasis transmitted by nocturnal *Anopheles* mosquitoes with a generalized distribution similar to that of malaria, *urban* filariasis transmitted by *Culex*, with a tendency to invade new areas, and the Polynesian Island variety, which has a homogenous (rural) distribution, but is transmitted by day-and-night biting *Aedes* mosquitoes.

W. bancrofti is found in the tropical regions of the world, but with only a few foci in South America and the Caribbean. *B. malayi* is restricted to East and Southeast Asia, overlapping with *W. bancrofti* in part of its range. *B. timori* is only found in the islands of Timor, Flores, Alor and Roti (Fig. 15.11). There are more than a billion people at risk in 80 countries.

Control and prevention A similar process to that used for malaria for identifying the best strategies for control can also be applied to filariasis. The various places at which control can be implemented are:

- reduction of the number of infective bites by mosquitoes;
- decreasing the number of microfilariae in the human host;
- reduction of the mosquito's expectation of life;
- decrease the mosquito density;
- alteration of the mosquito biting time;
- reduction of the number of adult worms.

REDUCING THE NUMBER OF INFECTIVE BITES   Multiplication does not take place when the larva enters the host, so the disease process and its severity depends upon repeated entry of parasites into the body, many of which will be unsuccessful. The transmission process is surprisingly inefficient, requiring some 15,500 infected bites to produce a reproducing adult. This means that for *Anopheles* mosquitoes, approximately eight bites per person per day can take place without the disease being transmitted.

The number of bites can be reduced by taking simple precautions of personal protection – mosquito nets, repellents, protective clothing, etc. ITMN or LLIN should be effective in nocturnally periodic filariasis, transmitted by anopheline mosquitoes. This would be an additional benefit of a malaria control programme.

DECREASING THE NUMBER OF MICROFILARIAE (MASS CHEMOTHERAPY)   Mass drug treatment is the main method used in the filariasis elimination programme, given as an annual single dose treatment to all the population for at least 5 years, preferably 7 years. Two regimes are used:

- albendazole 400 mg+DEC 6 mg/kg, or
- albendazole 400 mg + ivermectin 150–200 mcg/kg.

An alternative is to use diethylcarbamazine (DEC)-fortified salt (or fortified soy sauce in China) for 6–12 months, if total compliance can be assured. DEC cannot be used in an area that also has onchocerciasis.

This strategy is likely to work in areas in which filariasis is transmitted by *Anopheles* mosquitoes, if the number of microfilariae can be maintained below the critical threshold (I in Fig. 15.10). One estimate suggests that this level is about 12 microfilariae/ $60 \, mm^3$. However, as the *Anopheles* is also a vector for malaria, reducing the number of parasitizing microfilariae, which cause damage to the mosquito, will increase the mosquito's expectation of life and improve its chance of transmitting malaria. Precautions should, therefore, be taken at the same time to prevent this from happening by the use of ITMN or LLIN.

In areas in which culicine mosquitoes are the vectors, it is unlikely that MDA alone will succeed in eliminating filariasis, as can be seen in Fig. 15.10 and from past experience in control programmes in Samoa and Tahiti. Control of the mosquito also needs to take place, a simple strategy being the use of expanded polystyrene beads, as was used in latrines in Zanzibar and soakage pits in South India (see also below).

Before mounting a mass drug treatment control programme, a complete survey is needed. Follow-up surveys of samples of the population are made at annual intervals. Thirty percent of the treated population should be sampled. Children less than 1 year of age, pregnant and nursing mothers, the sick and the very old should be excluded from mass treatment. Side-effects, especially itching, can be most unpleasant and a pilot control study should precede the main campaign. Considerable care should be taken in areas where both filariasis and onchocerciasis co-exist.

REDUCTION OF THE MOSQUITO'S EXPECTATION OF LIFE (VECTOR CONTROL)   By reducing the lifespan of the mosquito to below that of the developmental period of the parasite within the mosquito (range 10–15 days), transmission of infective larvae will be halted. This can be done by spraying residual insecticides inside houses or by treating mosquito nets.

Where the same vectors transmit both malaria and filariasis, then a joint control programme is cost-effective. ITMN or LLIN are particularly suitable for filariasis control, where there is an anopheline vector and could be used as the only strategy or combined with MDA (see above). The degree of mosquito reduction required is much less for filariasis than it is for malaria; however, mosquito control needs to be for a prolonged period, at least for 7 years and preferably for 10 years.

DECREASE MOSQUITO DENSITY (LARVICIDING)   The number of mosquitoes able to bite man is dependent upon the number of larvae that develop into adults, so by reducing the number of larvae, mosquito density is also diminished. This is a supplementary method of malaria control and has also been covered in the section on vector control (Section 3.4.1). Various methods can be used, such as larvicides, genetic modification, environmental or biological control. These methods are particularly appropriate to culicine-transmitted urban filariasis, although the degree of larval reduction required is often difficult to achieve. In enclosed areas of water, such as latrines and septic tanks, expanded polystyrene beads are very effective.

B. malayi is transmitted mainly by *Mansonia* and *Anopheles* mosquitoes, the *Mansonia* being particularly difficult to control because the larvae attach themselves to the underside of water plants (especially *Pistia*), where they are immune to surface oils and larvicides. Removal of these water plants by hand or with herbicides has had some effect.

ALTERATION OF MOSQUITO BITING PATTERN   The parasite has developed a periodicity of its microfilariae which coincides with the biting pattern of the vector mosquitoes. If it is possible to alter the time mosquitoes bite, then the chance of them taking up microfilaria will also be reduced. This has happened in some places due to the prolonged use of residual insecticides and although it is probably not possible to utilize this as a main control method, it could be of subsidiary value.

REDUCTION OF THE NUMBER OF ADULT WORMS   Unfortunately, there is no specific drug which kills adult worms, although DEC causes substantial mortality, a valuable secondary action to killing microfilariae. The worms lie embedded in the lymphatics so cannot be removed surgically, as practiced in onchocerciasis control.

Adult worms live for approximately 10 years (range 7–12 years), so if re-infection can be prevented for this period, they will die off and there will be no reservoir of infection. It is maintaining control methods for this period of time that is crucial with filariasis.

Treatment for established elephantiasis is unsatisfactory with mutilating surgical

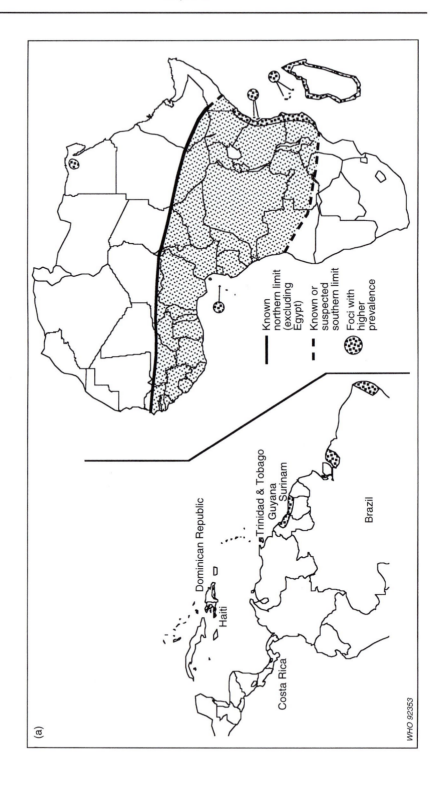

WHO 92353

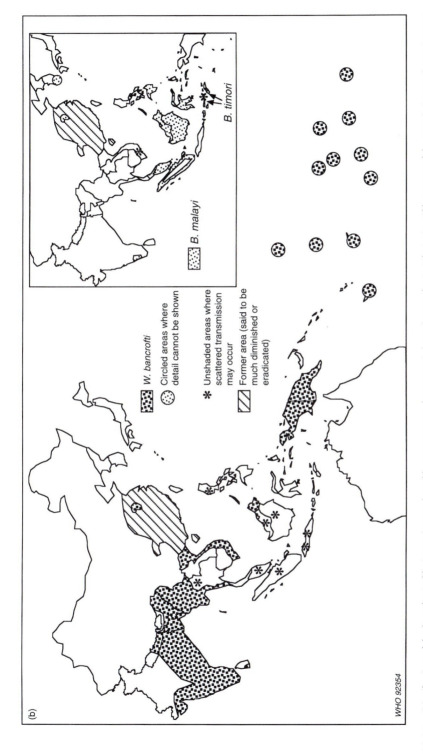

Fig. 15.11. Distribution of the lymphatic filariases. (Reproduced by permission, from WHO (1992) *Lymphatic Filariasis: Fifth Report of the WHO Expert Committee on Filariasis.* World Health Organization, Geneva, pp. 3–4.)

procedures. If discovered in its early stages of intermittent swelling, before tissue damage has occurred, then pressure bandages can prevent gross elephantiasis from developing. In *B. timori,* repeat doses of DEC reduce lymphoedema and to a certain extent elephantiasis.

Surveillance Hydrocele or lymph node surveys can be of value in rapidly defining the area of filariasis. Detailed blood surveys are then made.

15.8 Onchocerciasis

Organism *Onchocerca volvulus*, a nematode worm that has a predilection for the skin and eye, is transmitted by *Simulium* flies. Microfilariae are taken up by the fly when it bites humans and then undergo larval changes within the thoracic muscles, migrating to the head of the fly as infective larvae. When the fly bites again, microfilariae break out on to the skin to enter via any abrasion, especially the bite wound.

Clinical features The microfilariae as they migrate through the skin cause itching and damage resulting in skin changes, such as hanging groin and discoloration, the so-called 'leopard skin'. They migrate through the skin and also enter the eye, where the reaction caused by their death leads to eye damage, the person in the course of time becoming blind, giving onchocerciasis its other name 'river blindness'.

Diagnosis is made by taking skin-snips, which are placed in saline and the liberated microfilariae identified (Fig. 15.9). Taking a measured area of skin with a special punch allows density measurements to be made. A slit-lamp examination of the eye may reveal microfilariae in the anterior chamber or characteristic eye damage. The adult worms live in palpable nodules in the skin, so their presence and characteristic skin changes can suggest a clinical diagnosis.

Transmission The vector *Simulium*, also called the black fly, breeds in fast-flowing streams where it is found in large numbers. The female fly attaches its eggs to the leaves of water plants on which they develop. The larvae require high oxygen levels, so are found only in fast-flowing water (Fig. 15.12). The fly has a painful bite and is persistent making it a considerable nuisance, but it is also a powerful flier and assisted by the wind can travel up to 100 km in search of a blood meal.

The *Simulium* vectors and their usual breeding places are listed in Table 15.4, the African flies preferring to bite the lower body, whereas the South American flies attack the upper part of the body. Although they can fly great distances, maximum density is at the breeding place, resulting in focal infection. They are outdoor, daytime biters, but each species prefer different times of day to seek their blood meal. South American *Simulium* have pharyngeal armatures, whereas African species do not, but mortality due to super-infection by *Onchocerca* is not important. The adult flies live for 2–3 weeks (with a maximum of 3 months), but prefer to feed on animals rather than humans. However, people need to collect water so it is when they have to come to the river, to wash or collect drinking water that they stand the greatest chance of becoming infected.

O. volvulus only infects humans (and epidemiologically insignificant chimpanzees and gorillas). Eye and skin pathology is related to the proximity of the nodules, so when there are more nodules on the upper part of the body, there is a higher prevalence of blindness. In Africa, the savannah infection produces more blindness than that acquired in forests.

Microfilariae are found only in the skin, a high density leading to the more severe clinical manifestations as well as producing greater opportunity to infect flies. They survive for up to 2.5 years and have a periodic cycle with a peak at 1600–1800 hours, but this is relatively unimportant.

Incubation period is prolonged, normally taking about 1 year for symptoms to start following infection.

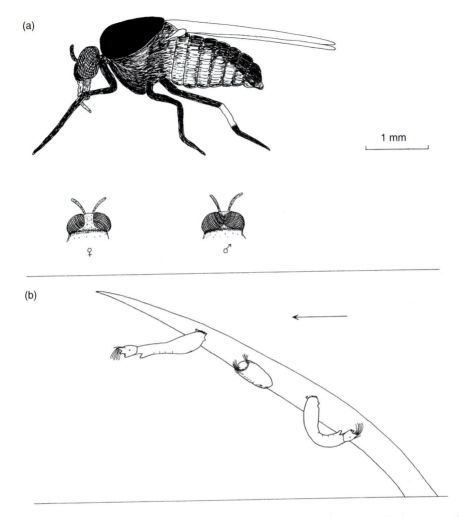

Fig. 15.12. *Simulium* the vector of onchocerciasis. (a) Adult. (b) Larvae and a pupa attached to a water plant, the stream flowing in the direction of the arrow.

Period of communicability is for some 16–17 years, adult worms producing microfilariae into old age. *Simulium* becomes infective after 6–13 days, depending on temperature.

Occurrence and distribution Onchocerciasis is found only in tropical Africa, Yemen and in South and Central America, with well-marked foci in much of this area (Fig. 15.13). In West and much of Central Africa, the infection is more widespread with the most westerly part of the region covered by the Onchocerciasis Control Programme (see below).

Repeat infection and progressive damage from dying microfilariae means that blindness is more common in adults, children then having to lead them around until their turn to become blind. Because of these severe consequences, abandonment of good village sites close to rivers has frequently resulted, although control programmes have largely reversed this trend.

Table 15.4. *Simulium (S.)* vectors of onchocerciasis. CAR, Central African Republic.

Geographical area	Species	Breeding place	Habitat
West Africa, CAR, Sudan, Uganda, Ethiopia, (Yemen?)	*S. damnosum* species complex	Large rivers	Savannah, but sometimes forest
West Africa, CAR, Sudan	*S. sirbanum*	Large rivers	Savannah
West Africa, CAR, Congo	*S. squamosum*	Small to medium-sized rivers in hilly areas	Forest savannah, mosaic
West Africa	*S. soubrense*	Large rivers	Forest, savannah
West Africa	*S. sanctipauli*	Large rivers	Forest
West Africa	*S. yahense*	Small watercourses	Forest
Cameroon, CAR, Tanzania	*S. mengense*	Large rivers	Forest
Congo, Burundi, Uganda, Tanzania, Malawi	*S. kilibanum*	Large rivers	Forest
Congo, Burundi, Rwanda, Uganda, Sudan	*S. naevi* species complex	Heavily shaded small permanent rivers in forest	Forest
Ethiopia	*S. ethiopiense*	Heavily shaded, small permanent rivers in forest	Forest
Tanzania	*S. woodi*	Heavily shaded, small permanent rivers in forest	Forest
Guatemala, Mexico	*S. ochraceum*	Small mountain streams	Highlands
Guatemala, Mexico, Venezuela	*S. metallicum*	Small streams	Highlands
Colombia, Ecuador, Venezuela	*S. exiguum*	Large rivers	Lowlands
Brazil, Venezuela	*S. guianense*	Large, fast-flowing rivers	Highlands
Brazil, Venezuela	*S. oyapockense*	Large rivers	Lowlands

Control and prevention Similar to lymphatic filariasis, various approaches to control can be tried. These are:

- reducing the fly density;
- avoidance of fly breeding places;
- reducing the microfilarial density;
- reduction of the number of adult worms;
- reduction in the number of *Simulium* bites.

REDUCING THE FLY DENSITY (LARVICIDING)   The larvae breed in water, so insecticide is sprayed on streams and rivers. The larvae are relatively sensitive to insecticides so low-dose applications, 0.05–0.1 mg/l are effective. Temephos (Abate) is suitable as it is effective in a very low dose, is relatively non-toxic to fish and retains some residual action. It exerts its effect for some 20–40 km downstream in the wet season. The main

difficulty with larviciding is to ensure that every water course is treated. Owing to the flies' ability to cover large distances, re-colonization soon takes place when insecticidal applications are discontinued. Although expensive, the extra cost of using aircraft and helicopters can be justified if many water courses, spread over large areas of countryside, have to be covered.

Unfortunately, insecticidal resistance has occurred in a number of areas, so biological control with *B. thuringiensis* is an alternative. This does not have the spreading power of insecticides and greater concentrations need to be used (in the order of 0.9 mg/l) and has to be mixed with water before it can be applied.

AVOIDANCE OF FLY BREEDING PLACES   Maximum contact between humans and flies occurs near rivers where *Simulium* breed, but

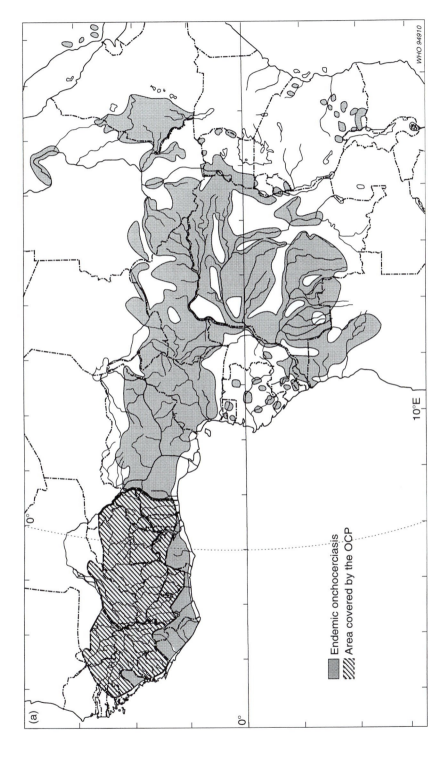

WHO 94910

■ Endemic onchocerciasis
▨ Area covered by the OCP

10°E

0°

(a)

Fig. 15.13. Distribution of onchocerciasis. (a) Africa and Yemen. *Continued Overleaf.*

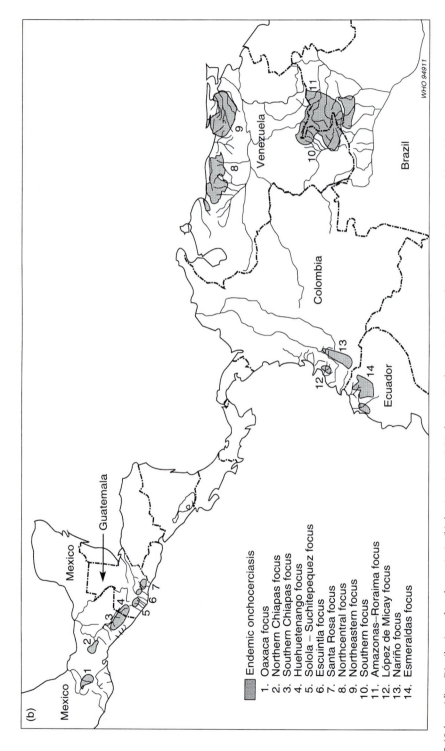

Fig. 15.13 (cont'd).   Distribution of onchocerciasis. (b) the Americas. OCP, former Onchocerciasis Control Project area. (From World Health Organization Technical Report Series (1995) *Onchocerciasis and Its Control*, No. 852. Reproduced, by permission of the World Health Organization, Geneva.)

these can be avoided by providing alternative water sources, such as wells or a piped supply to nearby villages.

REDUCING THE MICROFILARIAL DENSITY   Ivermectin immobilizes microfilariae, which are flushed out of the skin and eye and killed in the lymph nodes. As microfilarial death occurs away from the skin and eye, irritation is minimized and ocular reaction reduced. It can be given as a single dose of ivermectin 200 mcg/kg with re-treatment at 6- and 18-month intervals. This means that mass therapy for onchocerciasis can be used as an adjunct to vector control.

REDUCING THE NUMBER OF ADULT WORMS   Since the adult worms live for a considerable period of time, during all of which they are producing microfilariae, specific attack on the adult parasites can reduce both the symptoms and potential for transmitting infection. Nodulectomy or the surgical removal of adult worms from skin nodules can be a relatively effective procedure, practised particularly in the Guatemala onchocercal areas where nodules, more common in the upper parts of the body, are likely to produce ocular lesions. Moxidectin, used in veterinary medicine, has been found to kill adult worms, so is likely to be used in the treatment of the individual and community if free of side-effects.

REDUCING THE NUMBER OF *SIMULIUM* BITES   Personal protection is less effective against *Simulium* than with mosquitoes, with nets being inappropriate, although repellents have some effect. The wearing of long-sleeved shirts and long trousers with a hat and net can be used by individuals investigating the disease, but are not methods that can be developed for mass use. Avoiding passage through breeding sites will reduce fly biting.

ONCHOCERCIASIS CONTROL PROGRAMMES   Adult *O. volvulus* can live for 15–17 years, so any control programme would need to be maintained for this length of time before eradication can take place. However, most programmes seek to reduce the intensity of infection to a level where symptoms are absent. The criteria used in the Onchocerciasis Control Project (OCP) in West Africa were:

- less than 100 infective larvae/person/year;
- annual biting rates of less than 1000.

After many years of operation, the OCP programme finished in 2002, with delegation to individual countries to detect and treat all new cases.

The main method of control is larviciding, which can be extremely effective if carried out thoroughly. Species eradication of *S. naevi* was achieved in Kenya by methodically treating every water course with DDT. Where the disease covers a limited area, such an intense programme could be considered. In a more diffuse focus, the borders of control need to be extended sufficiently to prevent re-invasion by *Simulium* flying in from outside. While resistance is a serious problem, resistant *Simulium* are less important in transmission.

Mass drug therapy, or selective treatment to persons with heavy infections, can be given right from the start of the programme. This will rapidly reduce the microfilariae level and the potential for infecting flies. Preventing blindness (with ivermectin) has been particularly valuable in obtaining the cooperation of people. As lymphatic filariasis and onchocerciasis occur in the same areas in a number of countries (mainly in West Africa) and ivermectin is used to treat both diseases, joint programmes (with the addition of albendazole) are cost-effective. Moxidectin, which remains in the plasma for a much longer period (20 days as opposed to ivermectin's 2 days), could permit more flexible treatment regimes.

Treatment Ivermectin has been very effective, especially in the reduction of blindness, but moxidectin with its killing effect on adult worms may produce a more radical cure.

Surveillance Skin and nodule surveys can be used to indicate areas that need more intense skin-snip examination (see also the OCP programme above).

15.9 Loiasis

Organism *Loa loa*, a nematode worm. The life cycle of the parasite is essentially the same as *W. bancrofti,* except that the vectors are Tabanid flies.

Clinical features The disease is characterized by Calabar swellings (named after a town in Eastern Nigeria), which are transient, itchy and found anywhere on the body. Fever and eosinophilia suggest they have an allergic aetiology. *L. loa* is often confusingly called the eye worm (to be differentiated from *O. volvulus*), as the worm is sometimes seen migrating across the conjunctiva, but produces no pathology in the eye.

Diagnosis *L. loa* is diurnally periodic and diagnosis is made by examining daytime blood in which the microfilaria (Fig. 15.9) will be found. *Mansonella ozzardi, M. perstans* and *M. streptocerca* are also commonly found in blood and skin smears in the same area and need to be differentiated from *L. loa* as well as *W. bancrofti* and *O. volvulus.*

Transmission The vector is *Chrysops*, a large, powerful fly which inflicts a painful bite, attacking either within the forest or forest fringe.

Incubation period Although microfilariae may appear in the blood after about 6 months, the first symptoms may take years.

Period of communicability Like *O. volvulus*, the adult can live for up to 17 years, producing microfilariae all this time. *L. loa* takes 10–12 days to produce infective larvae in the fly.

Occurrence and distribution Loiasis is found in the West and Central African rain forests, especially the Congo River basin.

Treatment Both adults and microfilariae are killed by DEC, but caution needs to be exercised as allergic reactions can be profound. Low dosages of 0.1 mg/kg can be used to initiate treatment, gradually building up over 8 days to 6 mg/kg, which is continued for 3 weeks. Steroid cover may be required in those with more than 30 microfilariae/mm^3. Ivermectin will reduce the microfilarial stage and produces less reaction, so is more suitable for mass control programmes. However, reactions do still occur, especially in those in whom the worm is seen crossing the eye. So a useful preliminary examination is to show people a picture of the worm in the lower eye and exclude those in which it has been seen.

Control and prevention Extensive control measures are generally not warranted, the main preventive action being against the bites of *Chrysops* with protective clothing and repellents. Clearing the forest canopy, oiling of pools and mass treatment (with ivermectin) are methods that have been practised in areas of high transmission.

Surveillance Surveys for Calabar swellings or a history of them will indicate the area in which to take a blood smear survey.

15.10 African Trypanosomiasis (Sleeping Sickness)

Organism There are two forms of human sleeping sickness in Africa – one due to *Trypanosoma brucei gambiense* and the other caused by *T. b. rhodesiense*. A third form *T. b. brucei* is found in cattle, causing considerable economic loss.

The trypanosome exists in several different forms during its life cycle (Fig. 15.18). When seen in human blood, the trypomastigotes are long and slender, short and stumpy, or intermediate between the two, probably representing a cycle of antigenic variation (Fig. 15.18). They are introduced into the blood by the bite of the tsetse fly and multiply locally. After being disseminated round the body, they continue to multiply, rapidly in *T. b. rhodesiense*, less so in *T. b. gambiense*. They are infective to any tsetse fly when the fly bites, being taken up into the mid-gut. They multiply, migrate into the space between the peritrophic membrane and the gut wall and pass forward to the salivary glands. The epimastigote developmental form changes into a trypomastigote to infect the next person who is bitten.

Clinical features The bite of a tsetse fly generally causes a local reaction, but 7–10 days after it has subsided, it can become red and inflamed, which is the first sign of infection. Trypanosomes multiply at the bite site and aspirated fluid will contain the dividing forms. In *T. b. gambiense*, an enlargement of the lymph glands takes place, especially those in the cervical region. This rarely occurs in *T. b. rhodesiense*, the disease progressing rapidly to involve the CNS, with invariably a fatal outcome. The main clinical signs are fever and protracted headaches. In *T. b. gambiense*, the course is much more prolonged and personality changes may be the indication of infection, but inevitably the disease leads to progressive lethargy, emaciation, coma and death.

Diagnosis is by finding trypomastigotes in the blood, CSF or gland puncture. The blood smear should be repeated several times before a negative diagnosis is made. Parasite concentration techniques, such as capillary tube centrifugation or minianion exchange centrifugation, are valuable. Antibodies may be detected by serological techniques, while circulating antigen using the Card Agglutination Test (CATT) in which a drop of finger prick blood is mixed with a suspension of trypanosomes has revolutionized diagnosis. This technique is particularly useful for surveys in the field.

Transmission is from the bite of the tsetse fly in which the parasite goes through a devel-opmental stage. However, as the infective form for the fly and the human is the same (trypomastigote), mechanical transfer can occasionally happen if a contaminated fly bites another person within a short space of time.

The tsetse fly (*Glossina*) is easily recognized by its characteristic stance and behaviour. It is a large, powerful fly and rests on a surface with wings folded like a pair of scissors. Within the venation of these wings, a characteristic hatchet cell (Fig. 15.14) can be defined which helps in identification. However, when passing through 'fly' country, there is normally no doubt about its presence, as tsetse flies attack any moving object in large numbers, rendering the most painful bite. They are attracted by movement and will cling to the side of a vehicle travelling at 30–40 km/h without being dislodged. They prefer dark colours and if there is a large object, they will fly to that in preference. They are more abundant near their preferred breeding place in the sandy soil beside rivers.

Distribution of tsetse flies is shown in Fig. 15.15, where it will be noticed that distinct species are often related to particular sleeping sickness areas (compare with Fig. 15.16). Table 15.5 is a simplified guide for assistance in identifying the species of *Glossina*, but professional confirmation should always be obtained.

Incubation period 3 days to 3 weeks in *T. b. rhodesiense*, months to years for *T. b. gambiense*.

Period of communicability The trypanosome takes 12–30 days to complete its developmental stage in the tsetse fly, and depending on temperature, the fly then remains infected for life. Humans can be infected for many years with *T. b. gambiense*, but due to the shorter history with *T. b. rhodesiense*, the animal reservoir is probably more important.

Occurrence and distribution *T. b. gambiense* mostly occurs to the west of the Central Rift Valley of Africa, containing the lakes of Tanganyika, Kivu, Edward and Albert,

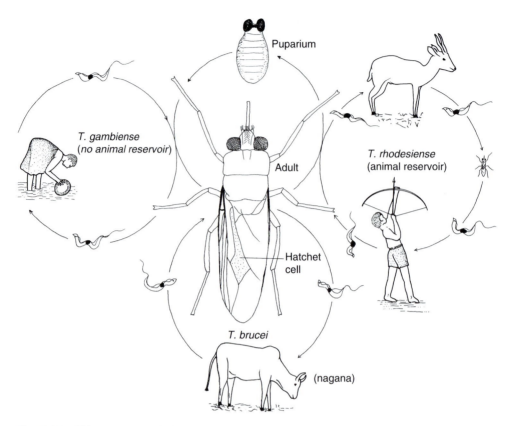

Fig. 15.14. African trypanosomiasis.

while *T. b. rhodesiense* is to the east (Fig. 15.16). *T. b. gambiense* infection is particularly prevalent in Congo (formerly Zaire) and *T. b. rhodesiense* in Tanzania. These two diseases differ markedly in their epidemiology and control.

15.10.1 Gambian sleeping sickness

Sleeping sickness as with other vector-borne diseases is determined by the habits of the vector. In the gambiense type, the tsetse fly breeds in the tunnel of the forest, along the course of rivers (Fig. 15.17). Although powerful flyers, they do not range far from this shaded protection, but travel extensively through this tunnel of forest in search of blood meals. Any mammals, including humans, that come to the river to drink or cross are attacked and fed upon.

Humans are the main reservoir of *T. b. gambiense* infection (although the domestic pig may be involved) and people whose jobs brings them into contact with the infected fly are more likely to succumb to infection. Since women are involved in the collection of water for domestic use, the preparation of food and the washing of clothes, they are more commonly infected with Gambian sleeping sickness.

The disease can occur in both endemic and epidemic forms. There are well-known foci from which people become infected at a constant rate (Fig. 15.16), but movements of infected flies or more commonly people, into new areas can initiate epidemics. Generally, infected flies are comparatively few in number, so that a large number of bites are required before a person becomes infected. Where the community that is fed upon is small and stable (less than ten persons/km^2), only a few cases will occur. When

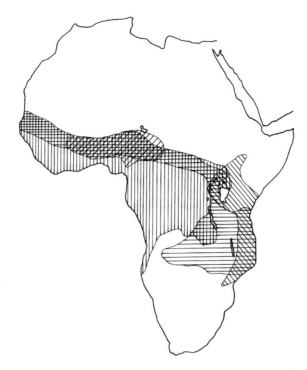

Fig. 15.15.   Tsetse fly distribution in Africa: = = , *Glossina morsitans*; \\\\\, *G. pallidipes*; |||||, *G. palpalis* and *G. fuscipes*; /////, *G. tachinoides*.

the community is much larger (above ten persons/km^2), as when an infected person travels to a more densely populated area, the infection can be transmitted to other people, who in turn form a reservoir to infect more flies and an increasing number of cases occur. Epidemic sleeping sickness is more likely in *T. b. gambiense* infection, as it is a more chronic disease and cases provide a reservoir (to infect flies), before symptoms cause them to seek medical attention. While endemic foci are difficult to eradicate, control measures should prevent epidemics from occurring.

15.10.2 Rhodesiense sleeping sickness

The principal vector of *T. b. rhodesiense* is *G. morsitans*, which breeds along water courses, but then travels widely throughout the extensive shade cover provided by the forest belt. This open type of forest, commonly called *miombo* (mainly *Brachystegia*

and *Julbemardi* spp.), is found in large areas of East Africa. Smaller wild animals inhabit it, especially the bushbuck that forms a reservoir of infection. Towards the margins of this forest belt, it breaks up into thickets separated by savannah grassland in which large numbers of wild animals are found. The tsetse fly ranges widely over these areas, feeding mainly on animals and using the thickets for cover and shade. It is, therefore, humans who travel through the forest fringing savannah in their occupational pursuit and the hunter and honey collector who become infected. Adult males are then the main victims in rhodesiense sleeping sickness.

   T. b. rhodesiense infection is not a focal disease and because of its short clinical course, epidemics are uncommon. However, movements of people, such as the development of new settlements in forest areas, will expose a large number of people to infected flies all at the same time, so allowing an epidemic to start. The first signs that this is

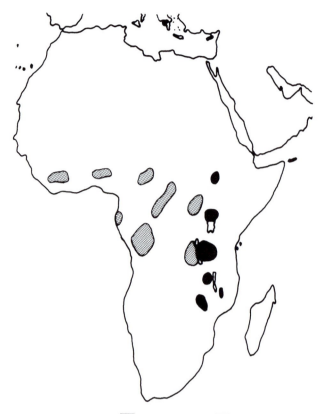

Fig. 15.16. Sleeping sickness foci in Africa. ▨ *T. b. gambiense;* ▆ *T. b. rhodesiense.*

happening are where women, and especially children, become infected.

Although these are the main patterns of the two diseases, sometimes a riverine tsetse fly becomes the vector of rhodesiense sleeping sickness.

Control and prevention

VECTOR CONTROL.   Knowledge of the habits and behaviour of the local vector is necessary before embarking on methods of vector control. The principal method is to modify the environment so that it is unsuitable for the fly, but not to cause so much damage that the water table is affected or soil erosion results. With the riverine type of habitat, areas of the forest tunnel are cleared removing all the dense undergrowth, but leaving the big trees with their extensive root systems to prevent erosion of the river bank (Fig. 15.17). Clearance should be continued for 0.5 km on either side of a river

crossing, water collection place or inhabited area.

In East Africa, where extensive forest provides a habitat for the fly, the forest margin is pushed back from any place of habitation. A band of at least 1 km, preferably 2 km, should be left between the area of habitation and the forest. This must also include any cultivated area and regulations are required to prevent people from moving into the cleared part to start new cultivation. Ring barking is a more economical method of forest clearance than cutting down every tree.

Where forest clearance is impractical, insecticides can be used. This is easiest along the course of substantial rivers using a boat, spraying the forest on either side. In the savannah-type habitat, isolated thickets can be treated. Extensive insecticidal application to *miombo* forest is inappropriate. Insecticides have to be repeatedly used, whereas forest clearance is permanent and

Table 15.5. A simplified key to Glossina of medical importance and their favoured habitats.

Hind tarsi	All segments dark above	G. palpalis group (1)
	Only two distal segments dark above	G. morsitans group (2)
1.	Abdomen obviously banded dorsally	G. tachinoides
	Abdomen dark, unbanded dorsally	G. palpalis (W. Africa)
		G. fuscipes (E. Africa)
2.	Distal two segments of front and middle tarsi without dark tip	G. pallidipes
	Last two segments of front and middle tarsi with dark tip	(3)
3.	Bands of abdomen very distinct and sharply rectangular	G. swynnertoni
	Bands on abdomen rounded medially and less distinct	G. morsitans

In summary, the vectors of *T. b. gambiense* are

G. palpalis
G. tachinoides
G. morsitans

and of *T. b. rhodesiense*

G. morsitans
G. pallidipes
G. fuscipes
G. swynnertoni
G. tachinoides in SW
   Ethiopia

Favoured habitats are:	
a. Lake and riverside, fringing forest	G. palpalis
	G. tachinoides
	G. fuscipes near Lake
	Victoria
b. Fringing forest without permanent water	G. pallidipes
c. Miombo woodland, thickets and 'game' savannah woodland	G. morsitans
d. Restricted to northern Tanzania 'game' savannah woodland	G. swynnertoni

the relative costs of these two techniques needs to be considered.

Trapping can also control the vector. A well-designed trap will collect enough flies to considerably reduce the biting risk. An effective trap has a fine metal mesh treated with insecticides, which is shaded to attract tsetse flies. These are rapidly killed when they touch the screen, but this must be cleaned regularly to work efficiently.

The fly can bite through thin clothing, so taking preventive action from being bitten in a tropical climate is difficult.

ALTERATION OF THE HUMAN HABITAT   Sleeping sickness has been responsible for large movements of people from their traditional homelands, either by choice or by government action to avoid an epidemic. Moving people away from the sleeping sickness areas is the ultimate method of control, but one to be taken only when all else fails.

The preferable alternative to moving populations is to modify the habitat so that it is unsuitable for transmission. Methods of forest clearance have already been described, while providing water supplies will remove the reliance on obtaining water from rivers.

The density of population largely determines the endemicity, as mentioned above. Two different approaches can be taken:

- keep the population close together and clear an area of forest around them;
- encourage the people to spread out very widely so that they partially clear a large area of forest.

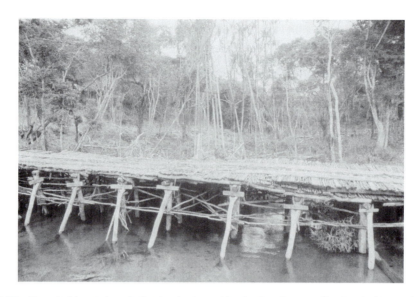

Fig. 15.17.   Tunnel of forest along the banks of a river with selective clearance (leaving the big trees).

In the first method, the people are safe as long as they remain within the village, but once they pass through the forest, they are subjected to a considerable number of bites. In the second alternative, people will become infected in the initial stages of forest clearance, but once this has been done, then protection will be much greater and more use can be made of the land. In the initial period of forest clearance, a surveillance service will be required to find these pioneer cases. The most unsatisfactory solution is a moderately large population spread evenly over the area; this is the potential situation for an epidemic.

PARASITE REDUCTION   A surveillance service should be set-up and all cases treated (see below). Finding cases in the early stages of the disease, not only increases the chance of successful treatment, but also removes a potential source of infection to tsetse flies.

Another approach to reducing the parasite reservoir in *T. b. rhodesiense* is to destroy the animal population. This used to be practised on a wide scale, but animal conservation has now questioned the wanton slaughter of animals. In most cases, it will be found that the human reservoir is more important than the animal, but where there is evidence that flies are becoming infected

from this alternative source, then game can be killed or driven off.

Treatment of cases requires hospitalization as the drugs are highly toxic. Suramin is effective in early and intermediate cases of both *T. b. rhodesiense* and *T. b. gambiense*. When the CNS is involved, Melarsoprol is the drug of choice. Eflornithine is very effective in all stages of *T. b. gambiense* infection (including cerebral), but is not effective in *T. b. rhodesiense*. Pentamidine has been used as a prophylactic against *T. b. gambiense* to people at special risk. There is no prophylactic against *T. b. rhodesiense* infection.

Surveillance In a sleeping sickness area, a surveillance service should be set up. Sleeping sickness workers are recruited more on their knowledge of the local community than their medical skills, as the simple techniques of gland puncture or making a blood slide can easily be taught. The workers cover a set area and take slides from people with symptoms of persistent fever and headache, or those who pursue a particular occupation, such as hunters, honey collectors or wood-cutters. In *T. b. gambiense* infection, palpation for neck glands can provide a useful estimate of prevalence. In an epidemic of *T. b. rhodesiense*, a mass blood slide examination can be performed in the worst-affected areas to detect asymptomatic cases.

The illness in animals is more extensive than in the human population and veterinary services often set-up extensive surveillance and control programmes, so combining efforts with them can be of value.

15.11 American Trypanosomiasis (Chagas' Disease)

Organism *Trypanosoma cruzi.* The trypanosome in American trypanosomiasis undergoes a development cycle both in the vector bug and the vertebrate host, with trypomastigotes, the infective form and pseudocysts forming in the muscle. These contain amastigotes, which grow a flagellum to become promastigotes and epimastigotes (Fig. 15.18) when the pseudocyst ruptures, finally developing into infective trypomastigotes (Fig. 15.19). The trypomastigote of the American disease has a larger kinetoplast and is more curved than the African one. The infection differs in that repeat cycles take place in the host's muscles producing a chronic disease state.

Clinical features American trypanosomiasis presents as an acute infection, generally in children, with fever, local swelling at the site of inoculation and enlargement of the regional lymph nodes. Muscular tissues are attacked so that in adult life, chronic conditions such as enlargement of the heart, oesophagus or colon develop. Heart failure and cardiac irregularities are common manifestations that lead in the course of time to disability and early death. In HIV infection, acute myocarditis or meningoencephalitis can occur.

Diagnosis is by finding the organism in the blood in the acute stage. Methods of concentrating the erythrocytes or xenodiagnosis (feeding of laboratory-reared clean bugs on the patient) are often required. In the chronic case, serological tests may be positive.

Transmission is by *Reduviidae* bugs, differing from area to area according to the species of the *Reduviidae* and the reservoirs of infection. The main genera of bugs are *Triatoma*, *Rodnius* and *Panstrongylus*, which can be differentiated from each other by their antennae and mouth parts (Fig. 15.19). Essentially, there are two cycles, one wild and the other domestic, which are illustrated in Fig. 15.20.

In the wild cycle, armadillos, opossum, raccoons and a number of other animals have been found infected, living in close proximity to their burrow-inhabiting bugs. This infection remains as a zoonosis until disturbed by a domestic animal, commonly a dog ferreting around the burrows of these wild animals. They are attacked by the bugs and acquire the infection. On returning to the house, the dog becomes a reservoir for the domestic bugs, which transmit the infection to any humans living or staying in the house.

In Central America, the cycle is semi-domestic with the reservoir maintained in the domestic rat (*Rattus rattus*), from which house-haunting bugs pass on the infection to people in the house. Although the bugs feed on people, it is the passage of trypanosomes in the bug faeces, which are rubbed into the wound or conjunctiva that produces the infection.

The bugs live in cracks in the walls and floors and within the thatch in the roof. The mud and wattle type of structure is particularly suited to the conditions required. The number of bugs hiding within the cracks and crevices can be several hundreds.

Infection can also be transmitted by blood transfusion, and small epidemics in a group of people sharing the same food suggests that contamination of food by bug faeces could lead to transmission by the oral route.

Incubation period 5–14 days.

Period of communicability Bugs become infected after 8–10 days and remain so for life, which lasts about 2 years. Infected persons have circulating trypanosomes in the acute and early chronic stages of the disease,

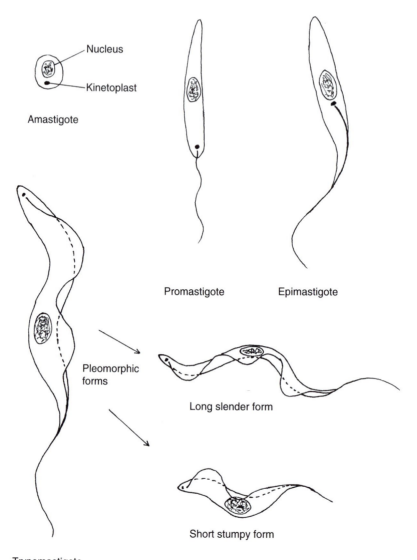

Fig. 15.18. Different forms of the trypanosomidae.

and this may persist in small numbers for the life of the individual.

Occurrence and distribution Chagas' disease is found throughout Central America and in most countries of South America. Considerable progress has been made in controlling the disease, Uruguay being declared free of infection in 1997, Chile in 1999 and Brazil in 2000. Argentina and Venezuela will probably be declared free very soon.

Control and prevention The methods of control are to reduce the number of bugs that can come into close proximity with humans and the reservoirs of disease. These requirements are both satisfied by improvements to housing. Unfortunately, trypanosomiasis is a disease of poverty, and building new and better houses is rather impractical in this segment of the population. If assistance can be given, then proper foundations and cement walls will not only deny a place for

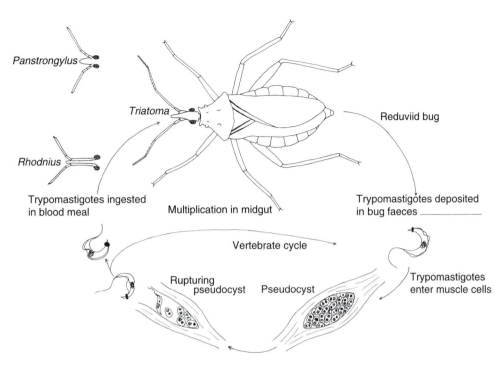

Fig. 15.19. Life cycle and vectors of American trypanosomiasis (Chagas' disease).

the bugs to live, but also prevent rats and armadillos from making their burrows underneath them. Even with existing houses, much can be done by applying a layer of mud plaster to walls and erecting a simple ceiling. Where cost prohibits any of these methods, residual insecticides can be sprayed on the walls and ceilings. This can effectively be carried out as a control programme using a similar methodology to malaria.

First a pyrethrum spray is administered, which draws the bugs out of their hiding places and marks the infected houses. In the attack phase, a residual insecticide is sprayed on all houses in an infected locality (not just to infested houses). A second spraying is made 90 days after the first, to houses where bugs have been found either in the preliminary or attack phase. Spraying continues at this time interval until the number of infested houses falls below 5%. Maintenance is achieved by regular house searches, instituting focal spraying when re-infestation is discovered.

The use of pyrethroid fumigant cans which release insecticide when lit, and insecticidal paints are simpler methods than residual spraying.

An alternative is to protect the individual from being bitten by the use of ITMN (see further under malaria discussed previously).

The dog is probably the most important domestic reservoir and householders should question the value of maintaining such animals if they are proving a threat to the health of the family. Good hygiene, trapping and poison will keep down rats. Control of the wild reservoir is unlikely to be successful.

In areas of high endemicity, screening of blood donors is required and gentian violet can be added to the blood.

Treatment Nifurtimox and benznidazole are effective in the acute and early chronic phase of the disease.

Surveillance Regular monitoring of houses for signs of infestation or re-infestation should be maintained (see above).

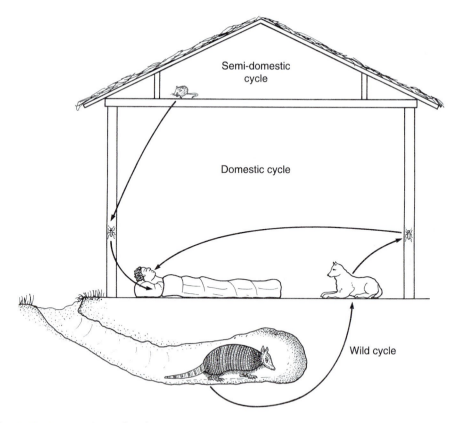

Fig. 15.20. Transmission cycles of American trypanosomiasis.

15.12 Leishmaniasis

Organism. There are seven species of *Leishmania* and a number of subspecies:

Visceral leishmaniasis	*L. donovani* (*donovani, infantum, chagasi, archibaldi*)
Mucocutaneous	*L. braziliensis* (*braziliensis, peruviana*), *L. guyanensis* (*guyanensis, panamensis*)
New world cutaneous	*L. mexicana* (*mexicana, amazonensis, pifanoi, garnhami, venezuelensis*)
Old world cutaneous	*L. major*
Old world cutaneous	*L. tropica* (*killicki, tropica*)
Old world cutaneous	*L. aethiopica*

They are all transmitted by the bite of the sandfly and undergo the same simple life cycle. Promastigotes enter man with the bite of the sandfly, change into amastigotes (Fig. 15.18), and are engulfed by macrophages. They multiply and finally rupture the cell, invading other macrophages. When the sandfly takes a blood meal, they change into promastigotes. These multiply continuously so that the number produced can be so large as to block the fore-gut. When the insect next bites, it is forced to regurgitate promastigotes into the host before it can take a blood meal (Fig. 15.21).

In cutaneous leishmaniasis, the amastigotes remain at the site of introduction, contained by the macrophages of the skin. In visceral leishmaniasis, large mononuclear cells and polymorphonuclear leucocytes become invaded, which subsequently carry the parasites to the viscera, especially

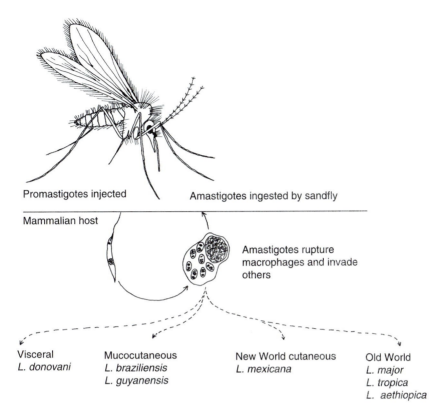

Promastigotes injected   Amastigotes ingested by sandfly

Mammalian host

Amastigotes rupture
macrophages and invade
others

Visceral	Mucocutaneous	New World cutaneous	Old World

Visceral
L. donovani

Mucocutaneous
L. braziliensis
L. guyanensis

New World cutaneous
L. mexicana

Old World
L. major
L. tropica
L. aethiopica

Fig. 15.21. Leishmania vector, parasite and life cycle.

the liver, spleen and bone marrow. The mucocutaneous form is intermediate, the parasite restricting its attack to the reticulo-endothelial system of the mucus membranes of the mouth, nose and throat.

Clinical features There are three main clinical forms of the disease – cutaneous, mucocutaneous and visceral (kala-azar). The cutaneous infection starts with a papule and enlarges to become an indolent ulcer, which either heals or persists for many years. In the New World infections, a more aggressive form of mucocutaneous leishmaniasis (espundia, Chiclero ulcer) results in nasopharyngeal destruction and hideous deformities. The visceral form is a chronic infection with fever, hepato-splenomegaly, lymphadenopathy and anaemia. There is progressive emaciation and weakness with generally a fatal outcome if not treated. Post-kala-azar dermal leishmaniasis can occur after apparent cure of the visceral case.

Like leprosy, host response largely determines the outcome of the disease and in any condition in which this response is minimized a more florid disease results. Cutaneous leishmaniasis is normally a self-limiting condition, but in some individuals diffuse cutaneous leishmaniasis, in which metastatic lesions are disseminated around the body can occur. The resulting nodular lesions resemble lepromatous leprosy and respond poorly to treatment. So any condition that compromises the host response, such as HIV infection, may lead to reactivation of latent disease or cutaneous disease progress to visceral illness. Leishmaniasis, like tuberculosis, is intertwined with HIV infection so that in areas where leishmaniasis is found, both conditions have a more serious outcome.

Diagnosis is by the detection of the intracellular-infected macrophages (Leishman–Donovan bodies) in liver, spleen, bone marrow or cutaneous lesions by stained smear or culture. PCR techniques can also be used.

Transmission is by the minute and fragile phlebotomine sandflies, *Phlebotomus* and *Lutzomyia*. They are weak fliers, utilizing a hopping flight that only carries them a short distance from their habitat. This requires conditions of high humidity as found in animal burrows and moist tropical forests. Typical habitats are tree holes, new or old animal burrows, termite hills, rock crevices, foliage clumps and fissures that

develop in the ground during the dry season.

The life cycle from oviposition to emergence of the adult can take 30–100 days depending on species and temperature, while the adult lives for approximately 2 weeks. Only the female sucks blood, but lizards, birds and mammals are satisfactory alternative food sources to humans.

Most species feed out of doors during the evening and night, or in the day when there is shade or the weather is overcast. If it is windy, they are unable to fly. They are not able to bite through clothing and mainly attack the lower parts of the body. The main vectors are summarized in Table 15.6.

Table 15.6. The vectors and reservoirs of leishmaniasis.

Type and parasite	Geographical area	Main vector	Reservoir
Visceral			
L. donovani (including infantile)	Mediterranean, SW Asia	*Phlebotamus peniciosus, P. ariasi, P. major syriacus, P. longicuspis*	Dogs, foxes
	Central Asia	*P. major syriacus, P. smirnovi, P. longiductus*	Dogs, jackals, foxes
	China	*P. chinensis*	Dogs
	India, Bangladesh	*P. argentipes, P. papatasi*	Humans
	Sudan, Chad	*P. orientalis, P. martini*	Wild rodents and carnivores
	Kenya	*P. martini*	Dogs
	Central and South America	*Lutzomyia longipalpis*	Dogs, foxes
Mucocutaneous			
L. braziliensis *L. guyanensis*	Central and South America	*L. wellcomi, L. umbratilis, L.trapidoi*	Rodents and forest animals
Cutaneous (New World)			
L. mexicana	Mexico, Belize, Guatemala	*L. olmeca*	Forest rodents
	Amazon Basin	*L. flaviscutellata*	Forest rodents
	Peru	*L. peruensis, L. verrucarum*	Dogs
Cutaneous (Old World)			
L. major	Mediterranean	*P. papatasi*	Rodents, dogs, gerbils
	Southwest Asia	*P. papatasi, P. sergenti*	Dogs, rodents
L. tropica	Central Asia	*P. papatasi*	Rodents, gerbils
	India	*P. sergenti*	Dogs
	West Africa	*P. duboscqi*	Dogs, rodents
L. aethiopica	Ethiopia	*P. longpipes*	Hyrax
	Kenya	*P. pedifer*	Rodents

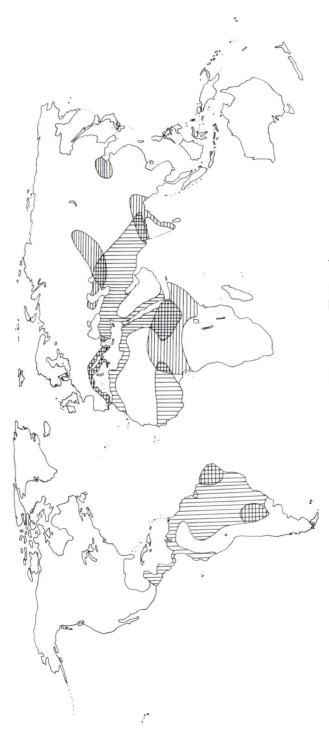

Fig. 15.22. The global distribution of cutaneous and visceral leishmaniasis. ▨, Cutaneous; ▦, visceral.

A range of reservoirs is found in this complex of diseases. In Central Asia, cutaneous leishmaniasis is a zoonosis, the gerbil being the main reservoir. In India, there is a domestic reservoir, mainly dogs, but direct human-to-human transmission also occurs. These are summarized in Table 15.6.

Transmission can also take place directly through needles and other instruments contaminated with blood of an infected person. Sadly, this is also the method by which HIV is transmitted in many developing countries.

Incubation period 2 weeks to 6 months, but can be years.

Period of communicability The untreated case can remain infectious to sandflies for up to 2 years.

Occurrence and distribution Leishmaniasis is found in Central and South America, north of the equator in Africa , in the Mediterranean, Southwest, Central and South Asia and part of China as shown in Fig. 15.22 and Table 15.6. Population movements, both of persons from endemic rural areas into towns and large man-made projects, such as dams in endemic foci, have brought an increasing number of people into contact with leishmaniasis. Also, the spread of HIV infection has made what was largely a curable condition into a persistent source of parasites for the vector sandfly and as a result, a more serious disease.

Immunity develops following infection with the parasite, but there is little cross-immunity. *L. tropica* has been used for a long time as an inoculum to induce a sore on a hidden part of the body so as to prevent a more disfiguring lesion developing on the face. *L. major* will protect against *L. tropica* as well as *L. major* lesions, and suspensions of living organisms have been prepared for this purpose. There is no cross-immunity with kala-azar and the other species of *Leishmania*, but an attack of kala-azar will protect against developing kala-azar in any other part of the world.

Control and prevention Cases of the disease are normally sporadic, so should be treated to prevent flies from becoming infected. Repellents and personal protection adequately protect the individual from being bitten. Sandfly nets can be used, but a more effective solution is ITMN or LLIN (see Malaria above). Because of the fragile nature of the vector, it is easily attacked with insecticides, either with a residual house spray if the vector comes indoors, or by insecticide powder blown into mammal burrows, ant hills and similar micro-habitats. A long-term solution is to alter the micro-environment, such as by the destruction of termite hills and killing of rodents. Proper control of domestic animals, especially dogs, can be effective where they are important reservoirs. Low-dose inocula and attenuated vaccines have been developed to minimize the severity of disease in some endemic areas. The concomitant problem of HIV infection has added to the seriousness of dual infection, so a simultaneous programme of STI control is required and information produced on how to avoid both diseases.

Treatment is with sodium stibogluconate or meglumine antimonate, but pentamidine or amphotericin B may be required in cases that do not respond, especially mucocutaneous leishmaniasis. Because of the toxicity of the preparations, treatment should be undertaken in hospital. Miltefosine maybe useful in the treatment of visceral leishmaniasis.

Surveillance Outbreaks should be reported to neighbouring countries so that they can take control measures in border areas. Patients with HIV infection should be examined for reactivated leishmaniasis.

16

Ectoparasite Zoonoses

Ectoparasites are non-flying vectors of disease, such as fleas and lice. They are responsible for an important group of infections, which are often associated with animals in which the reservoir of infection is found. Because of the close inter-relation between the ectoparasite and the animals on which it feeds, focal zoonoses (or exoanthropic zoonoses) result. Humans are often the accidental victims of these zoonotic infections, and a knowledge of the biology and how to avoid these foci can often be all that is needed to prevent being infected. At other times, specific methods against the ectoparasite, the animal or both are required.

16.1 Plague

Organism *Yersinia pestis*, the fragile organism that causes plague is a small oval-shaped bacillus that stains negative with Grams stain. It is sensitive to heat above 55°C, 0.5% phenol for 15 min and exposure to sunlight. *Y. pestis* occurs in three varieties, *orientalis*, *antigua* and *mediaevalis*, separated by their ability to ferment glycerol and reduce nitrates, which can be useful in elucidating the particular organism involved in an epidemic.

Clinical features The disease in humans, due to the bite of an infected flea, is called bubonic plague, after the bubo or swelling that develops at the regional lymph nodes draining the site of inoculation. It is commonest in the groin and secondly in the axilla, while it can also occur in the cervical lymph nodes. This latter site is more likely in the case of sylvatic plague as infection can result from ingesting the organism when eating the reservoir rodent. (Some people eat rodents as a normal item in the diet, while in famine conditions, others may be driven to eat whatever they can find, including rats.)

The bubo is painful and tender, becomes fluctuant and often breaks down to discharge pus. There is an associated high fever, confusion, irritability and signs of haemorrhage may develop. These may be subcutaneous, into the stomach or intestines, leading to prostration and shock with death soon after.

In a few cases, the disease may be overwhelming from the start with septicaemic plague. All the signs are more severe and develop so rapidly that a bubo is not formed and the patient is dead within a few days. In the generalized spread of the organism around the body, it can invade the lungs and should a case of bubonic or septicaemic plague start coughing out bacteria, then transmission can occur via the respiratory route. This leads to pneumonic plague, where spread is from person-to-person contact and the flea is not involved. It is highly infectious and lethal, so stringent protective action must be taken. About 5% of bubonic patients develop terminal pneumonia and transmit infection via the respiratory route. The onset of pneumonic plague is very quick with shallow, rapid breathing, watery blood-stained sputum, high temperature, pulmonary oedema and shock. Death occurs between the third and the fifth day.

A mild form of the disease with swollen glands and slight rise in temperature can occur as pestis minor, but many cases go undiagnosed and tend to occur towards the latter part of an epidemic. During an epidemic, routine throat swabs may detect *Y. pestis*, but there is no good evidence that transmission can occur from these cases.

Diagnosis Fresh aspirate from a gland or sputum stained with Gram stain will show the bipolar staining organism in preliminary field investigations. Culture on to blood agar or desoxycholate can be made from blood, throat swabs, sputa and material aspirated from buboes. Fluorescent antibody or antigen-capture ELISA is a specific confirmatory test. Asymptomatic cases of plague are common during epidemics and can be detected near foci by the passive haemagglutination test (PHA).

Transmission Figure 16.1 illustrates the different transmission cycles of plague, the trio of bacillus, rodent and flea, into which humans can be fatally drawn. In the established focus of wild rodent plague, infection is maintained in a comparatively resistant colony of animals, which suffer little from the disease. If a person strays into this focus as a hunter or trapper, then fleas from a wild rodent they have killed may bite them and cause plague. This is sylvatic plague and is generally an isolated case with little epidemiological significance. The more important event is when some change takes place in the wild rodent focus and domestic rodents become involved. Wars of nature

are similar to wars of man and a replacement of one group of plague-resistant rodents by another of no resistance could cause a change in the ecological balance. On the other hand, an increase in the domestic rodent population may expand into the wild rodent one. Whichever of these alternative mechanisms takes place, the deprived flea seeks a new host and settles on a domestic rodent. The domestic rodent being highly susceptible to plague is rapidly killed, which brings the flea of the domestic rodent in search of a new host and because of their proximity, humans are likely to become the next victims.

In Africa, the multi-mammate rat (*Mastomys natalensis*) acts as an intermediary between the feral rodent reservoir and the domestic rat, feeding on the remnants of the harvest. However, when the rains come, it is driven to look for alternative stores of food and enters the home bringing it in contact with the occupants. This makes a seasonal pattern of plague. If there is a drought, the situation is even more serious because there is no food for the desperate multi-mammate rat, which is forced early into conflict with the domestic rat and an epidemic occurs in the dry season as well.

A focus of plague is determined by three factors: (i) the organism, (ii) the reservoir host and (iii) the flea vector. Many fleas have been incriminated as possible vectors, but species of *Xenopsylla* are the most important (*X. cheopis*, *X. brasiliensis* and *X. astia*). In identifying fleas, they can either have a comb on the top of the head or they are combless. *Xenopsylla* is combless, differentiating it from *Ctenocephalides*, which is the common dog and cat flea. The common human flea *Pulex* is also a combless flea, but lacks the other distinguishing feature of *Xenopsylla*, i.e. the presence of a meral rod (these important features are illustrated in Fig. 16.1).

Fleas are able to survive for considerable periods without taking a blood meal (6 months) and the larval and pupal stages are well adapted to changing conditions. If there is a limited food supply or low temperature, then the larva may prolong this stage from 2 weeks to more than 200 days

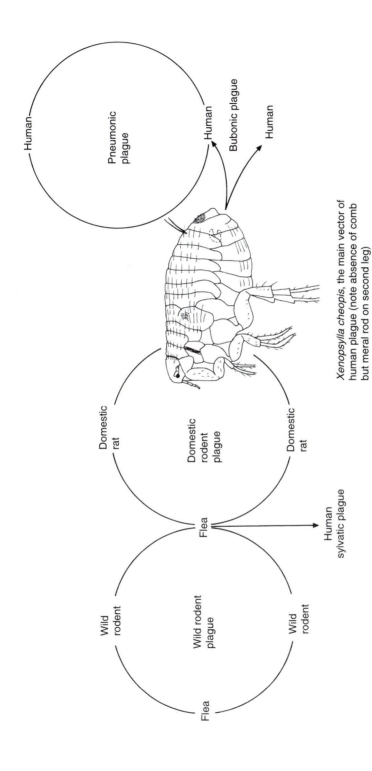

Fig. 16.1. Plague vector and life cycles.

and the pupae remain cocooned. When vibrations in the habitat, the emission of carbon dioxide or a rise in humidity indicate that an inhabitant has returned, the larva rapidly develops and the emergent flea feeds on the new host. Fleas are not specific, but prefer their normal host species and fertility may be reduced if they cannot feed on them. Fleas rapidly abandon a dead host and use their powerful hind legs to help them hop on to a new one. Once re-established, they tend to crawl around and settle to a regular feeding pattern. If fleas take in *Y. pestis* with their blood meal, these multiply in the proventriculus and lead to a blockage of the feeding apparatus. When the flea tries to feed again, it regurgitates bacteria into the blood stream while trying to take up blood. It is unsuccessful, so moves to a new host and tries again. Blocked fleas are important in rapidly infecting many people.

Over 340 species of mammals have been found susceptible to plague including rabbits, monkeys, dogs, cats and camels, but the main reservoir is in rodents, particularly rats. They differ in their susceptibility so that a focus will die out where there is a highly susceptible colony, but persist where resistance is high. While it is the resistant rodents that maintain a focus, it is the movement of susceptible animals, which is responsible for extending plague. Where the speed of mortality is high and the pool of susceptible animals limited, then the exacerbation will collapse and the focus return to its original boundary, but when a coincidence of susceptible rodents abuts domestic rodents, then the stage is set for an epidemic in the human population. Foci of infection have been delineated (Fig. 16.2), some of which have given rise to plague outbreaks, while others have all the potential, but human disease has not occurred.

Incubation period 2–6 days.

Period of communicability An unblocked infected flea can remain alive for several months able to transmit infection. Pneumonic plague is highly infectious and can spread rapidly within a concentration of people although infected individuals will remain alive for only a few days.

Occurrence and distribution Plague is a classic example of an ectoparasite zoonosis, the greatest of all epidemic diseases. It has ravaged the Orient, Asia and Europe, altering the course of history. Today it is confined to established foci (Fig. 16.2) from which it erupts from time to time, but fortunately effective control now prevents the uncontrollable pandemics of the past.

Plague is a disease of civil disturbance and war. In recent history, the largest human focus has been in Vietnam. Persistent endemic foci in Madagascar and East Africa continue to produce cases, while a worrying exacerbation was an outbreak of pneumonic plague in Ecuador in 1998.

Control and prevention The methods of control depend upon the transmission cycle involved (Fig. 16.1).

Wild rodent plague foci are often extensive and harmless, and to try and destroy them a considerable task. If they are localized and close to habitation, then it might be feasible to alter the environment by cultivation or in a way that discourages rodents. Precautions need to be taken that a plague epidemic is not generated by such activity. Where hunters or soldiers have to pass through a plague focus, then personal protection can be obtained from long trousers tucked into socks, treated with repellents or insecticides. Warnings should be given about the danger of touching or eating any animals killed.

Domestic rodent plague depends upon the two components of the rat and the flea, but the order in which they are attacked is crucial according to the stage of the disease. To kill rats during a plague epidemic only makes the infected fleas search for a human host and increase spread. In the presence of plague, the fleas must be controlled first. Using insecticide powder (permethrin, bendiocarb, carbaryl or fenitrothione), burrows can be insufflated and rat runs liberally dusted. Rats pick up insecticide on their fur and take it into their nests with them. Fleas do not like cleanliness and

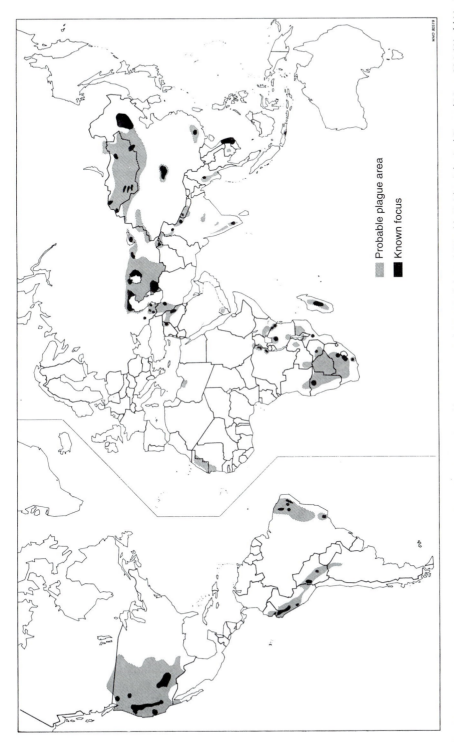

Fig. 16.2. Known and probable foci of plague, 1959–1979. (Reproduced by permission, from WHO (1980) *Weekly Epidemiological Record* 32, p. 234. World Health Organization, Geneva.)

people should be encouraged to wash with soap and warm water. Clothes can be searched and fleas picked off, but it is preferable to boil clothing (see Box 16.1 for the control of rats).

Plague vaccine will protect persons at risk for several months, but should not be relied upon. Chemoprophylaxis with tetracycline 250 mg four times a day or doxycycline 100 mg a day for a week should be given to close contacts of cases and medical workers at risk.

Quarantine of all cases is required by international health regulations for a period of 6 days. All persons should be dusted with insecticides to remove fleas and precautions taken to prevent aerosol spread from pneumonic cases. Any cases dying of plague should be buried or burnt with aseptic precautions.

Treatment Effective treatment depends upon the speed of making a diagnosis and treating early. If plague has already been diagnosed in the area, then a confirmatory test should not be awaited. The clinical presentation of fever and bubo in a severely ill patient is sufficient and treatment needs to be started immediately. This is either by:

- Streptomycin 1 g followed by 0.5 g every 4 h, up to a total of 20 g;
- Tetracycline 3 g immediately, followed by 1 g three times a day for 12 days;
- Doxycycline 100 mg every 12 h for 7 days;
- Chloramphenicol 500 mg every 6 h for 7–10 days.

Gentamicin and co-trimoxazole have also been used.

Streptomycin is the treatment of choice, but can cause a Herxheimer reaction, so tetracycline is preferable in the critically ill. Resistant strains have occurred and the sensitivity of the organism should be monitored.

Isolation of cases is mandatory and the terminal bubonic case with pneumonia or pneumonic plague is highly infectious and, therefore, extreme precautions should be taken. Gowns and full-face masks should be worn, while goggles are required to protect the eyes as *Y. pestis* can be absorbed through the conjunctiva.

Surveillance of foci should be maintained with regular trapping of rodents to examine them for infection and their flea populations. Notification of any confirmed or suspected case of plague must be made to WHO and neighbouring countries. Any person travelling from an area where there have been cases of plague should be placed under surveillance for 6 days.

16.2 Typhus

There are many similarities between the epidemiology of typhus and plague, and it is convenient to approach the disease in the reverse order to which it is normally described in order to assist in its description. While plague is a composite disease of three different cycles utilizing the same organism and vector, there are three different forms of typhus (scrub, murine and epidemic), each with its own organism and vector (Fig. 16.3).

Organism The causative organism of typhus is a *Rickettsia* or *Orientia*, an intracellular bacteria which requires cellular tissue of the host or ectoparasite to develop and reproduce. It can survive in the environment if suitable conditions prevail (e.g. in louse faeces); otherwise, it is sensitive to heat (being killed by a temperature of 60°C for 30 min) and easily by antiseptics.

The typhus-producing organisms and their ectoparasites are as follows:

Scrub typhus	*Orientia tsutsugamushi*	Trombiculid mites
Murine typhus	*Rickettsia typhi (R. mooseri)*	Flea, *X. cheopis*
Epidemic typhus	*R. prowazekii*	Human louse

Clinical features Typhus was confused with typhoid for a considerable period of time because they both produced fever, prostration and a rash. Indeed, typhoid obtained its name only when it was finally separated from typhus as being a less infectious disease, with markedly abdominal symptoms and a milder rash.

In the most severe form, epidemic typhus, there is a sudden onset with headache, pains, rigours and malaise as the temperature rapidly rises to 40°C or more; where it remains for the duration of the illness. The characteristic rash appears between the fourth and seventh day and consists of petechial haemorrhages on the trunk and limbs, but sparing the face, palms and soles. As the disease progresses, the patient becomes semi-stuporous with confusion, anxiety and considerable dullness. The patient appears unable to hear, talks nonsense and has to be fed. By the third week, if treatment has not been given, the patient will progressively recover or else sink further into heart failure, bronchopneumonia and death.

In scrub typhus, the illness similarly commences with fever, progressive prostration and a macular rash, but after a few days, the infective mite bite develops into an eschar. This is a red indurated area with central vesicle that subsequently breaks down to leave a black scab. The severity of the disease varies markedly from area to area, being a severe and fatal illness, similar to epidemic typhus in some places, while in others, so mild and innocuous that it passes as 'flu'. I remember visiting a school near a well-known mite island, which expected all new students to have a minor illness for a day or two and then be immune for the rest of their academic stay.

In murine typhus, there is fever, followed by a rash, but the illness is milder than epidemic typhus, mortality is low and complications rare so that most people fully recover in 7–10 days.

Diagnosis will probably be on clinical grounds, the escar of scrub typhus being characteristic, but where available, the indirect fluorescence antibody test, labelled enzyme with ELISA, latex agglutination or PCR can be used.

Transmission

SCRUB TYPHUS   Like wild rodent plague, scrub typhus is a zoonosis in which humans are not involved. Well-defined areas, called mite islands, harbour rodents, mites and the *Orientia*, which is transmitted between them. A large number of rodents have been incriminated, including rats, and it is their system of burrows, runs and range of activity that determines the limit of the mite island. The rodents are fed upon by the larval stage of various *Leptotrombiculid* mites that need to take blood so that they can develop into a nymph and subsequently an adult. The larva climbs up on to grass or vegetation and awaits the passage of a rodent or any other passing mammal to which it attaches itself. Once it has fed, it drops off and continues its development in the soil. If during its feeding it sucks up *O. tsutsugamushi*, these develop in the nymph and adult and are passed on transovarially to infect the next generation of blood-sucking larvae. The mites appear unaffected by this infection, acting as a reservoir, hardly requiring the mammalian host except to provide a blood meal for their own continuity. Such is the balance of this arrangement that a mite island can persist undisturbed, causing harm to no one unless accidentally entered by humans. The larval mite will attack people just as it will attack birds and other mammals that come crashing through its hunting ground, transmitting the infection to its unusual host.

Scrub typhus is the disease of the wandering farmer, hunter or travelling army, passing through or camping in mite islands. These can be very small and localized or cover extensive areas, but generally, they are associated with transitional vegetation or fringe habitats, such as areas separating different vegetation zones (e.g. forest and grassland). Mite islands are nearly always the result of human activity, where forest is destroyed either for timber or in 'slash and burn' agriculture. The land regenerates as secondary growth, rats

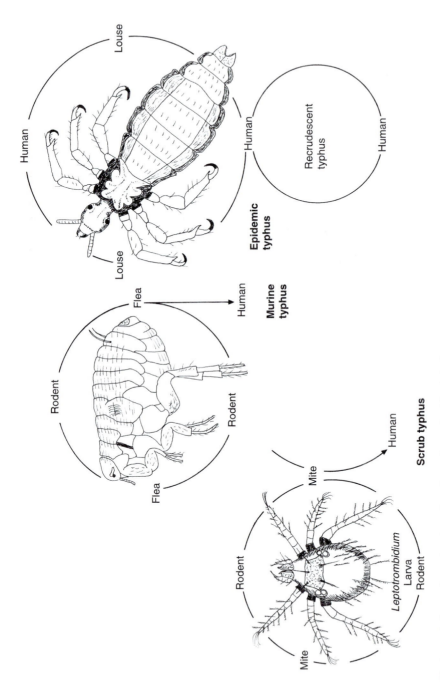

Fig. 16.3. The transmission cycles and vectors of scrub, murine and epidemic typhus.

and other rodents move in and provide suitable conditions for the *Leptotrombiculid* mites.

MURINE TYPHUS   Scrub typhus has been given the alternative name of rural typhus, which adequately distinguishes it from urban typhus, the main characteristic of the flea-borne disease. Murine typhus is then a disease of towns and habitation, maintained there by domestic rodents, *Rattus rattus* and *R. norvegicus*. In contrast to scrub typhus, the mammal in murine typhus is the reservoir of the disease and the common rat flea *X. cheopis* acts only as a transmitter. Many other mammals have been found infected – mice, cats, opossums, shrews and skunks – but the key in all these alternative sites is always the domestic rat.

The flea becomes infected by biting the host, the infection appearing not to have any effect on the flea and does not shorten its lifespan. *R. typhi* is not transmitted by the bite of the flea, but is passed in its faeces. If infected faeces are rubbed into an abrasion or inhaled as an aerosol, other rats become infected. The body of the flea is also highly contagious and if crushed, the organism is liberated. While *X. cheopis* is the main vector, the organism has been isolated from *Pulex irritans*, the common human flea, lice, mites and ticks. These probably do not form an important means of transmission, but could explain epidemics where *X. cheopis* is not found.

Humans are infected by their close association with domestic rodents. When a flea is squashed or scratched into an abrasion, its tissue juices or faeces contaminate the wound. The habit of some people when catching fleas of crushing them between their teeth is also a potential method of infection. However, it would seem that the direct attack by the essentially healthy rat flea is uncommon and the more important method of transmission is from an aerosol of organisms in the flea faeces. These are carried on the rats' fur or sent into the air when disturbed. *R. typhi* can be inhaled, swallowed or enter through other mucus membranes, such as the conjunctiva. Murine typhus is common where rats live in constant contact with humans.

EPIDEMIC TYPHUS   While scrub typhus and murine typhus are zoonoses, epidemic typhus is an infection where only humans and the body louse, *Pediculus humanus corporis,* are involved. The louse can spend its entire life cycle on the same host, laying its eggs in the seams of clothing and finding all the food and shelter it requires. Female lice lay some 5–10 eggs per day, which hatch in 6–9 days depending on temperature. If the clothes are kept on the body, then the temperature is maintained and hatching takes place rapidly, but if they are removed and cooled down, development may take 2–3 weeks. One month is the maximum period they can survive, so clothes that are not worn for this length of time will be free of lice.

The egg hatches into a nymph, which in all respects resembles a small adult, and sucks blood. Three nymphal stages are passed through before it becomes an adult louse. Lice, both males and females, can only survive by taking blood meals and if deprived, can last no longer than 10 days. They are sensitive to temperature and will abandon a dead person as well as one with a high fever. The lifespan of an adult louse is about 1 month and during this time, a female may lay some 200–300 eggs.

R. prowazekii is ingested in the blood meal and can infect both males, females and all nymphal stages. The rickettsiae develop in the epithelial lining cells of the stomach, which they distend to such an extent that rupture takes place, liberating them back into the damaged gut lumen. These are then passed into the louse faeces in which they can survive for 100 days or more. The damage caused to the louse can be sufficiently severe to kill it within 10 days and this helps to explain why few lice are found on a person suffering from typhus.

Humans become infected by scratching the louse faeces into abrasions or the puncture wound left by the feeding parasite, or if the lice is crushed on the skin or in the mouth. Dried lice faeces can remain viable for a considerable period of time and fine particles that are inhaled or enter the conjunctiva can be a potential hazard to those not infested with lice.

Lice thrive in conditions of deprivation and poverty, where clothing is worn without changing and people live in close proximity to each other. Lice cannot travel far, or survive for long without a blood meal, so it is the crowding together of people that allows lice to crawl across and infest a new host. Where clothing is changed or washed, or the ambient temperature is high, body lice do not occur and typhus is not found. But, in times of human disruption brought about by war, famine or social upheaval, the crowding together of people, in conditions of poor sanitation, provides the stage for an outbreak of typhus. A similar situation can occur in the highland areas of tropical countries, where people live close to each other to keep warm.

Various claims have been made for non-human reservoirs of *R. prowazekii*, but humans appear to be an adequate reservoir and the louse an ideal vector. The difficulty is what happens to the organism when an epidemic has subsided? The probable answer is found in Brill–Zinsser disease, more suitably called recurrent typhus. In this condition, people are found to have *R. prowazekii* in their bodies long after they had the disease. The organism remains dormant until some event causes a breakdown in host resistance and overt disease reappears. Cases have been found 20 and 40 years after the person was in a typhus area and where lice have been absent for this length of time. But if lice are fed on these cases, they become infected and can transmit epidemic typhus.

Incubation period is 1–2 weeks (up to 3 weeks in scrub typhus). The incubation period is related to the infecting dose.

Period of communicability Lice can become infected during the febrile illness, which may last for 2 weeks, but since lice will leave a febrile person, it is probably only during the earlier part of the illness. A chronic carrier (with Brill–Zinsser disease) can infect lice for up to 40 years. Lice excrete rickettsiae 2–6 days after an infected blood meal, but continue to be a source of

infection for weeks after they have died. Fleas in murine typhus remain infected for life (about 1 year).

Occurrence and distribution Like plague, typhus is a disease of history, particularly associated with the conflicts of man. When the anger of man causes war, disruption of civilizations, famine and refugees, then the disease of war, typhus, enters into the attack. At the present time, it is a particular risk of refugee camps.

Epidemic typhus can occur in highland areas, particularly during the rainy season with outbreaks occurring in Rwanda, Burundi, Ethiopia, Guatemala, Bolivia and Peru. The three countries in Africa have reported the most cases in recent times.

Murine typhus is endemic in Pakistan, India and the Malaysian peninsula, but may become epidemic in any part of the world where rats are found, such as in ports.

'Mite or typhus islands' are found in East, South and Southeast Asia, including Siberia, China, Japan, Thailand, Pakistan, Australia and Pacific Islands.

Control and prevention of scrub typhus is by the wearing of clothing treated with repellents or insecticides to prevent the larval mite from attacking humans. Long trousers tucked into boots with high lace-up sides, or gaiters to cover the gap, impregnated with diethyltoluamide, dimethylphthalate or a synthetic pyrethroid. Repellents should also be smeared on to arms and necks because it is these sites that are attacked when working in the undergrowth. If an area of scrub typhus is known and it is desired to clear it permanently, then the undergrowth should be cut down and burnt, leaving the ground to thoroughly dry out before being safe to use. A less permanent method is to spray the area with insecticides. Tetracycline can be taken as a prophylactic by those at particular risk, but such methods are never reliable.

Control of murine typhus is the same as for plague (Section 16.1) where the subject is covered in more detail. Essentially, it is the control of fleas and rats with the use of insecticide powders to kill the fleas first,

---

Box 16.1 Rat control.

The control of rats can be by cats, traps or poisoning. Rat protection with shields and guards should be used after rats have been removed. A well-trained cat can be most efficient. Trapping is an effective means of rat control if carried out properly. Traps can be made out of scrap pieces of metal and are, therefore, simply manufactured in developing countries. A knowledge of the rat runs is gained and the trap left baited, but unsprung. Once the bait has been taken, then the trap is set. Traps must be visited regularly, all dead rats disposed of (by burning) and set again.

Poisoning can be either with acute or chronic poisons. The number of poisons is considerable and where available, it is preferable to solicit professional advice. Poisons strong enough to kill rats are also able to kill other animals that may consume them. They are also dangerous to humans, especially children, so proper safety precautions must be observed. Zinc phosphate is a useful acute poison. A good bait should be used, such as broken maize or rice mixed in a proportion of 1:10 using cooking oil to dissolve it. Alternatively, it can be mixed with water and bait, then dried out before applying to the traps. There is a danger from the dust and gases produced when preparing baits, so mask and gloves should be used. Copper sulphate is an antidote and can be administered in 0.25 g portions orally, every 10 min until vomiting is induced. The most commonly used chronic poison is Warfarin, which is mixed with bait in a ratio of 1:19. With chronic poisons, the bait should first be placed and only if it is taken, mixed with poison on subsequent applications. Gassing is very effective as it kills both rats and fleas at the same time, but strict precautions must be observed. Rodents living in burrows can be gassed, blocking all exits; hydrogen cyanide gas is most commonly used.

---

followed by measures against rats. Buildings should be protected against re-infestation and new structures built with rat-proofing (Box 16.1).

Control of epidemic typhus is control of the louse. In an epidemic, this is most effectively done by blowing an insecticide powder into people's clothing. This can be by a blower with a long nozzle that is pushed up the arms of clothing, down through necks and up trousers and skirts. The clothing should be thoroughly treated remembering that the lice live between the underclothing and body. Temephos (2%), propoxur (1%), permethrin (0.5%) or other synthetic pyrethroids can be used. Samples of lice should be tested for insecticidal resistance before and during mass treatments. Since it is conditions of overcrowding that generate epidemics, it is often not too difficult to disinfect large numbers of people in a comparatively short time. Dead bodies should be dusted with insecticides before burial. A long-term preventive method is to treat underclothing with insecticides in the same way as mosquito nets are treated, to give a target dose of 0.65–1 g/m² permethrin. Clothes can be washed, but treatment should be repeated every 6 weeks.

Prophylactic antibiotics, generally tetracycline, can be given to contacts to reduce the extent of the reservoir. Treatment centres should be set up to discover cases early and antibiotics given.

Vaccines have been successful in controlling epidemics, but they suffer from various disadvantages. A killed vaccine (Cox) is painful when injected and does not give complete immunity, whereas a live, attenuated vaccine appears to give solid immunity for over 5 years, but must be prepared carefully as virulence can increase. Vaccines can either be used for mass administration in the face of epidemics or be given to individuals at increased risk, such as medical personnel.

In the long term, typhus will only disappear when all lice are removed. People should be encouraged to wash themselves and their clothes. Clothes must be boiled or washed at over 70°C, which is a higher temperature than most washing machines achieve. Ironing clothes kills both adults and eggs.

Treatment should be commenced as soon as possible, even before the diagnosis is confirmed, as speed is of the essence if treatment is to be effective. A single dose of

200 mg doxycycline, irrespective of age, is the treatment of choice. Alternatively, tetracycline at a dose of 500 mg four times a day may be given, and where both of these are unavailable, chloramphenicol may be used. Careful nursing is of utmost importance.

Surveillance is the cornerstone of prevention by conducting louse surveys at clinics, prisons, institutions and collections of people. Cases of proven or suspect epidemic louse-borne typhus should be notified to WHO. All contacts of a case should be placed under surveillance for 14 days.

16.3 Louse-borne Relapsing Fever

Organism *Borrelia recurrentis*, a spirochaete indistinguishable from *B. duttoni* in stained preparations, and with some cross-immunity between the two.

Clinical features Louse-borne relapsing fever is an epidemic disease occurring in the same situations or even at the same time as epidemic typhus. The disease is very similar to tick-borne relapsing fever (see below), with periods of fever lasting for a few days and then recurring after 2–4 days, but the number of relapses is generally less. The onset of fever is sudden with headache, myalgia and vertigo. A transitory petechial rash can occur and other symptoms, such as bronchitis and hepatosplenomegaly, may develop.

Diagnosis is by darkfield illumination of fresh or stained blood taken during a pyrexial episode.

Transmission *Pediculus corporis humanus* is infected when it feeds on humans during the pyrexial period, the spirochaete invading the haemocoel of the louse. The spirochaete is not transmitted when the louse feeds, but when it is crushed, the *Borrelia* entering the bite wound or any abrasion. Crushing lice between the fingernails or teeth are possible ways of acquiring infection. The spirochaete can also enter through

mucous membranes and possibly even unbroken skin. The greatest risk then is to the attentive parent or acquaintance delousing a member of the family or a friend.

Sub-clinical infection must also occur because the lice are killed even though the person does not show any symptoms. Humans are the only reservoir of the louse-borne infection.

Incubation period 5–15 days, normally 8 days.

Period of communicability Humans are most infectious during periods of pyrexia, but as reservoirs, they can infect lice at any time. The louse becomes infectious 4–5 days after an infected blood meal.

Occurrence and distribution The disease is associated with poor personal hygiene and overcrowding, in which lice flourish. Distribution is similar to epidemic typhus, being found in the highland areas of Africa, India and South America. There is an endemic focus in Ethiopia from which epidemics appear to originate, all the conditions being favourable about once every 20 years.

Control and prevention is the same as for epidemic typhus above, with delousing and improvement of hygiene.

Treatment is with a single dose of procaine penicillin (300,000 units) on the first day, followed by tetracycline 250 mg on the next day. Severe reactions to antibiotic therapy are commoner in louse-borne than tick-borne relapsing fever.

Surveillance Cases of louse-borne relapsing fever must be notified to WHO and neighbouring countries. Routine inspections for lice should be carried out where facilities permit, such as in prisons, institutions and to new arrivals coming into refugee camps.

16.4 Tick-borne Relapsing Fever

Organism *Borrelia dutoni*, which is indistinguishable from *B. recurrentis* in stained blood films.

Clinical features Fever develops with a recurring or relapsing pattern as the name of the disease indicates. The period of fever lasts for a few days and then recurs after 2–5 days, with up to ten or more relapses occurring in the untreated case. The onset of fever is sudden with headache, myalgia and vertigo; a transient petechial rash can occur and a variety of other systems may be involved. There can be bronchitis, nerve palsies, hepato-splenomegaly and signs of renal damage.

Diagnosis Spirochaetes are found in the blood during febrile periods when blood slides should be taken and either stained or viewed by dark ground illumination. An improvement on this technique is the direct centrifugal method.

Transmission, occurrence and distribution Two different patterns of tick-borne relapsing fever occur; an endemic in Africa and epidemic in other parts of the world (Fig. 16.4).

In Africa, the vector *Ornithodorus moubata* is domestic in habit living in and around the home, transmitting the disease within the household. The reservoir is the tick, but humans act as a source of organisms. When a tick feeds on an infected person, spirochaetes are ingested with the blood, multiply in the gut and enter the haemocoel, where they increase to enormous proportions. The spirochaetes pierce all organs of the tick's body, including the salivary gland, the coxal organ and the reproductive system, leading to transovarial infection. Nymphal stages may already be infected when they take blood meals or can become so from their hosts. People are infected both by the bite of the tick and from the coxal fluid (see below), but not from the faeces. In *O. moubata* adults, the coxal fluid is the main source of spirochaetes, but in the nymphs and other species of *Ornithodorus*, it is the salivary glands.

Babies and young children are particularly susceptible to infection in endemic areas, with adults exhibiting immunity.

However, immunity is lost by pregnancy and congenital infection can occur. Relapsing fever is a cause of abortion, stillbirth and premature delivery. This is particularly the pattern in Central and East Africa.

In other parts of the world, the infection is a zoonosis with a transmission cycle maintained between rodents and their parasitic ticks. People enter this cycle as intruders or by accident in a similar way to sylvatic plague or scrub typhus. Rodent-inhabited caves or campsites near rodent burrows are areas where sporadic infection can occur. When temporary shelters or log cabins are erected near a zoonotic focus, rats invade these buildings and their ticks begin to feed regularly on humans. An endemic pattern, similar to that in Africa may then develop. Ticks responsible for transmitting relapsing fever in other parts of the world are *O. tholozani* in Asia, *O. erraticus* in North Africa, and *O. rudis* and *O. talaje* in Central and South America.

Soft ticks (*Argasidae*) have a retracted head and no scutum, which differentiates them from hard ticks (see below). As their name implies, soft ticks do not have a rigid structure, but a leathery body that looks like a collapsed bag. This hangs over the body structures, so viewed from above only the legs can be seen protruding from it (Fig. 16.4). When the tick takes a blood meal, its collapsed body fills and becomes greatly distended. The tick digests the blood meal utilizing a structure called a coxal gland, which is like a filter to remove excess fluid.

After hatching, there are several nymphs (four in *O. moubata*), each needing to take a blood meal before passing on to the next nymphal stage. Finally, the fourth instar changes into an adult and egg laying commences after the female has become engorged with blood. Ticks can live for several years so that many eggs can be laid in a lifetime. In contrast to hard ticks, the female does not die after egg laying, but is able to continue taking blood meals, laying eggs after each meal.

Ticks rest in cracks and crevices of poorly built houses, emerging at night to feed on sleeping occupants. They can

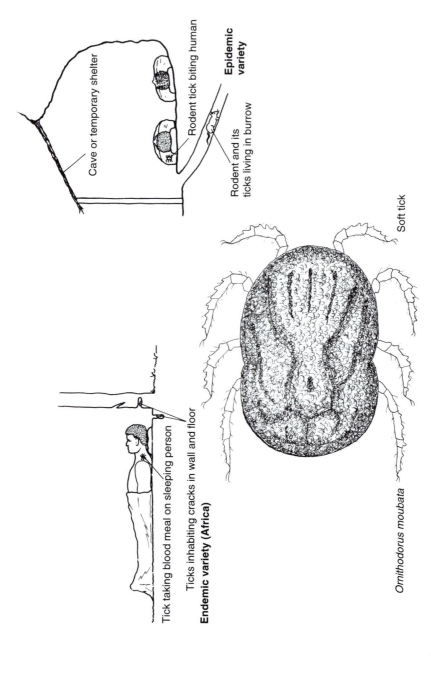

Cave or temporary shelter

Rodent tick biting human

Epidemic variety

Rodent and its ticks living in burrow

Tick taking blood meal on sleeping person

Ticks inhabiting cracks in wall and floor

Endemic variety (Africa)

Soft tick

Ornithodorus moubata

Fig. 16.4.   The vector and epidemiology of tick-borne relapsing fever.

remain alive for up to 5 years after a single blood meal and are able to attack again after the owner re-occupies a house following a prolonged absence. The eggs are coated with a waxy protective layer allowing them to remain viable for several months – laid in walls, floors and furniture, they will hatch in 1–4 weeks if conditions are suitable. Soft ticks once established are very persistent occupants.

Incubation period 3–10 days.

Period of communicability All stages of the tick are able to transmit infection and they remain infective for life.

Control and prevention Ticks can be controlled with insecticides, such as malathion, diazinon, permethrin or propoxur, sprayed around houses. Special attention needs to be paid to any cracks and crevices where ticks may hide. In addition, insecticides can be mixed with the floor or wall plaster during construction or repair work. BHC as 140 mg base/m^2 is a suitable preparation. Infants (and adults) can be protected from house-invading ticks by sleeping under a mosquito net. Repellents, such as DEET or dimethylphthalate smeared on skin or as a solution to impregnate clothing, are effective in preventing ticks from biting. Items, such as socks, can be treated with insecticides in the same way as mosquito nets (see Sections 3.4.1 and 3.4.4). Ticks are also deterred from entering rooms in which a night-lamp is glowing.

The rodent reservoir is of major importance in bringing ticks close to human habitation so all the methods mentioned in plague (Box 16.1) to control rodents should be used. Improved house construction will prevent rodents from burrowing underneath.

Treatment is with a single dose of 300,000 units of procaine penicillin immediately, followed the next day by tetracycline 500 mg four times daily for 10 days. This regime provides adequate treatment, while at the same time minimizes reactions.

Surveillance Mass screening using fresh or stained blood slides can be used to delineate the infected population prior to a control programme.

16.5 Diseases Transmitted by Hard Ticks

16.5.1 Hard ticks (Ixodidae)

Hard ticks are responsible for transmission of several different kinds of organisms including rickettsiae, *Borrelia* and arboviruses. The genera of medical importance are *Amblyomma*, *Dermacentor*, *Haemaphysalis*, *Hyalomma*, *Ixodes* and *Rhipicephalus*. A female *Dermacentor*, to characterize the group of hard ticks, is illustrated in Fig. 16.5. The feature that distinguishes hard from soft ticks is the presence of a scutum (shield) and protruding mouthparts. Care has to be taken in identifying the engorged specimen, for the body is so greatly distended as to obscure the head and mouthparts (Fig. 16.5). The female has a smaller scutum than the male, but since both males and females take blood meals, there is no need to distinguish between them.

Eggs are laid in a large mass on the ground, hatching after weeks or months into six-legged larvae. These larvae resemble mites, but are differentiated from them by prominent mouthparts and a scutum. The larvae climb on to grass or prominent vegetation to await a passing mammal on to which they cling. Once attached, they crawl around to find an area of soft skin, such as in the ears, eyelids or belly of an animal. On humans, they may surreptitiously climb up the leg and attach themselves to the scrotum or between the buttocks. Once in a favourable site, they pierce the skin with their powerful mouthparts, inject saliva and feed on the host's blood. Larvae will remain attached for 3–7 days, after which they drop to the ground and seek a place to moult. Developing into an eight-legged nymph, the nymph repeats the feeding pattern, being attached for 5–10 days and then falling to the ground once more for the final moult.

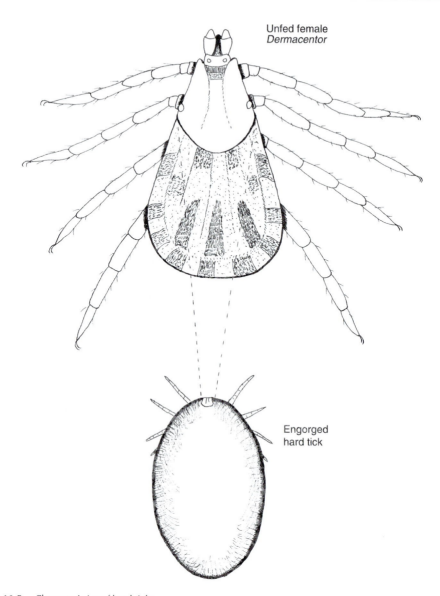

Fig. 16.5.   Characteristics of hard ticks.

From the nymph develops a male or female adult, which subsequently quests for a new host on which it remains for a considerable period of time (up to 1 month) becoming greatly engorged with blood. Finally dropping off, the female digests her blood meal and begins egg laying, after which she dies.

The life cycle of ticks is modified by temperature and humidity, such that if it becomes too cold, the cycle of development will be delayed until more favourable conditions return. Larvae and nymphs tend to feed on small mammals and humans, whereas adults prefer larger animals, such as cattle and game animals.

Control of ticks is mainly through the use of insecticides and repellents. Permethrin, malathion and propoxur are suitable insecticides, administered as dusting powders or solutions to infested animals. Cattle are commonly treated by making them swim through an insecticidal bath or dip. This should be carried out on a regular basis, with monitoring of ticks for insecticidal resistance. Dogs are important carriers of ticks and should be similarly treated by insecticidal baths, making sure that they are totally immersed as the ears are a common site for ticks to attach. Dogs should wear tick-repellent collars.

Repellents, such as diethyltoluamide or dimethylphthalate smeared on skin or as a solution to impregnate clothing, are effective in preventing ticks from becoming attached. Items, such as socks, can be treated with insecticides in the same way as mosquito nets (see Sections 3.4.1 and 3.4.4).

Ticks take nearly 2 h to attach themselves and start feeding, so a careful search of the body, paying particular attention to the upper legs, groin and buttocks, should be made after passing through tick-infested country. Larval and nymph stages can be very small. Ticks should not be pulled off directly as the mouthparts may be left behind, which will continue to cause irritation. Applying methylated spirit, ether, benzene or similar solutions will kill the tick and sterilize the wound.

16.6 Tick Typhus/Fever

Going under a host of names, Boutonneuse fever, Mediterranean-spotted fever, African tick typhus, Indian tick typhus, Siberian tick typhus, Queensland tick typhus, to give but a few, this similar group of infections has been reported from different parts of the world.

Organism *Rickettsia conori*, *R. africae*, *R. siberica* and *R. australis*.

Clinical features Generally, a mild illness of a few days, infection is characterized by an eschar at the site of the tick bite and regional lymphadenopathy. There is fever and a generalized maculo-papular rash, resolving spontaneously after about 1 week.

Diagnosis is usually on clinical appearance following history of a tick bite, but can be confirmed with serological tests or PCR.

Transmission The reservoir of infection is the dog tick (*Rhipicephalus sanguineus* in the Mediterranean area, and *Amblyomma hebreum* in Africa), which inadvertently moves from the dog to its human handler during their close association. Alternatively, humans acquire infection from passing through scrub forest inhabited by rodents and their ticks (*Ixodes holocyclus* in Australia, *Dermacentor* and *Haemaphysalis* in Siberia), the rodent serving as a secondary reservoir.

Incubation period 1–15 days (generally 5–7 days).

Period of communicability Not transmitted from human-to-human, the tick remaining infected for life.

Occurrence and distribution Found in slightly different forms in the Mediterranean region, Africa, Indian sub-continent, Australia and northeast Asia.

Control and prevention Where the dog is the carrier of ticks, they should wear tick-repellent collars and be inspected regularly to ensure the animal is tick-free. In Australia, Siberia, Mongolia and northern China where rodents and small marsupials are mainly responsible, repellents and insecticide-treated socks and trousers should be worn. Since it takes the tick about 2 h to fully attach itself, it is always a good practice to examine the body carefully after going through tick-infested country. When camping, people should sleep off the ground (e.g. on camp beds) and dogs should be kept away.

Treatment is with tetracycline, doxycycline or chloramphenicol.

Surveillance Make a regular habit of examining the body after walking through countryside.

16.7 Rocky Mountain Spotted Fever

Organism *Rickettsia rickettsii.*

Clinical features The illness commences suddenly with onset of high fever, headache, malaise, muscle pains and rash. Appearing about the third day, the characteristic rash is maculo-papular from numerous petechial haemorrhages and covers the whole body including the palms and soles.

Diagnosis is made clinically with the additional help of enzyme immunoassay and immunofluorescence tests containing the specific antigen.

Transmission Humans are infected by the bite of a tick although infection can also be acquired by scratching in tick faeces or crushing the tick on the skin or mucous membranes. Larval and nymphal stages, as well as adult ticks, can transmit the infection. Rickettsial infection is maintained by transovarial transmission and the tick acts as the reservoir.

Incubation period 3–14 days.

Period of communicability Since the tick is the reservoir of infection, it is not spread from person to person.

Occurrence and distribution First described in the Rocky Mountains of North America, the disease is also found in Mexico, Panama, Costa Rica, Brazil, Colombia and Argentina.

Control and prevention Prevention is by avoiding any known tick country or wearing protective clothing, treated with repellents or insecticides. The common vector in North America is the dog tick, *D. variabilis*, or the wood tick *D. andersoni* so the control of dogs and their ectoparasites

with tick-repellent collars is effective. *Amblyomma cajennense* is the main vector in the rest of the Americas.

Treatment is with doxycycline, tetracycline or chloramphenicol.

Surveillance Dogs and other animals should be checked regularly for ticks.

16.8 Lyme Disease

Organism *Borrelia burgdorferi*, *B. garinii* and *B. afzelii.*

Clinical features The herald sign is an annular expanding erythematous skin lesion, called erythematous migrans (EM), often accompanied by fever, muscle pain, arthralgia and signs of meningeal irritation. Infection may develop over weeks or months into aseptic meningitis, encephalitis, peripheral nerve signs, cardiac irregularities and polyarthritis.

Diagnosis is mainly clinical, the EM lesion exceeding 5 cm, aided by serological tests, more useful in the later stages of the disease.

Transmission is from the bite of an infected deer tick, *Ixodes scapularis* or *I. pacificus*, in North America or sheep tick *I. ricinus* in Europe. In Asia, *I. persulcatus* is the vector. The reservoir of infection is in the tick, which can transmit the *Borrelia* transovarially. Adult ticks largely feed on deer (sheep in Europe), while the nymphal stage is responsible for transmitting the infection to humans and other animals, such as dogs, which will often develop similar symptoms to humans.

Incubation period 3–32 days (mean 7–10 days).

Period of communicability Not transmitted from person to person.

Occurrence and distribution Found in well-defined areas of USA and Canada, largely related to the deer population. Limited range in Europe, Russia, China and Japan. Foci of infection can be delineated by looking for the vector tick.

Control and prevention are similar to other tick-borne diseases mentioned above with the use of repellents and insecticide-treated clothing when passing through known infected areas. Since transmission of infection takes in excess of 24 h after the tick has attached, careful search of the body should be made after walking through countryside. The nymphal stage is the main transmitter to humans so small black spots should be looked for, possibly with the aid of a lens (see Fig. 16.4).

A vaccine has been developed against lyme disease in North America, but is not effective in other parts of the world. It is only useful for persons at constant risk of infection, such as game wardens or camp attendants, but other precautionary measures should also be taken.

Treatment is effective with doxycycline or amoxicillin in the early EM stage of the disease. In the late arthritic, cardiac or neurological stage of the disease, treatment is with benzylpenicillin or ceftriaxone for up to 21 days.

Surveillance Infected areas should be delineated and warning signs posted.

16.9 Arboviruses

16.9.1 Kyasanur forest disease (KFD) and Omsk haemorrhagic fever (OHF)

KFD is named after the forest in Karnataka, South India where an epidemic was first identified in 1983. A very similar disease, OHF, is restricted to western Siberia. The organisms and clinical features are described with the other arbovirus haemorrhagic fevers in Section 15.2.

Transmission is by *Haemaphysalis spinigera*, with a reservoir in rodents and monkeys in KFD and *Dermacentor reticulatus* and *D. marginatus* in OHF. The muskrat is the reservoir, so hunters are the main victims from which they can also acquire infection directly.

Incubation period 3–8 days.

Control is the same as the other tick-borne diseases. Experimental vaccines are under trial.

16.9.2 Crimean–Congo haemorrhagic fever

Crimean–Congo haemorrhagic fever virus is related to dengue and yellow fever with which it shares a similar clinical presentation (Sections 15.4 and 15.5). It is found in a wide area stretching from west and southern Africa through central and northeast Africa into the Arabian peninsula, to west and central Asia (Iraq, Iran, Pakistan, Afghanistan, Russia and west China) and westwards into the Balkans and Greece.

Transmission is by *Hyalomma marginatum* and *H. anatolicum* ticks, which also serve as reservoirs, although birds, rodents and hares may be involved. Person-to-person infection can also occur from exposure to blood and other body fluids. The ticks feed on domestic animals (cattle, sheep and goats), so the disease is an occupational hazard of farmers and shepherds, who can also contract the illness by contact with animal tissues and fluids.

Incubation period 1–3 days, but can be up to 12 days.

Period of communicability During the entire period of illness, the patient is highly infectious from urine, blood and other body fluids.

Control and prevention All the precautions
mentioned above should be taken to prevent
being bitten by ticks, including insecticide
treatment of domestic animals. Strict barrier
nursing should be observed with all cases.
Gloves and overalls should be worn when
working with animals. People in high-risk
areas can be vaccinated.

16.9.3 Other arbovirus diseases

Hard ticks can also be responsible for
spreading other arbovirus diseases normally
transmitted by mosquitoes, such as Japanese
encephalitis and St Louis, Eastern and Western equine encephalitis (see Section 15.2).

17

Domestic and Synanthropic Zoonoses

A zoonosis is an infection that is naturally transmitted between vertebrate animals and humans. In the last chapter, a group of infections that were mainly zoonoses, but also involved a vector were covered, while this chapter includes infections in which a vector is not involved. Most of these infections are due to the close association humans have with their domestic animals, but there are also some zoonoses in which animals that live close to humans, but are not welcomed, such as rats, are involved in the transmission of disease. These are called synanthropic zoonoses. Some zoonotic infections have been covered in earlier chapters where the means of transmission and control are similar to other allied conditions, for example, the pork and beef tapeworms will be found in Section 9.8 under food-borne diseases.

The most important source of infection from which humans suffer is from other humans, but the animals on which people depend for their livelihood and companionship are responsible for many others. Paramount amongst these is the dog, which is involved directly in a number of diseases, or is a reservoir for many others (Table 17.1). Less important, except to people who have close association with them are cats, cattle and other domestic animals. The principal synanthropic vector is the rat, already

covered in some detail in the section on plague (Section 16.1), but also involved in several other infections mentioned in this chapter. Control depends upon an understanding of the contact with the animal and how best to reduce it.

17.1 Rabies

Organism Rabies is caused by a rhabdovirus in the genus *Lyssavirus*. There are seven related viruses, including Mokola and Duvenhage (found in Africa), which produce rabies-like illness. The virus withstands freezing temperatures for considerable periods of time, but is killed by boiling, sunlight and drying. It is not easily destroyed by disinfectants.

Clinical features The disease starts quietly with malaise, fever, sore throat and lack of appetite; paraesthesia develops and abnormal muscle movements occur. The patient then enters the excitable stage when they become anxious, there is difficulty in swallowing and frank hydrophobia and generalized convulsions may take place. The patient either dies in the convulsive stage or enters progressive paralysis as the terminal symptom. In the bat-transmitted

Table 17.1.   Infections transmitted to humans from dogs or in which the dog is a reservoir.

Viruses	Arboviruses
	Rabies
Rickettsiae	*R. rickettsii, R. conorii, R. africae, R. australis, R. siberica*
Bacteria	Anthrax
	Brucella canis
	Campylobacter jejuni
	Capnocytophaga
	Escherichia coli
	Leptospirosis
	Mycobacteria
	Pasteurellosis
	Salmonella
	Spirillum minus
	Tularaemia
Fungi	Ringworm
Protozoa	Chagas' disease
	Cryptosporidiosis
	Isospora belli
	Leishmaniasis
Helminths	*Ancylostoma* (larva migrans)
	Brugia malayi, B. pahangi, B. patei
	Diphyllobothium latum,
	Dipylidium caninum
	Dirofilaria immitis
	Dracunculus medinensis
	Echinococcus granulosus, E. multilocularis, E. vogeli
	Echinostoma
	Gnathostoma spinigerum
	Heterophyes heterophyes
	Metagonimus yokagawai
	Multiceps multiceps
	Opisthorchis sinensis, O. felineus
	Paragonimus westermani
	Strongyloides
	Schistosoma japonicum
	Toxocara canis
Arthropods	Fleas
	Ticks
	Pentastomids (*Linguatula*)

form of the disease, there is no excitable stage and the patient dies from respiratory paralysis.

Diagnosis The clinical picture following a history of an animal bite is usually sufficient to make the diagnosis, but the virus may be isolated from saliva, tears, CSF, urine and many other tissues if facilities exist to culture it. Immunofluorescence antibody staining of tissue smears (e.g. skin biopsy) is of value.

Transmission Virus enters the body through a bite or abrasion of the skin. Classically, it is a dog bite, but if an infective dog, cat or cow licks the abraded skin, then transmission can occur in this manner. The vampire bat also transmits rabies, but mainly to cattle, with humans only occasionally infected this way. People have contracted rabies by entering bat-infested caves where it is thought that fine particles of bat faeces contaminate the conjunctiva or enter the respiratory mucosa.

The virus has a special affinity for brain and mucous-secreting tissue, travelling along peripheral nerves to the CNS and salivary glands. Large quantities of virus particles are present in the saliva from 1 to 10 days before the development of symptoms in the animal, right up until it dies.

The disease in the dog occurs in two forms, the furious and dumb. In furious rabies, the animal becomes restless, wanders away from home and bites anybody or anything that comes in its way. It is unable to bark, may attempt to eat sticks and stones, but is foiled in the attempt by a difficulty in swallowing. It foams at the mouth and suffers from the progressive paralysis of dumb rabies and is dead within a few days. Sometimes the furious course is not followed and dumb rabies only is manifest.

While the disease is invariably fatal in domestic dogs, cats and cows, it would appear to have a more variable effect in wild dogs, such as foxes and wolves. Certainly, rabies controls fox populations, but individuals do recover from the disease. There is little evidence to support the finding of a reservoir in such canines, but this may not be the case in rodents and bats. Rabies virus has been found in mongooses and the multimammate rat, *Mastomys natalensis*. These animals suffer from rabies, but sub-clinical infections may occur. When canines feed on small mammals they can acquire rabies. Vampire bats have been shown to recover from the disease and rabies virus has also been isolated from insectivorous bats, which do not take blood meals. This suggests that rabies may exist in a mild and asymptomatic form for most of the time in these mammals, but when they bite or people enter their virus-contaminated habitat, they are at risk of losing their life (see further Section 18.3).

Incubation period depends upon the proximity of the point of introduction of the virus to the brain and the size of the infective dose. It is usually 2–12 weeks, but can be years in young children with a minor bite.

Period of communicability Theoretical transfer from person-to-person is possible, so barrier nursing should be instigated. Animals are infectious from 4 to 14 days before clinical signs start until they die or are killed, but their saliva remains infectious. Sixty per cent of persons bitten by a known rabid animal do not contract the disease.

Occurrence and distribution A disease that strikes terror into people, it is widely spread throughout the world, as important in temperate as tropical countries. It is common in Russia, Africa, Asia and South America. India reports 30,000 deaths per annum, more than half the total cases in the world, with other countries in Asia accounting for most of the rest. It is particularly dangerous to children aged 5–15 years who are the main victims.

It is mainly transmitted by dogs, including wolves, foxes, jackals and hyenas, but the cat and cow have also been responsible. Other infected wild animals are mongooses, skunks and raccoons. In South America, the vampire bat transmits rabies particularly to cattle, but insectivorous and fruit-eating bats have also been found infected.

Control and prevention Control measures can be aimed against the domestic dog, the reservoir in wild animals, and the protection of humans.

Domestic dogs should be licensed and vaccinated, destroying all the stray ones. Vaccination of all domestic animals with an approved vaccine should be mandatory in all endemic areas.

Control of the wild animal reservoir is a massive undertaking, but alteration of habitat and local destruction around dwellings or place of work can be practised. As rabies follows a natural cycle in many wild animals, their total destruction over large areas may upset this balance and produce a rebound increase, so it is preferable to try and maintain this balance by using vaccination. This has been effectively used in Europe and Canada by leaving vaccine baits for wild animals to take. With bat rabies, control of bats is largely unsuccessful and it is preferable to immunize cattle, which are the main victims.

People who are at special risk, such as veterinarians, animal handlers and those working with bats, can be vaccinated with human diploid cell vaccine (HDCV), Vero cell vaccine (VCV) or purified chick embryo cell vaccine (PCEC). Adverse reactions do occur so the vaccine should only be administered to those at risk of exposure to rabies. The vaccine is given on days 0, 7 and 28 with a booster after 1 year. If the risk continues, then boosters every 5 years are recommended, although protection probably is maintained for 10 years with HDCV and VCV.

Because children in the 5–15-year age group are at the greatest risk of dying from rabies, some countries may consider vaccinating children between 2 and 4 months of age. To save costs, three doses of 0.1 ml HDCV by the intradermal route at 2, 3 and 4 months of age may be more feasible.

Treatment Fortunately, rabies virus can be inactivated on its passage along the peripheral nerves and this is the main method of protecting the individual bitten by a rabid dog. The first procedure is to wash out the wound thoroughly with soap or detergent under running water, followed by a quaternary ammonium compound or 0.1% iodine. Any alcohol, such as whisky or gin, can be used if there is nothing else available. If there is a high suspicion of infection, then rabies antiserum should also be injected locally around the wound. Tetanus toxoid and penicillin should be administered, as tetanus is often a greater danger from a bite than rabies.

If the biting animal can be caught, then it should be tied up and observed for 10 days. After this time, it would either have died from the disease or remained well. If it

has died or was killed, then the head is severed with aseptic precautions (as the saliva is highly infectious), packed in ice and sent to a laboratory for viral antigen testing or histological studies. Section of the brain will show characteristic Negri bodies.

Post-exposure vaccination can be given with HDCV, VCV or PCEC immediately and on days 3, 7, 14, 28 and 90. If pre-exposure immunization was given, then give one dose immediately and a second in 3 days. The normal dose is 1 ml intramuscularly, but because of the high cost, money can be saved by giving much smaller doses (0.1 ml of HDCV) intradermally.

Hyper-immune anti-rabies serum is given as soon as possible, half around the wound and the rest intramuscularly. Human immune globulin is preferable, but if horse serum only is available, then a test dose must first be given. The dose is:

- human immune globulin, 20 IU/kg body weight;
- animal immune globulin, 40 IU/kg body weight.

Table 17.2 summarizes the procedure to be followed in treating a person who has been attacked by a rabid animal.

Surveillance Cases of rabies should be reported to WHO. Countries should work towards a system of vaccine certification of dogs using microchip implants or permanent collars containing vaccination details.

17.2 Hydatid Disease

Organism *Echinococcus granulosus*, a cyclophyllidean tapeworm of canines.

Clinical features Hydatid cysts, the intermediate stage of the parasite, have been recorded from all parts of the human body. The commonest site is the liver, with lung, abdomen, kidney and brain in descending order of frequency. As the cysts increase in size, they can cause serious problems some times fatally. The cyst contents are infective so if it ruptures either accidentally or at operation, then numerous new cysts are formed. The liberation of so much foreign protein in the body can result in a severe anaphylactic reaction.

Diagnosis of the disease is clinically, from enlargement of liver or discovery of a cyst on chest X-ray. Immunological methods are useful. A diagnostic aspiration of the cyst must never be made.

Transmission Eggs passed in the dog faeces contaminate pastureland and when eaten by sheep, pigs, goats, cattle, camels and horses develop into hydatid cysts (Fig. 17.1). The hydatid cyst is a fluid-filled sack containing enormous numbers of scolices, any of which can become an adult worm in the dog. The common means of infection is for dogs to be fed the offal of domestic animals. In the wild, jackals, wolves and wild dogs become infected by killing and eating infected herbivores.

Humans enter this cycle accidentally by swallowing the eggs either:

- through food items (e.g. fruit or vegetables contaminated by dog faeces);
- drinking water contaminated by dog faeces;
- close contact with dogs (e.g. by touching their fur or being licked by them; when a dog licks itself, it can spread eggs all over its body as well as sticking to its tongue).

Primary infection commonly occurs in childhood, with symptoms developing in adult life.

Incubation period Generally a period of several years.

Table 17.2. Post-exposure and anti-rabies guide. This is only a guide and should be used in conjunction with local knowledge of rabies endemicity and the animal involved.

Type of animal	Status of animal	Type of exposure	Treatment
Domestic	Healthy and remains so for 10 days	Any	None
Dog Cat Cow	Signs suggestive of rabies. Retain animal for 10 days	Mild, scratch or lick Bite	Rabies vaccine (discontinue if animal not rabid by day 5)
	Rabid or becomes so during retention	Mild, scratch or lick	Rabies vaccine
		Bite	Anti-rabies serum plus vaccine (discontinue if animal not rabid by day 5)
	Escaped, killed or unknown	Mild, scratch or lick	Rabies vaccine
		Bite	Anti-rabies serum, plus vaccine
Wild	Regard as rabid if unprovoked attack	Bite	Serum immediately followed by course of vaccine
Fox Wolf Raccoon Mongoose Bat, etc.			

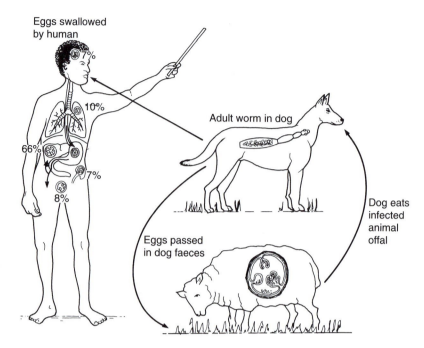

Fig. 17.1. Hydatid disease, the life cycle of *Echinococcus granulosus*.

Period of communicability Dogs are often repeatedly infected so continue to be a source of infection, especially to children.

Occurrence and distribution The disease is widespread, but occurs in concentrated pockets, such as sheep-rearing areas or where dogs live in close proximity to humans. A very high rate of infection is found in the Turkana people of northern Kenya where dogs are trained to care for young children.

Control and prevention can be implemented at several points in the life cycle:

Infected material should not be fed to dogs or if this cannot be avoided, it must be well cooked. Dogs can be treated with praziquantel to remove any adult worms. Measures should be taken to reduce faecal contamination, such as fencing water sources and food gardens or the general training of dogs. Ultimately though control will depend upon human attitude to dogs by keeping them in an appropriate place, not touching them or feeding them at meal times, destroying unwanted animals and observing personal hygiene. Children, in particular, should be taught to wash their hands before eating and after touching dogs.

Treatment Albendazole and mebendazole are effective, but where necessary surgical removal may be required, taking care to remove the entire cyst or if rupture seems likely to sterilize the contents with formalin. Praziquantel will prevent the development of secondary cysts if rupture of a primary cyst has taken place, so is a useful precaution during surgery.

A similar, but rare infection is *E. multilocularis*, which as its name suggests forms multi-loculated lesions rather than single cysts. These invade the body much in the same way as a neoplastic growth, including producing metastases. It is found in the colder regions of the world (Siberia, Alaska and northern Canada), a parasite of foxes and dogs, with voles, lemmings and mice being intermediate hosts.

Another variety, found in Colombia, Ecuador and Brazil, is *E. vogeli*, caught by dogs eating agoutis, pacas and spiny rats. A polycystic hydatid cyst results.

17.3 Toxocariasis

Organism The roundworms of dogs, *Toxocara canis* and less commonly cats, *T. catis*.

Clinical features Larvae unable to complete their development in the human body wander until they die. The body responds to this invasion by the production of eosinophils, but more serious is the tissue in which the larvae go to, an unfortunate site of predilection being the eye, which can result in blindness. In heavy infections, there is fever, cough, an urticarial rash and hepatomegaly.

Diagnosis can be made with larval antigen ELISA.

Transmission Eggs are accidentally ingested from the dog's fur, from contaminated soil or from vegetables contaminated by dog faeces. The typical picture is of the young child playing with soil frequented by pet dogs and putting the fingers in their mouth. The eggs are resistant to desiccation and remain in the soil for many months so that the soil in parks and other areas where dogs are taken for walks can be heavily contaminated.

Incubation period Transient infection may occur after a few weeks, but more serious eye complications will probably not present until the child is 5 years or older.

Period of communicability Although the infection is not transferred from one human to another, the eggs may be from unhygienic habits.

Occurrence and distribution Worldwide, wherever dogs and cats are found living in close association with humans, especially as pets.

Control and prevention Dogs should be prevented from promiscuous defecation of playgrounds, streets, parkland and vegetable gardens. Owners of pets should scoop-up faeces and dispose of them safely. Stray animals, especially unwanted puppies, should be destroyed. Dogs and cats should be dewormed at 6-month intervals starting when the animal is 3 weeks old. Young children should not play with pets and should be taught personal hygiene from a young age.

Treatment Albendazole and mebendazole are used in treatment of the acute case, but will not cure eye damage.

17.4 Larva Migrans

Organism The larval form of several animal parasites wander aimlessly in the human body, if they enter it by mistake. Examples are the cat and dog hookworms, *Ancylostoma brasiliense*, *A. stenocephala* and *A. canium*, producing a condition called creeping eruption; and the cat and dog filariae, *Dirofilaria immitis*, *Brugia pahangi* and *B. patei*, which cause the more serious disease of visceral larva migrans. *Bayliscaris procyonis*, a roundworm of raccoons, can result in fatal encephalitis.

Clinical features Creeping eruption is often visible as serpiginous tracks just underneath the skin, which contain wandering larvae. These are painful and red at the advancing end, causing intense pruritus, and advancing a little each day, sometimes continuing for several years.

In larva migrans the body reacts to the wandering parasites, especially when they pass through the lungs, with a profound eosinophilia, one of the causes of the condition known as pulmonary eosinophilia. Symptoms are a paroxysmal cough, not unlike asthma, with the production of large quantities of sputum, sometimes streaked with blood. A diagnosis of tuberculosis can mistakenly be made.

Diagnosis is largely made on clinical grounds, but the filaria antigen of *D. immitis* can be used as a skin test in larva migrans.

Transmission The animal hookworm larvae are contracted in the same way as human *Ancylostoma* infection (Section 10.3), walking without adequate foot covering in an area of soil contaminated by dog and cat faeces. The filarial worms are transmitted by culicine mosquitoes, but as with human disease repeated infection is required. The raccoon roundworm is deposited in frequently used defecation areas, which can be associated with urban structures, such as rooftops, attics, woodpiles and in gardens close to trees, where humans, especially children, inadvertently pick up the eggs and swallow them.

Incubation period Variable, weeks to months.

Occurrence and distribution Found in the tropical and temperate regions of the world in areas where dogs and cats are kept as pets or for hunting. Raccoons are progressively moving into urban areas where they pose a risk to children in particular.

Control and prevention Animal hookworms are prevented in the same way as human infection with the wearing of adequate footwear (Section 10.3). Efforts can be made to reduce cat and dog fouling by restraining them and keeping animals to designated parts of the village. Children should be taught to wash their hands before eating.

The same methods as are used to reduce mosquito bites in lymphatic filariasis (Section 15.7) are applicable for the dog and cat filarial infections; especially the use of repellents and insecticide-treated nets.

Treatment Larva migrans responds dramatically to DEC, while albendazole or ivermectin can be used in creeping eruption.

A localized form of visceral larva migrans occurring in Thailand and China results from *Gnathostoma spinigerum*, an intestinal parasite of cats and dogs. People are infected by the larval stage, through eating raw fish. The disease presents as a single migratory swelling, either superficially or in the deeper tissues, cerebral lesions being not uncommon. It causes intense itching and eosinophilia. If the larva comes near the surface of the body, its surgical removal can result in cure, otherwise albendazole, mebendazole and DEC have been reported to have some effect. Ensuring that fish are properly cooked is the easiest method of control.

17.5 Toxoplasmosis

Organism The coccidian protozoa *Toxoplasma gondii*, found in the cat.

Clinical features The toxoplasma, which develop from the oocysts, disperse to many parts of the body including the CNS where they form small inflammatory foci (pseudocysts). They result in surprisingly little pathology to their host occasionally producing lymphadenopathy and a low-grade fever, but congenital infection can result from an acutely infected mother. The infant may have hepatosplenamegaly, corioretinitis or mental retardation and quite often dies. Toxoplasmosis can also become reactivated in the immunocompromised (e.g. in the HIV-infected individual), causing pneumonia, myocarditis or fatal encephalitis.

Recent evidence has suggested that far from the pseudocysts causing little pathology when they attach to the brain of the non-neonate, they might produce some alteration in human response. Experiments in mice show that by the parasite selectively attacking the brain, it disables the animal's response to the presence of a predator so making it more easily caught and the parasite being transmitted. In the human, the effect is to prolong the reaction time making the victim more likely to have a road-traffic accident.

Diagnosis can be made by a rise in specific IgM during the first 8 weeks, IgG over several years or by lymph node biopsy.

Transmission Oocysts are passed in cat faeces and if accidentally swallowed by humans they become infected. Children are commonly infected when playing with pets, or sand and soil in which cats defecate. Adults are more commonly infected from swallowing pseudocysts in undercooked meat (generally mutton or pork). Congenital infection occurs when the mother becomes infected during the early course of her pregnancy. Oocysts can be inhaled or drunk in contaminated water, and toxoplasma tachyzoites are passed in cow and goat milk.

Incubation period 10–20 days.

Period of communicability Mothers can pass on infection to their fetus anytime during pregnancy, but the more serious disease results from infection in the first few months. Oocysts remain viable in moist soil or water for at least a year and in raw meat until it is cooked.

Occurrence and distribution Exposure to toxoplasmosis is common and widespread, with up to 40% seropositive in some countries. Infection is also found in birds and other mammals including sheep, cattle, goats, pigs, chickens and rodents. All members of the cat family can produce oocysts, often becoming infected from eating rodents or birds.

Control and prevention is by personal hygiene especially hand-washing after touching cats. Cats should be banished at meal times and when food is being prepared. The habit of giving cats scraps of food during the course of a meal should be strongly discouraged. All meat should be properly cooked and milk pasteurized. Children's play areas, especially sandpits, should be protected from cats.

Treatment Pyrimethamine, with or without sulphonamides, can be used for treatment.

Surveillance In high-incidence areas, pregnant women can be asked questions on contact with cats or eating undercooked meat during the antenatal visit.

17.6 Brucellosis

Organism is a Gram-negative bacillus, *Brucella melitensis*, *B. abortus*, *B. suis* and *B. canis*. *B. melitensis* causes the disease in goats that was first investigated in Malta (Melita was the Roman name for the island). *B. abortus*, as its name implies, causes abortion in cattle. *B. suis* is an infection of pigs. Both pigs and sheep are often infected with *B. melitensis* and *B. abortus*. *B. canis* is restricted to dogs.

The organism is killed by heating at 60°C for 10 min and by 1% phenol for 15 min. It survives well in milk and cream cheeses that have not fermented or gone hard. In places contaminated by the faeces and urine of infected animals, survival can be for months and even years, especially at lower temperatures. With temperatures above 25°C, survival time is reduced.

Clinical features The severity and duration of the disease is very variable and may go undiagnosed for a considerable period of time. Characteristically, there are intermittent or irregular fevers (undulant fever) with generalized aches and pains. The patient is unduly weak and tired, often retiring in the second half of the day. There may be depression, a cough, lymphadenopathy and splenomegaly. Recovery may occur spontaneously, or the disease become chronic, with the undulant pattern of fever and fatigue more pronounced. If not treated, this can continue for 6 months to 1 year, after which 80% of patients fully recover. Abortion is more frequent in women with the disease.

Diagnosis is difficult, but isolation of the organism from blood, bone marrow or urine should be attempted. Serum agglutination tests can be used, but a rise in titre is required.

Transmission Humans are infected by drinking raw milk or milk produce. *B. melitensis* is mainly spread by unpasteurized goat's milk or the consumption of cream cheeses prepared from it. *B. abortus* has less invasive power and virulence when consumed in cow's milk and so asymptomatic infection from drinking cow's milk can occur. In people whose occupations bring them in close proximity to animals, infection can occur through the skin, probably via an abrasion, the mucous membrane, the conjunctiva or as an aerosol through the respiratory tract. Such persons as farmers, shepherd, goat herds, vets and abattoir workers are at greater risk. Animal handlers can contract the much rarer *B. canis* infection from dogs.

Incubation period is 5–60 days, but may be up to 7 months.

Period of communicability Not transmitted from person to person.

Occurrence and distribution The disease is mainly one of animals, resulting in economic losses to the society and ill health to those involved in looking after animals. Brucellosis is common in South and Central America, Africa, the Mediterranean, South, Southwest and Central Asia. It is often not recognized, being found in a large number of animals if looked for. In Sudan and Nigeria, 60% of cattle were found to be infected.

Cattle become infected from eating placentae, licking a dead fetus or close contact with contaminated surroundings, such as cattle paddocks, barns or shelters. The young can obtain infection through the milk of their mothers.

Control and prevention is by pasteurization or boiling of cow and goat milk. Where pasteurization is not a legal requirement, people should be told of the risks of drinking raw milk and advised to boil it.

Anybody working with animals, especially those concerned with slaughter of animals, or coming into contact with products of abortion, should wear overalls and gloves that are frequently washed and sterilized. Proper animal husbandry reduces areas of contaminated pastureland that perpetuates infection.

Where facilities permit, herds or flocks can be rendered *Brucella*-free by diagnosis and slaughter of infected animals. A useful test for this purpose is the milk-ring test on cow's milk. Haematoxylin-stained *Brucella* antigen is added to a sample of cow's milk and if positive, a blue ring appears at the interface. By removing infected animals from a herd and preventing them from coming into contact with others, whole areas of land, and even complete countries, have been made *Brucella*-free. This is a large and expensive undertaking and beyond the means of many developing countries. An alternative is to vaccinate herds. The live, attenuated vaccine Rev-1 or recombinant RB51 can be given to calves at 6–8 months. Vaccination can also be given to adult animals, but should not be administered if an eradication programme is envisaged as it then becomes impossible to tell whether an animal is infected or not.

Treatment is with doxycycline 100 mg every 12 h combined with either rifampicin 600 mg daily, or streptomycin 1 g daily, for 6 weeks.

Surveillance of cattle using the milk-ring test (see above). Brucellosis is a notifiable disease in countries in which it has been eliminated, such as in northern Europe, USA and Japan.

17.7 Anthrax

Organism *Bacillus anthracis* is a rod-shaped organism occurring in pairs or chains and staining positively with Gram's stain. In the vegetative state in the animal or where there is a low oxygen content, the bacillus is surrounded by a capsule. If the dead animal's tissues become exposed to the air or the organism is cultured aerobically, then spores develop, which appear as round-filling defects in the stained rods.

The vegetative form is killed by heat at 55°C for 1 h, or if the carcass is not opened, putrefaction will raise the internal temperature sufficiently (30°C for 80 h) to render it free of organisms. However, if it is butchered or a post-mortem performed, then exposure to the air encourages the development of highly resistant spores, which are one of the most persistent forms of life known. They have survived 160°C for 1 h and −78°C despite thawing and re-freezing, while in pastures they have been found viable after 12 years and possibly up to 60 years.

Clinical features Essentially an infection of cattle, anthrax ranks with rabies and plague as a much feared and fatal disease. Infection commences with a small papule at the site of inoculation. By the second day, a ring of vesicles surrounds the lesion, which are at first clear, but then become blood-stained. The central papule then ulcerates and enlarges to form a depressed dark eschar, which increases in size and darkens to the black coal colour that gives the disease its name (anthrax is coal in Greek). Pus is never present despite the development of oedema around the lesion. The oedema is extensive and may cause respiratory embarrassment if around the neck. The associated lymph nodes are often enlarged, but must be left to resolve spontaneously. The primary lesion commonly occurs on the head or face, while the neck and forearm are also often affected. Surprisingly, the fingers are rarely involved.

As well as the primary lesion and its surrounding oedema, there are systemic symptoms of varying severity. The patient feels unwell although the temperature is normal or only slightly raised. A high temperature or weak pulse is a serious sign, generally indicating pulmonary disease, which results from the inhalation of a large dose of spores. Illness sets in rapidly with cough, dyspnoea and cyanosis. Lymph nodes enlarge and there is splenomegaly. This passes into a stage of cardiovascular collapse and the patient is dead within 2–3 days.

Intestinal anthrax is another uncommon, but severe form of the disease resulting from people eating infected meat. The primary lesion occurs in the intestines and the massive oedema that results produces intestinal obstruction as well as systemic symptoms. However, cutaneous anthrax is the commonest form even in people who butcher and subsequently eat an animal that has died from anthrax.

Diagnosis is made by examination of the fluid from the vesicle in a person who gives a history of contact with an animal that recently died. A smear is made on to two slides, one being stained by Gram and the other fixed by heat and stained with methylene blue or Giemsa. The first shows Gram-positive rods and the second demonstrates the red capsule surrounding the blue bacilli. This finding can be confirmed by culture on selective media.

Transmission Anthrax spores are ingested or become accidentally inoculated through the skin, such as by thistle scratches around the muzzle or legs of an animal close grazing in an infected pasture. Biting flies have also been incriminated. The spores germinate into the vegetative form, which rapidly invades, increasing in virulence. A local lesion grows at the point of inoculation and extensive oedema develops around it. The capsulated bacilli produces a lethal factor, which causes anoxic hypertension or cardiac collapse, resulting in sudden death of the animal. After death, the animal appears black from tarry blood that is slow to clot.

People are infected by contact with the deceased animal, either in butchering and handling of the infected meat, or at a place far removed from the death of the animal from spores in its hide, hair or bones.

Incubation period is less than 7 days, with as short as only 2 days in the rapidly fatal pulmonary form.

Period of communicability Not transmitted from person to person.

Occurrence and distribution The disease commonly affects cattle, sheep, goats and horses, but has occurred in dogs and cats. It is probably widespread in the wild and has been found in elephants, hippopotamuses and on the claws and beaks of vultures and other scavenger birds. Widespread in the bovine populations of the world, its persistence in the environment and in the produce of cattle makes it an ever-present threat both in the developing and developed world. It is a particular problem in Africa, Southwest Asia, Russia, South and Central America.

Control and prevention is difficult due to the persistence of the organism in the environment, but once an outbreak starts, it should be possible to bring it to an end by vigorous control of animals and their slaughter. No animal that dies from anthrax should be allowed to be butchered and sold for meat. Its hide and bones are also infectious, so should be deep buried with lime or burnt. Anthrax is a common disease in pasturalists. For fuel, they often conserve dried cow dung, which also makes an ideal material to incinerate the carcass as it burns slowly but continuously.

The animal should not be cut open to obtain specimens or perform autopsy, but cutting off an ear is quite sufficient for diagnostic purposes.

Once anthrax is recognized, then all animals should be vaccinated with a live, attenuated vaccine. Due to the persistence of the organism in the soil, especially at a site where an infected animal has been buried, anthrax is likely to recur year after

year at the same site, so-called anthrax districts. Hot, moist areas are particularly liable to offer the right conditions for continuous sporulation and germination, leading to a steady infectious state throughout the year. In contrast, hot arid areas encourage spore formation and when the vegetation dries out, close grazing brings the animal into proximity with the spores in the dust, so a dry season outbreak is more common. This can be anticipated and cattle vaccinated prior to the anthrax season.

Anthrax is an occupational disease in those persons who deal with hides, hair (including wool) and bones of animals. The spores can persist almost indefinitely in these animal remains and when tested are found to be present in a large proportion. Pasturalists particularly will not waste an animal that dies and taking off its skin and leaving the bones to dry in the sun encourages formation of spores which remain with these products when they are shipped all over the world. It is an impossible task to identify these infected animal products and because of the high proportion involved, an uneconomical process to destroy them. Quite surprisingly, people who handle infected hides and products only rarely develop anthrax, but they should, of course, be warned and provided with facilities to be examined and treated. Protective clothing should be provided and a ventilation system to remove spores from the air when unpacking, beating or a similar process occurs. Many industrial processes disinfect the animal products, but where this does not occur, sterilization can be introduced. With persons at increased risk of developing anthrax, vaccination can be offered. The vaccine is from a sterile filtrate of *B. anthracis* and is given in 0.5 ml doses at 6 weeks after the initial dose, then 6 months and thereafter at annual intervals. Modified anthrax can occur in the vaccinated.

Treatment is with penicillin to which the organism is very sensitive. Benzylpenicillin 4 million IU every 4–6 h for 7 days or if still available, procaine penicillin 1 mega unit daily for 3 days can be used. No local treatment is required and surgical removal of the eschar or incision of oedema only leads to unpleasant scarring and development of intractable sinuses. Ciprofloxacin or doxycycline can be used for respiratory and intestinal cases. Supportive measures need to be given for shock and tracheostomy may be required when there is severe oedema of the neck.

Surveillance Anthrax is a notifiable disease in many countries. Where no animal source can be shown, then bioterrorism should be considered (Section 18.5).

17.8 Leptospirosis

Organism *Leptospira interrogans* with a large number of serovars, the most important of which is *icterohaemorrhagiae*. It is passed in rat's urine and can contaminate any area that they frequent. For the survival of the organism, there must be moisture, such as a canal or sewer, or else in damp soil, the washings of abattoirs or similar conditions. The pH of the soil or water is important and the *Leptospira* cannot survive in an acid environment. Leptospirosis is, therefore, commoner in places where the soil is alkaline. Salt water and chlorine solutions rapidly kill the organism.

Clinical features Commencing with fever, malaise, vomiting and myalgia, jaundice subsequently develops and there may be haemorrhages into the skin, mucous membranes and internal organs. The disease may progress to a more serious form with liver failure, renal failure or meningitis. However, many people only have mild infections and the vast majority do not exhibit any symptoms at all. In endemic areas, children are probably most commonly infected.

Diagnosis is by finding the motile organism by dark field illumination in a wet blood film during the first week of the disease. After this time, serological tests or animal inoculation can be used, whereas *Leptospira* may be found in the urine from the third week onwards. Culture of the organism can take up to 1 month.

Transmission The *Leptospira* enters the skin of humans through minor abrasions or mucous membranes, although it does appear to be able to enter unbroken skin as well. Infection results from exposure to contaminated moist areas, such as swimming in canals, or walking barefoot over damp rat-infested soil. A direct rat bite can transmit the disease, as also an aerosol of contaminated fluid or ingestion of contaminated food.

Other animals can become infected with different serovars: cattle and water buffalo with *hardjo*, dogs with *canicola* and pigs with *pomana*. These domestic animals subsequently excrete *Leptospira* in their urine, contaminating the surroundings.

Incubation period is 4–19 days, usually 10 days.

Period of communicability *Leptospira* are excreted in the urine for several months, but person-to-person spread is rare.

Occurrence and distribution Where rats are common and conditions are favourable, the infection is widespread. In many areas surveyed, *Leptospira* antibodies have been found in a large percentage of the population, endemic in the community with the occasional severe case. It is common in the tropics particularly where the soil is alkaline or irrigation is used for agriculture. Infection is, therefore, common in rice paddy areas and sugarcane estates. This association of the disease with certain occupations is helpful in making the diagnosis. Such occupations as mine workers, farmers, canal cleaners, sewer workers, people employed in the cleaning and preparation of fish or in abattoirs, are at greater risk.

Flooding can widen the area of contamination leading to outbreaks in people not normally at risk. Disasters and any alteration in conditions that leads to an increase in the rat population will have a similar, but more long-term effect.

Leptospirosis is a very widespread zoonotic infection of animals, endemic in many rodents, especially rats. The organism has been found in a variety of other animals, opossums, mongooses, skunks, hedgehogs, squirrels, rabbits and dogs, to name but a few, but the two domestic rats *Rattus rattus* and *R. norvegicus* are by far and away the most important reservoirs.

Control and prevention is the avoidance of areas contaminated with rat and animal urine, often a difficult thing to achieve. Various measures are:

- the reduction of rats by extermination and protection of buildings, especially those used for preparing meat, fish and housing domestic animals (rat control in Box 16.1);
- burning of sugarcane fields after harvest and the drying out of rice fields;
- wearing of protective clothing to reduce abrasions and contamination;
- avoiding canals, lakes and bodies of water known to be infected;
- controlling the number of dogs;
- providing proper pens with drainage for domestic animals so that urine does not collect and make the surroundings sodden;
- wash down food premises with a solution of chlorine or salt water.

Vaccination of persons at risk has been achieved in some countries using the specific serovar. Doxycycline prophylaxis can be used where short-term exposure is expected (e.g. in troops).

Treatment is with benzylpenicillin 2 million IU every 6 h or doxycycline 100 mg for 7 days, preferably within the first week of the illness.

Surveillance Leptospirosis is a notifiable disease in many developed countries. Where outbreaks occur, the cause should be investigated and specific control measures instituted.

17.9 Lassa Fever

Organism Lassavirus is an arenavirus.

Clinical features There is a gradual onset with fever, malaise, sore throat, cough, vomiting, diarrhoea and general aches and pains. By the second week, lymphadenopathy, pharyngitis and a maculo-papular rash on the face or body develops. In severe cases, pleural effusion, encephalopathy, cardiac and renal failures can occur with a mortality of 15–20%.

In endemic areas, 80% of cases are mild or asymptomatic so that serological investigation will find a large number of people with past history of infection.

Diagnosis is often made on clinical criteria once the first case has been identified, with, in particular, inflammation of the throat and white tonsillar patches. Confirmatory diagnosis is made by testing IgM or IgG in urine, blood or throat washings, with ELISA, PCR or IFA, using extreme care.

Transmission is primarily through contact with the excreta (urine and faeces) of infected rodents, deposited on floors, beds or other surfaces, or through rat contamination of food or water. The main reservoir is the multi-mammate or grey rat, *M. natalensis*. This is probably the method of spread in the endemic area resulting in a large number of asymptomatic cases. However, in the severe case, all human body fluids are highly infectious so that secondary spread commonly occurs through contact with blood, urine, throat secretions and the aerosol produced by a coughing bout. The semen remains infectious for a considerable period of time so transmission via the sexual route can occur long after the person has recovered from their clinical illness.

Incubation period 6–21 days.

Period of communicability All body fluids are infectious from the start of the illness and up to 9 weeks for urine and 3 months for semen.

Occurrence and distribution Lassa fever is found in West and Central Africa including the countries of Guinea, Sierra Leone, Liberia, Nigeria and Central African Republic, but serological testing has found evidence of infection in Senegal, Mali, Guinea Bissau and the Congo.

All ages and both sexes are susceptible, but pregnant women have a severe infection with high mortality and loss of the fetus.

Control and prevention is by control of the rats and careful isolation of patients. *M. natalensis* lives in close proximity to humans in the home, fields where people tend their crops, and in mines and similar industrial sites. Rats should be controlled (see Box 16.1) and prevented from entering the home. Food and drinking water should be protected with covers and a state of cleanliness observed to minimize rat excreta contamination.

All cases must be hospitalized and:

- rigorous isolation of the patient by the most secure means possible;
- careful sterilization of syringes, needles and all re-used equipment with 0.5%

sodium hypochlorite, 0.5% phenol with a detergent, autoclaving or boiling;

- extreme precautions with any oral secretions, blood, faeces and urine. Blood must be handled with the utmost precaution using, as a minimum, holeless rubber gloves. Faeces and urine should be placed in plastic bags, which are boiled or burnt;
- terminal disinfection with formaldehyde fumigation to all articles used by the patient.

Treatment is with ribavirin intravenously for 10 days within the first 6 days of illness.

Surveillance All close contacts of a case should be identified and followed up for 3 weeks with twice daily temperature, and hospitalized if it becomes more than 38.3°C. With air travel, it is possible that an incubating case may travel to another country before showing symptoms, so if there is any indication, such as coming from an infected area, then the person should be admitted to hospital with strict barrier nursing procedures. Any known or suspected case should be reported to WHO and neighbouring countries.

18

New and Potential Diseases

Biology is not static – evolutionary forces will always look for opportunities to exploit new situations and no more so than in the field of communicable diseases. Humans have always waged a continuing war against organisms that attack them and although many might now be prevented, new organisms will seek to exploit any weakness in our defences. This chapter, therefore, looks at new and emergent diseases, plus what might be termed potential diseases – infections that could attack us, but have not shown any sign of doing so yet.

The term 'conflict' has been used above not only because our battle with parasitic organisms is like an arms race, but also because the horror of using infectious organisms by terrorist organizations in a purposeful way to attack people is now a possibility. This will probably be with organisms that are known to us, but in a way that would ensure that they are particularly potent. The last section of this chapter, therefore, looks at possible bioterrorist-induced diseases.

This chapter more than any other in this book will require constant updating, which can be done with much useful information now freely available on the Internet. The best source of information on epidemics and new diseases, with good updates on major health problems, is the *Weekly Epidemiological Record,* published simultan-

eously in English and French by the WHO and available on www.who.int/wer/2004/en/ where back copies can be found. A choice of the year in the address is available to get information, or if the latest copy is required, it can be obtained by subscription or a week later on the Internet. Also available from the Centres for Disease Control (CDC) is the *Journal of Emerging Infectious Diseases* on www.cdc.gov/ncidod/eid/past-con.htm in which research and general articles are published.

18.1 The Animal Connection

In the 1970s, it seemed as though the battle against the communicable diseases was won, we had all the weapons we needed to control most of them, all that was required was to have sufficient resources to combat the diseases in the developing world. Smallpox had been eradicated and the development of vaccines promised a similar fate for polio and other immunizable diseases, but then in 1981, there was a rude shock.

In June 1981, CDC in the USA reported five cases of *Pneumocystis carinii* pneumonia. In the following month, 15 more cases of this normally rare disease were reported as well as 26 cases of Kaposi's sarcoma, an unusual tumour. The common feature was that all these cases were in homosexual men. By the end of 1981, acquired immune deficiency syndrome (AIDS) as it was called, was also being reported from countries in Europe. In Belgium and France, an AIDS-like illness was observed amongst people originating from Africa. These observations led to investigations in Rwanda and Zaire (now Congo) where many AIDS patients were found. At the same time, an aggressive form of Kaposi's sarcoma was reported from Zambia and a new disease, called slim disease, described in Uganda. These were all found to be manifestations of AIDS. The African infection was transmitted heterosexually, starting its relentless course that has continued unabated until the present time.

The appearance of HIV infection alerted the world to new communicable diseases, several more (e.g. Lassa, Ebola and Marburg), of which have appeared in the last few years. Where had they come from and why were they appearing at this time? The first clue came with the discovery of a virtually identical retrovirus to HIV in simian monkeys called simian immunovirus (SIV), suggesting that HIV originated from a monkey source. Then in 1986, a disease appeared in cattle in England called bovine spongiform encephalopathy (BSE), which was shown to be due to cattle being fed the remains of sheep in their feed, some of which had the similar sheep disease called scrapie. This had not been transmitted from sheep before, so somehow the organism had crossed the species barrier and if this had happened from sheep to cattle, then why not from cattle to humans when they ate infected meat? Sure enough the first case of a new variant Creutzfeldt–Jakob disease (vCJD) appeared linking this condition to the consumption of beef. Since BSE had a 4–5-year incubation period, the potential for human infection was enormous and there was much speculation as to what would happen.

CJD is one of the group of transmissible spongiform encephalopathies (TSEs) which, as well as BSE in cattle and scrapie in sheep, is also found in other animals such as mink, elk and North American mule deer. The only other human disease is kuru,

found in the Fore people of Papua New Guinea who traditionally eat the brains of the recently dead in the belief that they will obtain the wisdom and prowess of their ancestors.

The TSEs have been shown to be due to a new kind of organism, a self-replicating protein called a prion, which produces a clinical picture of depression in humans followed by organic brain disease, including cerebella ataxia, cortical blindness, localized weakness and progressive intellectual deterioration. Speech is lost, swallowing becomes difficult and a rigidity of limbs develops as the patient sinks further into a hopeless state of debility and death. Unfortunately, it is difficult to confirm the diagnosis of vCJD (tonsillar biopsy and magnetic resonance scans are useful) until after death, indicating that there had been 142 cases by the end of 2003. This fortunately suggests that the epidemic will not be as large as was feared, and as all offal-based ruminant feeds were banned in Europe in 1994, there should be few if any more cases.

While the public health profession was recovering from BSE and vCJD, another new communicable disease, severe acute respiratory syndrome (SARS) was reported from Vietnam in February 2003. A businessman who had been travelling in China was admitted to hospital in Hanoi with a history of high fever, cough and difficulty in breathing. His condition worsened, so he requested to be transferred to Hong Kong, where despite ventilatory support, he died. In the hospital in Hanoi, several health care workers contracted a similar illness and the attending doctor and a nurse died. Search was made for the organism, which at first was thought to be a new strain of influenza, but subsequently was identified as a coronavirus. An incubation period of 1–14 days, but more commonly 3–5 days and period of communicability of 3–14 days from the start of symptoms was subsequently calculated. Fortunately, the household secondary attack rate was between 6% and 15% in Singapore and Hong Kong, especially low if the initial case was a healthcare worker. This contrasted with hospitals, especially if their barrier nursing was deficient, which were found to be potent sources of transmission.

Tracing the case back, it was discovered that there had been a number of cases of a severe and highly contagious pneumonia in Guandong Province (Canton), southern China, in which one in 30 had died. The attending specialist travelled to Hong Kong for a wedding where in the early stages of the illness, he himself infected all the people in a lift in the hotel in which he was staying. One of these persons was the case that came to Hanoi, another was a person from Singapore and the third a lady returning to her home in Toronto, Canada. Hong Kong, southern China, Singapore, Vietnam and Canada then became the centres of epidemics, which demanded strict quarantine measures to contain them. After draconian measures, especially in China, the last case recovered at the end of July 2003. By that time, there had been 8422 cases and 916 deaths.

Coming back to the original question of what was the link between the three epidemics – HIV, BSE/vCJD and SARS – it seems likely that the organism, originally in animals had crossed the species barrier into humans. HIV from simian monkeys, BSE from scrapie-infected sheep and subsequently via beef to humans, while SARS possibly also had an animal connection. Southern China enjoys a culinary custom of eating almost any kind of animal, often held in cages or fish tanks, until required for the table. Such is the close proximity of people to all these animals and the general poor state of hygiene that all methods of transmission are possible. As well as the respiratory route, the SARS virus was found to be excreted in the faeces and urine of patients, possibly up to 23 days after symptoms first started. The original cases in southern China were in food handlers, 66 of whom were found to have antibodies, while of the animals tested masked palm civets, raccoon-dogs, ferret badgers, cynomolgus macaques, fruit bats, snakes and wild pigs were all found to be positive. Transmission in humans was through close human contact as the infection was in large

droplets rather than aerosol, and possibly also via sewage contamination in one area of Hong Kong. Several of these animals are regarded as delicacies and kept in cages so it seems quite possible that either of these methods could have been how the food handlers were infected. After the main epidemic had finished, a new case was found to be strongly associated with the masked palm civet; hence, it seems likely that this could have been how the epidemic started.

Although SARS has declined to negligible limits, its re-appearance must always be considered. It has been suggested that a clustering of pneumonia cases might be an early indicator, while persons of an older age are more likely to transmit infection. While there is no cause to restrict travel, suspect cases are more likely to come from the southern regions of China where there have subsequently been three cases (up to March 2004). Another case came from Henan Province in central China.

The so-called Asian flu epidemic of 1957 was found to have originated in chickens in Guandong province of southern China, followed in 1968 by the Hong Kong influenza epidemic, which also originated from the same area. Although the 1918 epidemic was termed Spanish flu, it is thought that this too might have started originally in southern China. The world waits in dread for the next major epidemic of influenza, possibly of a major antigenic shift (see Section 13.3), will it also originate here? There have been pandemics in 1889, 1918, 1957, 1968 and 1977 and the next one seems long overdue!

A recent cause for concern that a major influenza epidemic might be starting was the appearance of avian influenza H5N1 in January 2004. This is an infection predominantly of chickens and ducks, but can also occur in pigs. It is highly infectious and results in an almost 100% mortality of domestic fowl. The infection is probably maintained in wild waterfowl, sea birds and shore birds and can be spread over long distances when they migrate. However, the transport of birds, contaminated clothing and equipment are probably more likely causes, once infection in a fowl population has started. Bird droppings are highly infectious, so humans coming into contact with them or sick birds are at risk of infection. An outbreak occurred in Hong Kong in 1997 with 18 human cases, of which six died. The same virus was identified in fowls in 2002, resulting in a mass slaughter of chickens, but despite this action, there were four more human cases (two of which died) in 2003. In 2004, there was a more serious epidemic in Thailand and Vietnam that spread to domestic fowls in other countries in Southeast and East Asia (Cambodia, China, Indonesia, Japan, Laos and South Korea) with 34 human cases and 23 deaths. The main concern was that the avian flu could acquire genes from the human influenza organism and produce a potent infection that nobody would have any resistance to. Fortunately, this epidemic subsequently declined, but influenza remains the greatest threat of any emergent infection.

18.2 The Pox Diseases

The reason for including smallpox in the first edition was that there was a possibility that like the diseases already mentioned, one of the animal pox diseases could become serious in humans. Smallpox vaccination probably lasts for 10 years, possibly up to 30 years, but since smallpox vaccination was stopped in 1979, there is a decreasing number of people with any remaining immunity.

Monkey pox is a rare zoonosis, significant because it produces a disease similar to smallpox, localized to tropical rain forest areas of west and central Africa. Most cases have been reported from Congo (formerly Zaire). Although it is a disease of monkeys, it occasionally affects humans. It has a comparable case–fatality rate to smallpox although the secondary attack rate is much lower (15%).

The characteristics of smallpox and monkey pox are:

- clear-cut prodromal period of sudden onset of fever, headache and prostration;

- peripheral distribution of the rash (including soles and palms);
- lesions pass through the same stages at the same time;
- fever intensifies as the rash progresses to the pustular stage;
- lesions are deeply seated flat-topped and centrally depressed.

These features should be compared with chickenpox (Section 12.1).

Smallpox vaccination (vaccinia virus) also protects against monkey pox, so the waning level of vaccination poses the theoretical possibility of it spreading. However, the well-defined distribution, and the low secondary attack rate in close contacts, makes it unlikely to develop into such a serious disease and smallpox vaccination can be used to prevent it.

There are also other animal pox virus diseases which have infected or could infect humans. Examples are cowpox, camelpox, tanapox, yabapox, buffalopox and goatpox. There is very little evidence to suggest that any of these diseases can cause an infection in people that is likely to be spread from one person to another to any marked extent, but their importance is to recognize that they can occur and to differentiate them from smallpox.

18.3 Nipah and the Lyssa Viruses

In 1999, a severe encephalitic illness occurred in Nipah, Malaysia, caused by what has now become called Nipah virus, closely related to Hendra virus, first reported in the town of this name in Australia. They are members of the virus family *Paramyxoviridae*. The illness commences with fever and muscle pains, then progresses to encephalitis with a 50% mortality. The incubation period is 4–18 days. Another new virus disease called Manangle was discovered in 1997 also originating from pigs, but as it consisted of only two cases of an influenza-like illness and rash, little notice was taken of it.

Nipah is a zoonosis of pigs with the possible involvement of dogs and cats also, and transmission probably occurs from close contact with body fluids or tissues of the animal. However, the risk of transmission to humans is low, although all precautions, with the wearing of gowns and gloves, should be taken when handling animals. Hendra is a similarly transmitted disease of horses. Epidemics of Nipah occurred in Malaysia in 1998–1999 (265 cases, 105 deaths), Singapore in 1999 (11 cases, one death) and Bangladesh in 2001 (30 cases, 18 deaths).

The Nipah, Hendra and Manangle viruses are found in insectivorous and fruit-eating bats (including flying foxes) that are not made ill by them. Infected bat colonies have so far been found in Malaysia, Indonesia, the Philippines, Australia and some of the Pacific Islands, but how the infection is transmitted from the bats to either pigs or horses is not known. Also, examination of bats has shown a number of lyssa viruses (related to rabies), including Australian bat lyssavirus and a newly discovered candidate called Tioman. So far, no human illness has been reported, but the place of the bat as a reservoir of disease is becoming ever more important and greater precautions may need to be taken in places where they are common, for fear of a new infection originating from this source.

18.4 Arboviruses

The arboviruses (Section 15.2) have a propensity for producing new diseases unmatched by any other organism. At quite regular intervals, new arboviral diseases appear or those normally restricted to small areas of the world spread to new areas or become more important as human diseases. Examples are West Nile virus, which has appeared for the first time in North America, Rift Valley fever, which was normally confined to Africa, but has now spread to Asia (Section 15.2) and Crimea–Congo disease, which now has a worldwide distribution (Section 16.9.2).

The number of arbovirus infections in the world is enormous (Chapter 19) and new ones are likely to appear at any time. Although they are mainly transmitted by mosquitoes or ticks, it is likely that the reservoir will be in birds or mammals, as new-species adaptations, similar to the diseases mentioned above, seems to be how new diseases generally arise in the human population.

18.5 Bioterrorism

The idea of using biological substances for warfare is not new. In 1347, when the Mongols laid siege to Caffa (now part of the Ukraine), they catapulted the bodies of plague victims over the walls at the Genoese defenders. Escaping in their ships, the soldiers accidentally carried the bacillus back with them to Mediterranean ports, so starting the devastating epidemics of plague that became known as the Black Death. Since then, there has been such a horror of biological warfare that treaties and understandings, even in the midst of world wars, has prevented their use to any large extent. Sadly, unscrupulous persons have resorted to these methods to terrorize people in this modern age, raising the question as to what they are likely to use and with what results?

The most highly infectious disease of humans is smallpox and this would be the disease of choice if one wanted to produce the most devastating effect. Of the last two remaining colonies of variola virus left in the world, one is in the USA and the other is in Russia and were due to be destroyed in 2002, but this has now been changed to regular inspections. So unless the virus was stolen or in any other way obtained from either of these sources, the risk is minimal. Even if an outbreak did occur, then the means to control it by vaccination is readily available and it would then just depend upon the time it took to produce enough vaccine and vaccinate people. As mentioned above, anyone born before 1979 is likely to have been vaccinated and even though their immunity would have waned, they would probably have a milder form of the disease.

Plague is a more likely contender as the bacillus is readily obtainable and as shown above, can be spread with devastating results. However, it is an infection that is well known and reasonably easy to contain within well-circumscribed areas, as mentioned in Section 16.1. To make an effective weapon, the bacillus would need to be formulated in such a way that it was spread by the respiratory route, which without first passage through a human as septicaemic or pneumonic plague might not be possible. A vaccine is available which could be utilized in an emergency and treatment is effective if given soon after symptoms develop.

Similar to plague and easy to obtain would be *Francisella tularensis*, the organism that produces the disease tularaemia. Found in the northern part of the world (Russia, China and the USA), it is transmitted by almost every conceivable method – from the bites of ticks, mosquitoes and the biting fly *Chrysops*, in contaminated water or uncooked meat, by the inhalation of dust and hay from contaminated areas and through handling small animals, either by their bite or contact with their tissues. It presents as an ulcer at the site of introduction of the organism, with lymphadenopathy, then spreads to many sites in the body including the lung. It is this respiratory form, like pneumonic plague, that would make it a possible weapon. Sprayed in an aerosol, the cause would probably go unrecognized. Fortunately, tularaemia can be treated with streptomycin or gentamicin and a vaccine has been used in Russia, so providing the cause could be identified reasonably quickly, preventive action could be taken.

Anthrax is probably the most likely candidate and was used in the USA in 2001 in an attempt to target certain individuals through the postal system. A special formulation, probably obtained illegally from a biological warfare establishment was used, and this would be necessary if it was to be tried again. Cutaneous anthrax is generally a non-fatal disease, readily responding to treatment (Section 17.7) and the commonest form of the disease. For anthrax to be a deadly weapon, the organism needs to be inhaled or swallowed without first touching the skin, as in natural infections where people consume meat from an animal that has died of anthrax, nearly all of them develop cutaneous rather than intestinal disease. For it to be effective, anthrax would, therefore, need to be administered as a fine powder or in an aerosol.

Probably the easiest biological substance to use as a terrorist weapon is botulinum toxin. The toxin is produced by *Clostridium botulinum* in foods that have been poorly processed in any preserving method, particularly home preservation of fruit and vegetables that have not been held at a high enough temperature for sufficient length of time. When these foods are eaten, the patient, after a brief incubation period of 12–36 h, develops a dry mouth followed by blurring of vision, difficulty in swallowing, weakness and in the severe case a flaccid paralysis, with mortality of about 10%. It would, therefore, be quite easy to produce the toxin and introduce it as a foodstuff to the unsuspecting recipients or administer it as an aerosol in a direct attack. So if there is no obvious source of botulism in a food source, then bioterrorism should be suspected.

Any case of botulism should be reported to the local medical authority responsible and the suspect food item sent for analysis prior to destruction by prolonged boiling or incineration. The patient should be purged, the stomach washed out and if seriously ill, given polyvalent botulinum antitoxin. The usual cause of death is respiratory failure; so facilities, including intubation, should be made ready in case of need. Everybody else who might have eaten from the same food source must be contacted and observed.

With any biological weapon, it is the preparation and means of administration that are the key factors, so unless the terrorist has resource to laboratories and some sophisticated equipment, it is likely to be by theft or purchase that substances will be obtained. Hopefully, these are being carefully guarded against.

19

List of Communicable Diseases

Communicable diseases are listed in alphabetical order by the most commonly used name. Other names will be found in the index. Diseases printed in **bold** are covered in the text.

Incubation periods are the usual range, but exceptions to these limits do occur. Agents are: arboviruses (A), bacteria (B), ectoparasites (E), fungi (F), helminths (but not nematodes) (H), nematodes (N), prion (O), protozoa (P), rickettsiae (R), spirochaetes (S), toxins (T) and other viruses (V). Methods of control are: animal elimination, vaccination and the wearing of gloves and protective clothing (An), testing of donors and treatment of blood for transfusion (Bl), chemotherapy where this is used as a method of control (Ch), food hygiene, cooking and refrigeration (Fo), personal hygiene (Hy), vaccination/immunization (Im), sterilization of needles, instruments and blood giving sets (Ne), rat control (Ra), sanitation (Sa), water supply (Wa), vector control (Vc) and methods for controlling STIs (Xe).

Disease	Clinical features (agent)	Means of transmission (control method)	Incubation period
Absettarov	Fever (A)	*Ixodid* ticks (Vc)	–
Acanthamoebiasis	Granulomatous amoebic encephalitis (P)	Through skin lesion or conjunctiva	Weeks
Actinomycosis	Sulphur-granule lesions in jaw, thorax or abdomen (F)	Oral-to-oral (dental hygiene)	Months–years
Acute respiratory infections	Fever, cough, pneumonia (B, V)	Airborne and oral (Ch, Im)	1–3 days
Aeromonas	Diarrhoea, vomiting (B)	Contaminated food or water (Fo, Hy, Wa)	–
Alenquer	Sand fly fever (A)	*Phlebotomus* (Vc)	3–6 days
Amoebiasis	Diarrhoea and systemic abscesses (P)	Faecal-contaminated water and food (Wa, Sa)	2–4 weeks

(*Continued*)

Disease	Clinical features (agent)	Means of transmission (control method)	Incubation period
Angiostrongylus	Meningeal, CNS and abdominal signs (N)	Uncooked snails and slugs, rat reservoir (Fo, Ra)	1–3 weeks
Aniskiasis	Intestinal abscess (N)	Uncooked fish (Fo)	Hours
Anthrax	Skin, intestinal or respiratory lesions (B)	Contact with infected animal tissues (An, Ch)	2–7 days
Apeu	Fever (A)	*Aedes* and *Culex*, mosquitoes, rodent reservoir (Vc)	3–12 days
Apoi	Encephalitis (A)	Vector (unknown)	5–15 days
Armillifer	Calcified nodules (E)	Eating raw snakes or snake-contaminated water (Fo, Wa)	–
Ascaris	(N), malnutrition, intestinal symptoms	Ingestion of soil or food (Fo, Hy, Sa)	10–20 days
Aspergillosis	Bronchial obstruction and eosinophilia (F)	Airborne from compost, hay or stored grain	Days–weeks
Babesiosis	Fever and haemolytic anaemia (P)	*Ixodes* ticks, blood transfusion (Vc, Bl)	1–8 weeks
Bacillary dysentery	Diarrhoea with blood (B)	Faecal–oral, water, milk, flies (Hy, Wa, Sa)	1–7 days
Balantidiasis	Diarrhoea (P)	Faecal–oral, food, water (pig reservoir) (Hy, Fo, Wa)	Days
Bangui	Fever and rash (A)	Vector (unknown)	4–5 days
Banzi	Fever (A)	*Culex* mosquito (Vc)	5–15 days
Barmah Forest	Fever, arthritis (A)	Culicine mosquito (Vc)	–
Bartonellosis	Fever or skin sore (B)	*Lutzomyia* sand flies (Vc, Bl)	16–22 days
Batai	Fever (A)	Culicine mosquito (Vc)	4–5 days
Bhanja	Fever, encephalitis (A)	Tick (Vc)	–
Blastomycosis	Pneumonia, skin lesions (F)	Airborne in spore-laden dust	Weeks–months
Bluetongue	Fever (A)	*Culicoides* midge (Vc)	3–12 days
Botulism	Paralysis (B, T)	Preserved food (Fo)	12–36 h
Brazilian purpuric fever	Conjunctivitis, meningitis (B)	Contact with conjunctival discharges (Hy)	1–3 days
Brucellosis	Undulant fever (B)	Milk, cheese and contact with animal fluids (An, Fo)	5–60 days
Bunyamwera	Fever (A)	*Aedes* mosquito (Vc)	3–12 days
Burkitt's L.	Lymphoma (V)	Associated with malaria (Vc)	–
Buruli ulcer	Skin and tissue loss (B)	Inoculation of organism possibly by aquatic insect	–
Bussuquara	Fever (A)	Culicine mosquito (Vc)	5–15 days
Bwamba	Fever and rash (A)	Culicine mosquito (Vc)	3–12 days
California E.	Encephalitis (A)	*Aedes* mosquito (Vc)	5–15 days
Campylobacter	Diarrhoea (B)	Food, milk, water or contact with animals (Fo, Wa)	1–10 days
Candidiasis	Thrush (F)	Contact with secretions (Ch)	2–5 days
Candiru	Fever (A)	*Phlebotamus* sand fly (Vc)	3–6 days
Capillariasis, hepatic	Hepatitis and eosinophilia (N)	Uncooked liver (Fo)	3–4 weeks
Capillariasis, intestinal	Malabsorption syndrome (N)	Uncooked fish (Fo)	Months
Capillariasis, pulmonary	Pneumonitis (N)	Ingestion of foods contaminated by soil (Fo)	3–4 weeks

(*continued...*)

(*Continued*)

Disease	Clinical features (agent)	Means of transmission (control method)	Incubation period
Capnocytophaga	Fever, meningitis (B)	Dog bite, scratch or lick (An)	1–5 days
Caraparu	Fever (A)	Culicine mosquito, rodent reservoir (Vc)	3–12 days
Cat-scratch fever	Fever, lymphadenitis (B)	Cat scratch bite or lick (An)	3–14 days
Catu	Fever (A)	Culicine mosquito (Vc)	5–15 days
Central European encephalitis	Encephalitis (A)	*Ixodes* tick or drinking raw milk (Fo, Im,Vc)	7–14 days
Chagas' disease	Carditis and megacolon (P)	*Reduviidae* bug, blood transfusion (An, Bo, Ra, Vc)	5–14 days
Chagres	Fever (A)	*Phlebotamus* sand fly (Vc)	3–6 days
Chancroid	Genital ulcer (B)	Sexual contact (Ch, Xe)	3–14 days
Chandipura	Fever (A)	*Lutzomyia* sand fly (Vc)	1–6 days
Changuinola	Fever (A)	*Phlebotamus* sand fly (Vc)	3–6 days
Chickenpox	Rash (V)	Skin or airborne contact	2–3 weeks
Chikungunya	Fever, rash, arthritis (A)	*Aedes* mosquito, reservoir in baboons and bats (Vc)	3–12 days
Cholera	Watery diarrhoea (B)	Faecal contamination of water or food (Hy, Sa, Wa)	1–5 days
Chromomycosis	Skin growths (F)	Penetrating wound, e.g. splinter of wood	Months
Clostridium difficile	Diarrhoea, colitis (B, T)	Faecal–oral (Hy and reduce antibiotic use)	2–5 days
Coccidioidomycosis	Disseminated abscesses (F)	Airborne from soil in endemic areas (dust control)	1–4 weeks
Cold, common	Respiratory infection (V)	Airborne droplets through nose, conjunctiva or swallowed (Hy)	1–3 days
Colorado tick	Fever (A)	*Dermacentor* tick, reservoir in small mammals (Vc)	4–5 days
Congenital cytomegalovirus	CNS and liver abnormalities (V)	From genital secretions or breast milk. Adults infected by sexual contact or blood transfusion (Bl, Xe)	3–12 weeks
Conjunctivitis	Sore eyes (B, V)	Contact with eye discharges, airborne, flies (Hy, Sa, Wa)	1–3 days
Creeping eruptions	Urticaria and eosinophilia (N)	Soil contaminated by dog and cat faeces (footwear, An, Hy)	Weeks to months
Creutzfeldt–Jakob disease	Encephalopathy and paralysis (O)	Infected meat and tissue contact (Fo)	4–5 years
Crimean-Congo haemorrhagic fever	Haemorrhagic fever (A)	*Hyaloma* ticks and body fluid contact with humans and animals (Vc, An)	1–12 days
Cryptococcosis	Meningitis and skin lesions (F)	Airborne from pigeon droppings? (An)	–
Cryptosporidiosis	Diarrhoea (P)	Faecal–oral and from animals and water (An, Hy, Sa, Wa)	1–12 days
Cyclospora	Diarrhoea (P)	Water and fruit (Hy, Fo, Wa)	5–10 days
Cytomegalovirus infection	Mononucleosis and congenital CNS lesions (V)	Contact with body fluids and congenital. Blood transfusion or transplant. (Bl, Xe)	3–12 weeks

(*Continued*)

Disease	Clinical features (agent)	Means of transmission (control method)	Incubation period
Dakar bat	Fever (A)	Vector (unknown)	5–15 days
Dengue	Haemorrhagic fever (A)	*Aedes* mosquito (Vc)	3–15 days
Dermatophagoides	Asthma (E)	Inhaled dust mites (reduce dust)	–
Dhori	Fever (A)	Tick vector (Vc)	3–12 days
Diphtheria	Pharyngitis, cutaneous lesions (B)	Airborne or skin contact from case or carrier (Im)	2–5 days
Diphyllobothrium	Macrocytic anaemia (H)	Eating uncooked freshwater fish (Fo, Sa)	3–6 weeks
Dipylidium	Tapeworm (H)	Swallowing infected flea (An, Hy, Vc)	3–4 weeks
Dirofilariasis	Pulmonary eosinophilia (N)	Culicine mosquito (Vc)	Weeks to months
Dugbe	Fever (A)	Tick vector (Vc)	4–5 days
Duvenhage	Rabies-like illness (V)	Animal saliva or bite (An)	–
Eastern equine E.	Encephalitis (A)	*Aedes* mosquito, bird and rodent reservoir (Vc)	5–15 days
Ebola	Haemorrhagic fever (V)	Contact with body fluids or tissues (barrier nurse)	2–21 days
Echinococcus	Hydatid cysts (H)	From dog via fur, licking or contaminated food or water (An, Hy, Fo, Wa)	Months to years
Echinostoma	Diarrhoea (H)	Food (raw snails, fish or freshwater plants) (Fo)	–
Edge Hill	Fever, arthritis (A)	Culicine mosquito (Vc)	–
Ehrlichiosis	Fever (R)	*Ixodes* and *Amblyomma* ticks (Vc)	1–3 weeks
Encephalitis lethargica	Fever, encephalitis (V)	Airborne	–
Enteritis necroticans	Gangrene of bowl (B)	Uncooked pork and beef (Fo)	6–12 h
Enterobius	Anal pruritis (N)	Faecal–oral and in dust (Hy)	2–6 weeks
Enteroviral carditis	Fever and myocarditis in neonates (V)	Faecal–oral or airborne (mucus or faecal material) (Hy)	3–5 days
Entomophthoramycosis	Granuloma in skin or nasal passage (F)	Organism found in soil and rotting vegetation	–
Epidemic haemorrhagic conjunctivitis	Conjunctivitis and conjunctival haemorrhages (V)	Contact with eye discharges, airborne and in water (Hy)	1–3 days
Epidemic kerato-conjunctivitis	Keratoconjunctivitis (V)	Contact with eye discharges or shared treatments (Hy)	5–12 days
Epidemic myalgia	Fever and pain in chest or abdomen (V)	Faecal–oral or airborne (Hy)	3–5 days
Erysipelas	Cellulitis of tissue (B)	Contamination of abraded skin; flies (Hy, Sa)	1–3 days
Erythema infectiosum	Rash, fetal damage (V)	Airborne, congenital, blood transfusion (Bl, Hy)	4–20 days
E. coli 0157	Haemorrhagic colitis (B)	From uncooked beef, milk, faecally contaminated water or vegetables (Fo, Hy, Wa)	2–8 days
Everglades	Fever, encephalitis (A)	Culicine mosquito (Vc)	5–15 days
Exanthem subitum	Fever, rash (V)	Salivary contact (Hy)	5–15 days
Fascioliasis	Liver damage (H)	Uncooked freshwater plants (Fo)	–

(*continued...*)

(*Continued*)

Disease	Clinical features (agent)	Means of transmission (control method)	Incubation period
Fasciolopsis	Intestinal ulceration (H)	Uncooked freshwater plants (Fo)	2–3 months
Filariasis, lymphatic	Lymphoedema (N)	Anopheline and culicine mosquitoes (Ch, Vc)	1 year+
Fish poisoning	Vomiting and parasthesia (T)	Eating toxic fish (Fo)	0.5–3 h
Food poisoning	Diarrhoea and vomiting (B, T)	Contaminated food (Fo, Hy)	
		Staphylococci	1–6 h
		Bacillus cereus	1–12 h
		Clostridium perfringens	12–24 h
		Vibrio parahaemolyticus	12–48 h
Fort Sherman	Fever (A)	Culicine mosquito (Vc)	–
Gan Gan	Fever, arthritis (A)	Culicine mosquito (Vc)	–
Gastrodiscoides	Diarrhoea (H)	Raw vegetables and water plants (Fo)	–
Gastroenteritis	Diarrhoea (B, V)	Faecal–oral, food, water and milk (Hy, Fo, Im, Sa, Wa)	12–72 h
Germiston	Fever, rash (A)	Culicine mosquitoes (Vc)	5–15 days
Giardia	Diarrhoea, bloating (P)	Faecal–oral, water and food (Hy, Fo, Sa, Wa)	3–25 days
Gnathostoma	Systemic abscess (N)	Uncooked fish or poultry (Fo)	–
Gonorrhoea	Urethral discharge (B)	Sexual contact (Ch, Xe)	2–7 days
Granuloma inguinale	Ano-genital ulcers (B)	Sexual contact (Ch, Xe)	1–16 weeks
Guama	Fever (A)	Culicine mosquito (Vc)	5–15 days
Guanarito H.F.	Haemorrhagic fever (V)	Inhalation or swallowing of cane rat excreta (Hy, Ra)	7–16 days
Guaroa	Fever (A)	Culicine mosquito (Vc)	5–15 days
Guinea worm	Leg worm (N)	Water (swallowing infected copepods) (Wa)	1 year
Haemorrhagic fever with renal syndrome	Fever, haemorrhage, shock, oliguria (V)	Aerosol transmission from rodent urine, faeces and saliva (Ra)	2–4 weeks
Hand, foot and mouth disease	Stomatitis and skin lesions (V)	Direct contact with mouth lesions, airborne and faecal–oral (Hy)	3–5 days
Hantavirus pulmonary syndrome	Fever, myalgia, respiratory distress and shock (V)	Aerosol transmission from rodent (deer mouse, pack rats, chipmunks) excreta (Ra)	1–6 weeks
Hanzalova	Fever (A)	*Ixodes* ticks (Vc)	–
Helicobacter pylori	Gastritis, ulcer and adenocarcinoma (B)	Faecal–oral or oral–oral (Ch, Hy)	5–10 days
Hendra	Encephalitis (V)	Contact with horses, reservoir in fruit bats (An)	4–18 days
Hepatitis A	Jaundice (V)	Faecal–oral, water or food (Hy, Im, Fo, Wa)	15–50 days
Hepatitis B	Jaundice (V)	Inoculation, blood transfusion, sexual contact, perinatal (Bl, Im, Ne, Xe)	6 weeks to 6 months
Hepatitis C	Jaundice, chronic active hepatitis (V)	Inoculation, blood transfusion, sexual contact (Bl, Ne, Xe)	2 weeks to 6 months
Hepatitis delta	Jaundice, associated with HBV (V)	Inoculation, sexual contact (Im (HB vac.) Ne, Xe)	2–8 weeks

(*Continued*)

Disease	Clinical features (agent)	Means of transmission (control method)	Incubation period
Hepatitis E	Jaundice, mortality in pregnancy (V)	Water-borne. Pig reservoir (An, Hy, Wa)	3–9 weeks
Herpangina	Pharyngitis (V)	Contact with nose and throat discharges, faecal–oral and airborne (Hy, Wa)	3–5 days
Herpes genitalis	Genital sores, in infants encephalitis (V)	Sexual, oral and perinatal contact (Xe)	2–12 days
Herpes simplex	Cold sores or systemic lesions in infants (V)	Contact with saliva or lesions, perinatal (Hy)	2–12 days
Heterophyes	Enteritis (H)	Uncooked freshwater fish (Fo)	–
Histoplasmosis	Pulmonary and systemic lesions (F)	Inhalation of spores from soil (decrease dust)	3–17 days
Hookworm	Anaemia (N)	Larvae penetrate skin (Ch, Hy, Sa, Wa, footwear)	8–10 weeks
Human immunodeficiency virus	(V) Fever, diarrhoea, weight loss, opportunistic infection	Sexual contact, blood transfusion, needle-transfer, perinatal (Bl, Ne, Xe)	1–18 years
Human papilloma virus	Genital warts (V)	Sexual or direct contact (Xe)	2–3 months
Hymenolepis	Enteritis (H)	Faecal–oral, food or water (Hy, Fo, Sa, Wa)	1–2 weeks
Ilesha	Fever and rash (A)	Vector (unknown)	3–12 days
Ilheus	Encephalitis (A)	Culicine mosquito (Vc)	5–15 days
Influenza	Respiratory infection(V)	Airborne droplets inhaled, swallowed or direct contact with mucous (Hy, Im)	1–5 days
Inkoo	Fever (A)	Culicine mosquitoes (Vc)	5–15 days
Isospora	Diarrhoea (P)	Faecal–oral and from dogs and cats (An, Hy, Sa, Wa)	–
Issyk-Kul	Fever (A)	Tick vector (Vc)	4–5 days
Itaqui	Fever (A)	Culicine mosquito, rodent reservoir (Vc)	3–12 days
Jamestown canyon	Encephalitis (A)	Culicine mosquito (Vc)	5–15 days
Japanese encephalitis	Encephalitis (A)	*Culex* mosquito, reservoir in birds and pigs (Vc, Im)	5–15 days
Junin haemorrhagic fever	Haemorrhagic fever (V)	Aerosol or contact with rodent excreta (Ra, Im)	7–16 days
Jurona	Fever (A)	Culicine mosquito (Vc)	–
Kaposi's sarcoma	Vascular neoplasia (V)	Sexual contact, associated with HIV infection (Xe)	–
Karshi	Fever, encephalitis (A)	Tick vector (Vc)	–
Kasokero	Fever (A)	Vector (unknown)	5–15 days
Kawasaki syndrome	Fever and rash in children (T)	Unknown, probably airborne	–
Kemerovo	Fever (A)	Tick vector (Vc)	4–5 days
Kokobera	Fever, arthritis (A)	Culicine mosquito (Vc)	5–15 days
Koutango	Fever and rash (A)	Culicine mosquito (Vc)	5–15 days
Kumlinge	Fever (A)	*Ixodes* tick. Reservoir in rodents and birds (Vc)	–
Kunjin	Encephalitis (A)	Culicine mosquito (Vc)	5–15 days
Kuru	Cerebella ataxia (O)	Eating human brain	4–20 years

(*continued...*)

(*Continued*)

Disease	Clinical features (agent)	Means of transmission (control method)	Incubation period
Kyasanur forest disease	Haemorrhagic fever and encephalitis (A)	*Haemaphysalis* tick. Reservoir in rodents and monkeys (Vc)	3–8 days
La Crosse	Encephalitis (A)	*Aedes* mosquito. Reservoir in *Aedes* eggs, birds, pigs (Vc)	5–15 days
Lassa fever	Haemorrhagic fever (V)	*Mastomys* excreta, human blood and excretions, sexual (Hy, Ne, Ra, barrier nurse)	6–21 days
Le Dantec	Encephalitis (A)	Vector (unknown)	3–12 days
Legionellosis	Pneumonia (B)	Airborne aerosol of water	2–10 days
Leishmaniasis	Cutaneous, mucocutaneous and visceral lesions (P)	*Phlebotomus, Lutzomyia* sand flies. Mammalian reservoir specific to locality. Blood transfusion and needles (An, Bl, Ne, Vc)	2 weeks to 6 months
Leprosy	Skin and nerve lesions (B)	Close personal contact and possibly airborne (Ch, Hy, Im)	1–20 years
Leptospirosis	Fever and jaundice (S)	Contact with rat, pig, cow or dog urine or in water (An, Ra)	4–19 days
Linguatula	Nasopharyngitis (E)	Eating raw liver of sheep, goats and cows (Fo)	–
Lipovnik	Meningitis (A)	Tick vector (Vc)	4–5 days
Listeriosis	Meningoencephalitis in adults and neonates (B)	Eating milk and cheese, contact with animals and perinatal (An, Fo, Hy)	3–70 days
L. loa	Calabar swelling (N)	*Chrysops* fly (Ch, Vc)	Years
Louping ill	Encephalitis (A)	*Ixodes* tick (Vc)	7–14 days
Lyme disease	Erythematous migrans, meningitis (S)	*Ixodes* tick. Reservoir in ticks and mammals (An, Im, Vc)	3–32 days
Lymphocytic C.M.	Choriomeningitis (V)	Excretions of mice in food, contact or aerosol (Hy, Fo, Ra)	8–13 days
Lymphogranuloma venereum	Ano-vaginal lesions (B)	Sexual and direct contact with lesions (Ch, Xe)	3–30 days
Lympho-nodular pharyngitis A	Lymphonodular lesions in pharynx (V)	Direct contact with nose, throat discharges and faeces or by aerosol (Hy)	5 days
Machupo H.F.	Haemorrhagic fever (V)	*Calomys* rodent urine in dust or through skin (Ra)	7–16 days
Madrid	Fever (A)	*Aedes* and *Culex* mosquito, rodent reservoir (Vc)	3–32 days
Malaria	Fever (P)	*Anopheles* mosquito, blood transfusion (Bl, Ne, Vc)	9–17 days 18–40 days
Manangle	Fever and rash (V)	Close contact with pig fluids and tissues (An, Hy)	14–18 days
Mansonella	Fever, joint pain (N)	*Culicoides* and *Simulium* (Ch)	–
Marburg disease	Haemorrhagic fever (V)	Contact with blood and body fluids (barrier nurse)	2–21 days
Marituba	Fever (A)	*Aedes* and *Culex* mosquito, rodent reservoir (Vc)	3–12 days

(*Continued*)

Disease	Clinical features (agent)	Means of transmission (control method)	Incubation period
Mayaro	Fever, rash, arthritis (A)	*Mansonia* and *Haemagogus* mosquito (Vc)	3–11 days
Measles	Fever and rash (V)	Airborne or contact with nose or throat secretions (Im)	10–14 days
Melioidosis	Pulmonary consolidation (B)	Ingestion, inhalation or broken-skin contact with soil	Months to years
Meningitis, viral	Fever and meningitis (V)	Airborne or contact with nose and throat secretions (Hy, Im)	Depends on organism
Meningitis, meningococca	Fever and meningitis (B)	Airborne or contact with nose and throat secretions (Ch, Im)	2–10 days
Meningitis, *Haemophilus*	Fever and meningitis (B)	Airborne or contact with nose and throat secretions (Ch, Im)	2–4 days
Meningitis, pneumococcal	Fever and meningitis (B)	Airborne or contact with nose and throat secretions (Ch, Im)	1–3 days
Metagonimus	Diarrhoea (H)	Uncooked fish (Fo)	–
Microsporidiosis	Diarrhoea (P)	Ingestion, inhalation? (Hy)	–
Mokola	Rabies-like illness (V)	Animal saliva or bite (An)	–
Molluscum contagiosum	Skin papules (V)	Direct contact with lesions. Sexual contact (Hy, Xe)	19–50 days
Monkeypox	Pox rash (V)	Close contact with animal or person-to-person (An, Im)	–
Mononucleosis, infectious	Glandular fever (V)	Swallowing infected saliva directly or on toys, etc. (Hy)	4–6 weeks
Morumbi	Fever (A)	Culicine mosquito (Vc)	–
Mucambo	Fever (A)	Vector (unknown)	3–11 days
Mucormycosis	Thrombosis and infarction (F)	Inhalation, ingestion or inoculation of spores (Ne)	–
Mumps	Parotitis (V)	Airborne and contact with saliva (Im)	14–24 days
Murray Valley E.	Encephalitis (A)	*Culex* mosquito, reservoir in birds (Vc)	5–15 days
Murutucu	Fever (A)	Culicine mosquito, rodent reservoir (Vc)	3–12 days
Mycetoma	Localized induration and sinuses (B, F)	Inoculation from soil or wood splinters or thorns (footwear)	Months
Mycoplasma	Pneumonia	Airborne droplets or direct contact with secretions (Hy)	6–32 days
Myiasis	Furuncle, wound or various sites (E)	Fly larvae (Vc)	–
Naegleriasis	Meningoencephalitis (P)	Stagnant water in nasal passages, e.g. swimming	3–7 days
Nairobi sheep	Fever (A)	Tick vector (Vc)	4–5 days
Nasopharyngeal cancer	Obstruction of naso-pharynx (V)	Epstein–Barr virus from saliva exchange	Years

(*continued...*)

(*Continued*)

Disease	Clinical features (agent)	Means of transmission (control method)	Incubation period
Negishi	Encephalitis (A)	Vector (unknown)	5–15 days
Nepuyo	Fever (A)	Culicine mosquito, rodent reservoir (Vc)	3–12 days
Nipah	Encephalitis (V)	Close contact with pig fluids and tissues (An, Hy)	4–18 days
Nocardiosis	Systemic abscesses(B)	Inhalation of soil dust	Weeks
Non-gonococcal urithritis	Urithritis and discharge (B)	Sexual contact (Xe)	1–2 weeks
Non-Hodgkin's lymphoma	Lymphoma (V)	Reactivated EBV infection due to immunodeficiency	–
Norwalk or Norovirus	Diarrhoea (V)	Faecal–oral, airborne or via food and water (Hy, Fo, Wa)	1–2 days
Nyando	Fever (A)	Culicine mosquito (Vc)	3–12 days
Omsk haemorrhagic fever	Haemorrhagic fever (A)	*Dermacentor* tick or contact with muskrat (Im, Vc)	3–8 days
Onchocerciasis	Blindness and skin damage (N)	*Simulium* fly (Vc)	1 year
Onyong-nyong	Arthralgia (A)	*Anopheles* mosquito (Vc)	3–12 days
Opisthorchis	Liver damage (H)	Uncooked freshwater fish (Fo)	4 weeks
Opthalmia neonatorum	Conjunctivitis in newborn (B)	Genital secretions of mother to infant (Ch, Hy, Xe)	1–12 days 6–19 days
Orf	Maculo-papular lesion (V)	Contact with mucous membranes of infected sheep and goats (An, Hy)	3–6 days
Oriboca	Fever (A)	*Aedes* and *Culex* (Vc)	3–12 days
Oropouche	Fever and meningitis (A)	Culicine mosquito, reservoir in monkeys, sloths, birds (Vc)	3–12 days
Orungo	Fever (A)	*Aedes* and *Anopheles* (Vc)	3–12 days
Ossa	Fever (A)	Culicine mosquito, rodent reservoir (Vc)	3–12 days
Osteomyelitis	Bone abscess (B)	Blood or wound infection (Ch)	4–10 days
Otitis media	Ear infection (B)	Secondary to respiratory or throat infection (Ch, Hy, Im)	1–4 days
Paracoccidioidomycosis	Mycosis of respiratory tract and skin (F)	Airborne soil dust	Months to years
Paragonimus	Lung damage (H)	Freshwater crab/crayfish (Fo)	6–10 weeks
Parainfluenza	Croup, pneumonia (V)	Respiratory or contact (Hy)	1–10 days
Paratyphoid	Diarrhoea and rash (B)	Faecal contamination of food and water (Hy,Fo,Im,Sa,Wa)	1–10 days
Pasteurellosis	Cellulitis (B)	Cat scratch or dog bite (An)	12–24 h
Pediculosis	Urticaria (E)	From infested person (Hy,Vc)	10–14 days
Pertussis	Whooping cough (B)	Airborne droplets (Im)	7–10 days
Pinta	Maculo-papular rash (S)	Contact with lesions or by flies (Hy, Ch, Sa, Wa)	1–3 weeks
Piry	Fever (A)	Vector (unknown)	3–12 days
Plague	Bubonic	*Xenopsyla* fleas (Vc, Ra)	2–6 days
	Pneumonic (B)	Airborne (barrier nurse)	1–4 days
Pneumococcal	Pneumonia (B)	Airborne droplets or direct contact with discharges (Im)	1–3 days

(*Continued*)

Disease	Clinical features (agent)	Means of transmission (control method)	Incubation period
Pneumocystis	Pneumonia (P/F)	Airborne or reactivated infection (Ch)	1–2 months
Pneumonia, chlamydial	Pneumonia in neonates and adults	To infant during birth; adult by direct contact (Hy)	1–12 weeks
Poliomyelitis	Paralysis (V)	Faecal–oral or respiratory (Im)	5–30 days
Pongola	Fever, arthritis (A)	Culicine mosquito (Vc)	3–12 days
Powassan	Encephalitis (A)	Tick vector (Vc)	7–14 days
Psittacosis	Pneumonia (B)	Inhale bird droppings (An,Hy)	5–15 days
Puerperal fever	Genital tract infection following delivery (B)	Droplets, hands or faecal contamination (Hy, Ch)	1–3 days
Punta Toro	Fever (A)	*Phlebotomus* sand fly (Vc)	3–6 days
Q fever	Fever, endocarditis (R)	Direct from animal fluids, airborne or milk (An, Hy, Fo)	2–3 weeks
Quaranfil	Fever (A)	Tick vector (Vc)	4–5 days
Rabies	Encephalomyelitis (V)	Animal saliva via bite or abrasion. Also bats (An, Im)	3–8 weeks
Rat-bite fever	Fever and rash (B, S)	Rat bite, also secretions (Ra)	1–3 weeks
Relapsing fever	Periodic fever, mainly children (S)	*Pediculus* louse (Hy, Vc) or *Ornithodorus* tick (Ra, Vc)	5–15 days 3–10 days
Respiratory syncytial virus	Fever, rhinitis, pneumonia (V)	Respiratory, contact or swallowed (Hy)	2–8 days
Restan	Fever (A)	Culicine mosquito, rodent reservoir (Vc)	3–12 days
Rheumatic fever	Cardiac damage (B)	Secondary to sore throat from respiratory (droplet) (Ch)	1–3 days
Rhinosporidiosis	Growth in nose (B)	Stagnant fresh water, swimming	19 days
Rickettsial pox	Fever and rash (R)	Mite vector, rodent reser (Vc)	3–13 days
Rift Valley Fever	Haemorrhagic fever (A)	*Culex* mosquito; contact with animal tissues (An, Vc)	3–12 days
Rio Bravo	Encephalitis (A)	Vector (unknown)	5–15 days
Rocio	Encephalitis (A)	*Culex* mosquito (Vc)	5–15 days
Rocky mountain spotted fever	Fever and rash (R)	*Dermacentor* & *Amblyomma* ticks (An, Vc)	3–14 days
Ross River	Arthritis (A)	*Aedes* & *Culex* mosquito (Vc)	3–11 days
Rotavirus	Diarrhoea (V)	Faecal–oral, respiratory, direct or water (Hy, Wa, Im?)	1–3 days
Rubella / CRS	Rash in adults, neonatal lesions (V)	Respiratory or direct to congenital (Im)	15–20 days
Russian spring–summer encephalitis	Encephalitis (A)	*Ixodes* tick (Vc)	7–14 days
Sabia haemorrhagic fever	Haemorrhagic fever (V)	Inhaled rodent excreta (Ra)	7–16 days
St Louis encephalitis	Encephalitis (A)	*Culex* mosquito (Vc)	5–15 days
Salmonellosis	Diarrhoea (B)	Meat, milk, eggs, faecal–oral and water (Hy, Fo, Wa)	12–36 h

(*continued...*)

(*Continued*)

Disease	Clinical features (agent)	Means of transmission (control method)	Incubation period
Sand fly fever	Fever (A)	*Phlebotamus* and *Lutzomyia* sand fly (Vc)	3–6 days
Sarcocystis	Diarrhoea (P)	Uncooked meat (Fo)	–
Scabies	Urticaria (C)	Direct contact (Ch, Hy, Wa)	2–6 weeks
Scarlet fever	Rash (B)	Repiratory (Ch, Hy, Wa)	1–3 days
Schistosomiasis	Liver or bladder damage (H)	Water contact (Ch, Hy, Sa, Wa, decrease water contact)	2–6 weeks
Semliki Forest	Encephalitis (A)	Culicine mosquito (Vc)	3–12 days
Sepik	Fever (A)	Culicine mosquito (Vc)	5–15 days
Serra Norte	Fever (A)	Vector (unknown)	–
Severe acute respiratory syndrome	Cough, pneumonia, difficult breathing (V)	Respiratory, close contact, faecal–oral? (Hy)	1–14 days
Shingles	Vesicular rash (V)	Reactivated chickenpox	2–3 weeks
Shokwe	Fever (A)	Culicine mosquito (Vc)	3–12 days
Shuni	Fever (A)	Mosquito, *Culicoides* (Vc)	3–12 days
Simian B	Meningoencephalitis (V)	Monkey bite or contact with saliva (An, Hy)	3 days to 3 weeks
Sindbis	Arthritis, rash (A)	*Culex* mosquito, reservoir in birds (Vc)	3–12 days
Sleeping sickness	Fever, headache, somnolence (P)	*Glossina* tsetse fly (An, Ch, Vc)	Weeks to months
Smallpox	Pox rash (V)	Respiratory, skin contact (Im)	7–19 days
Snowshoe hare	Encephalitis (A)	Culicine mosquito (Vc)	3–12 days
Sparganosis	Subcutaneous nodules (H)	Water, or eating frogs and other amphibians (Fo, Wa)	–
Spondweni	Fever (A)	Culicine mosquito (Vc)	3–12 days
Sporotrichosis	Skin nodules (F)	Percutaneous, inhalation from wood or sphagnum moss	1 week to 3 months
Staphylococcus	Skin, wound, bone or organ infections (B)	Autoinfection, contact with lesions or flies (Ch, Hy, Wa)	5–10 days
Streptococcal sepsis of the newborn	Pneumonia and meningitis (B)	Perinatal from genital tract infection (Ch, Hy)	1–7 days
Streptococcal sore throat	Inflamed throat and tonsils (B)	Respiratory or ingestion of food or milk (Ch, Hy, Fo)	1–3 days
Strongyloides	Creeping eruption (N)	Larvae penetrate skin, oral or autoinfection (Hy, Sa)	–
Syphilis, endemic	Skin and bone lesions (S)	Shared drinking vessels and direct contact (Ch, Hy, Wa)	2 weeks to 3 months
Syphilis, venereal	Skin, heart and CNS lesions (S)	Sexual or direct contact; via blood or congenital (Bl, Ch, Xe)	9–90 days
T cell leukaemia	Sarcoma, lymphoma or leukaemia (V)	Breast milk, blood, needles or sexual contact (Bl, Ne, Xe)	–
Tacaiuma	Fever (A)	*Anopheles* mosquito (Vc)	3–12 days
Taenia saginata	Tapeworm (H)	Eating uncooked beef (An, Fo)	8–14 weeks
Taenia solium	Tapeworm and cysticercosis (H)	Uncooked pork, autoinfection, swallowing eggs (An, Fo)	8–12 weeks
Tahyna	Fever (A)	Culicine mosquito (Vc)	–
Tamdy	Fever (A)	Tick vector (Vc)	4–5 days
Tataguine	Fever and rash (A)	Culicine mosquito (Vc)	5–15 days
Tensaw	Encephalitis (A)	Culicine mosquito (Vc)	3–12 days

Disease	Clinical features (agent)	Means of transmission (control method)	Incubation period
Tetanus (and neonatal)	Muscular contractions and rigidity (B, T)	Contamination of abraded skin or umbilicus (Hy, Im)	4–21 days
Thogoto	Meningitis (A)	Tick vector (Vc)	4–5 days
Tick-borne E.	Encephalitis (A)	Tick vector (Vc)	4–5 days
Tick typhus	Fever (R)	Dog tick vector and reservoir (An, Vc)	1–15 days
Tinea	Fungal skin and nail disease(F)	Direct skin contact, also animals (An, Hy, Wa)	4–14 days
Tonate	Fever (A)	Culicine mosquito (Vc)	3–12 days
Toscana	Meningitis (A)	*Phlebotamus* sand fly (Vc)	3–6 days
Toxic shock syndrome	Fever and shock (B)	Frequently associated with absorbent tampons and contraceptive in women (Ch)	4–10 days 1–3 days
Toxocara	Larva migrans (N)	Ingestion of earth or food contaminated with dog and cat faeces (An, Hy, Fo)	Weeks to months
Toxoplasmosis	Often asymptomatic in adult, but brain damage to neonate (P)	Eating uncooked meat, earth contaminated with cat faeces or direct from cat (An,Hy,Fo)	10–20 days
Trachoma	Red-eye, blindness (B)	Contact with eye discharges from fingers, wipes and clothing. Flies (Ch,Hy,Sa,Wa)	5–12 days
Trench fever	Fever, endocarditis (B)	*Pediculus* louse (Hy, Vc)	7–30 days
Trichinosis	Fever and systemic cysts (N)	Uncooked pork and other meat (An, Fo, Ra)	8–15 days
Trichomonas	Vaginitis (P)	Sexual contact (Ch, Xe)	5–20 days
Trichuris	Diarrhoea, debility in children (N)	Ingestion of soil and soil on vegetables (Hy, Fo, Sa, Wa)	2–3 months
Trivittatus	Fever (A)	Culicine mosquito (Vc)	–
Tropical spastic paresis	Myelopathy and spasticity (V)	Blood or sexual contact (Bl, Xe)	–
Tropical ulcer	Skin ulcer with tissue loss (B)	Contamination of abraded skin. Flies (Hy, Sa, Wa)	2–7 days
Trubanaman	Fever, arthritis (A)	Culicine mosquito (Vc)	–
Tuberculosis	Cough, weight loss and anaemia (B)	Respiratory, spitting Unpasteurized milk (Ch,Im,Hy)	4–12 weeks
Tucunduba	Encephalitis (A)	Culicine mosquito (Vc)	–
Tularaemia	Lymphadenopathy, systemic lesions (B)	Tick, *Chrysops*, *Aedes*, animal bite, from water and meat or inhalation (An, Hy, Fo, Vc)	1–14 days
Tunga	Foot furuncles (E)	Invasive flea (footwear)	–
Typhoid	Fever and bowl ulceration (B)	Faecal contamination of food, water. Flies (Hy, Fo, Im, Sa, Wa)	3–30 days
Typhus, epidemic	Fever, prostration and rash (B)	*Pediculus* faeces scratched-in or inhaled (Hy, Im, Vc)	1–2 weeks
Typhus, murine	Fever and rash, mild (B)	*Xenopsylla* flea faeces inhaled (Hy, Ra, Vc)	1–2 weeks

(*continued...*)

(Continued)

Disease	Clinical features (agent)	Means of transmission (control method)	Incubation period
Typhus, scrub	Fever, eschar and rash, mild-severe (B)	*Leptotrombidium* mite, reservoir in s. mammals (Vc)	1–3 weeks
Usutu	Fever, rash (A)	Culicine mosquito (Vc)	3–12 days
Venezuelan equine E.	Fever and encephalitis (A)	Culicine mosquito, reservoir in rodents and horses (Im,Vc)	2–6 days
Vesicular stomatitis	Fever, pharyngitis (A)	*Lutzomyia* sand fly (Vc)	–
Wanowrie	Fever and bleeding (A)	Tick vector (Vc)	4–5 days
Warts	Skin growths (V)	Direct contact, inoculation or indirect (e.g. floors) (Hy)	2–3 months
Wesselsbron	Fever (A)	Culicine mosquito (Vc)	3–12 days
West Nile	Fever (A)	*Culex* mosquito, reservoir in birds (Vc)	3–12 days
Western equine E.	Encephalitis (A)	*Culex* mosquito (Vc)	5–15 days
Wyeomyia	Fever (A)	Culicine mosquito (Vc)	3–12 days
Xingu	Fever, hepatitis (A)	Vector (unknown)	–
Yaws	Skin and bone lesions (S)	Contact with lesions and exudates. Flies (Ch,Hy,Sa,Wa)	2–8 weeks
Yellow fever	Haemorrhagic fever (A)	*Aedes* mosquito, reservoir in monkeys (Im, Vc)	3–6 days
Yersiniosis	Fever and diarrhoea (B)	Faecal–oral, contaminated food and water. Pig reservoir (An, Hy, Fo, Sa, Wa)	3–7 days
Zika	Fever (A)	Culicine mosquito (Vc)	5–15 days

Index

Diseases are listed by the name most commonly used, such as whooping cough rather than pertussis, but leptospirosis rather than Weil's disease. Cross-references are given to all other names of each disease. All countries where communicable diseases are commonly found are mentioned, except for European countries where they are all under the single heading of Europe.

303

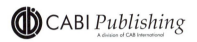
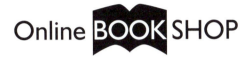

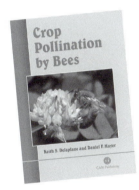
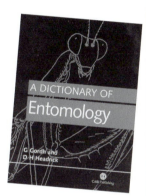
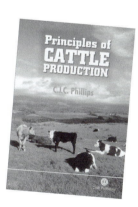
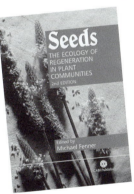